Making Healthcare Safe

Lucian L. Leape

Making Healthcare Safe

The Story of the Patient Safety
Movement

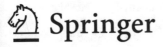 Springer

Lucian L. Leape
Harvard T. H. Chan School of Public Health
Boston, MA
USA

ISBN 978-3-030-71125-2   ISBN 978-3-030-71123-8   (eBook)
https://doi.org/10.1007/978-3-030-71123-8

This Springer imprint is published by the registered company Springer Nature Switzerland AG
The registered company address is: Gewerbestrasse 11, 6330 Cham, Switzerland

To:
James Reason and Charles Vincent
Pioneers, mentors, friends, and
colleagues who taught us about error
and its effects on patients,

and

To the nurses who take care of us
and strive to keep us safe

Foreword

I guess we all live history in some sense. But, for some of us, that phrase has a more specific meaning. For Lucian Leape, it has meant, not just witnessing the historic birth of the health care patient safety movement, but, arguably, creating it.

This book is an invaluable and unique account of the evolution of the evidence, concern, activities, and structures that inform the world's current understanding of how patients are injured too often by the care that is intended to help them and what can and should be done about that. For a topic of such enormous gravity, involving life-or-death consequences every year for tens of thousands of people in the USA, alone, and many hundreds of thousands globally, this story is remarkably recent. The modern scientific foundations for safety in every sector of human endeavor were laid first no earlier than the mid-twentieth century, and the application of those sciences to medical care, with just a few, slender exceptions, began only in the mid-1980s, barely 40 years ago as of this writing.

It is, of course, not at all the case that medical errors and injuries from care appeared de novo in the past half-century. We know now that hazards to patient safety have been with us as long as there have been patients at all – that is, for many millennia. Such hazards come part and parcel with any complex human activity, and even more when that activity includes invading the human body with sharp instruments and foreign chemicals and invading the human psyche with intimidating hierarchies and opaque rites. No count exists of the number of people killed by medical errors since Hippocrates and despite physicians' best intentions, but the toll, if known, would be staggering.

The culprits for that toll, we know now, would not be, for the most part, rogue clinicians or even incompetent ones, but rather the very designs of health care delivery, itself, in which even the best of the workforce get trapped. Or, to be clearer, they are the myriad interactions of those delivery system designs and the frailties of unaided human minds and manipulations – the so-called "human factors" that set up normal people – most of us – for slips, errors, and lapses, the familiar "oops" of daily life. When I forget to set my alarm clock, that's a nuisance; when I forget to give a medication to a critically ill patient, that can be a disaster. But the causes are the same; being human. Only when medicine ceases to rely on heroism for excellence can the pursuit of real safety begin effectively.

Modern safety sciences and their first cousins, the sciences of human error, first gelled in the 1960s and 1970s. The seeds were there in studies of cognitive psychology, social psychology, and general systems theory of the preceding century or so. But it was not until a group of engineers and psychologists began to name the problems of human error and system safety beginning in the 1960s that the field of safety science coalesced. Among the founders was Professor James Reason, from the University of Manchester, whose 1990 book, "Human Error," was and remains the leading monograph on that topic.

Lucian Leape became a student of these emerging sciences of safety not long after Reason's book first appeared. He was primed for the field, having participated as a highly regarded pediatric surgeon in the groundbreaking Harvard Medical Practice Study, which was the brainchild of Dr. Howard Hiatt and New York State Commissioner of Health David Axelrod. That study set out in commanding detail empirical findings about injuries to patients in New York hospitals, defining "adverse events," and convincingly showing that the vast majority of those injuries could be seen as preventable, not inevitable.

Streams converged: the evidence of errors and their consequences, the growing awareness of the value of systems thinking regarding health care quality, the maturation of the safety sciences in other industries, and the self-education of Lucian Leape. The result was a turning-point publication: Lucian's magisterial December 1994, article in the *Journal of the American Medical Association*: "Error in Medicine." Not often can we trace a change in the consciousness of an entire industry to a single treatise; but this time, we can. Within just a few years of Lucian's call to arms, massive shifts were underway in health care's awareness of and concern about patient safety and its defects.

In this book, Lucian recounts the key events and actors preceding and following his seminal article. With dignity and generosity, he describes the contributors to the development of the field he helped to found. Some were conferences, in many of which Lucian had a big role: the "Annenberg Conferences" where the actual voices of injured patients and families first rang out as loudly as they must; the Salzburg Seminar on Patient Safety, which first brought together a truly international group of patient safety scholars, and which incorporated leading scholars from outside health care, including Jim Reason, himself. Some were action collaboratives, such as IHI's Breakthrough Series Collaborative on Medication Safety, which Lucian, himself, chaired.

Some were new structures, most importantly the National Patient Safety Foundation, and its daughter, the Lucian Leape Institute, which gave formal homes to the movement and whose sponsors included the needed range of public and private sector organizations. Most important of all was the decision of the Institute of Medicine, and especially its courageous President, Dr. Ken Shine, to establish a Committee on the Quality of Care in America, whose first report, "To Err Is Human," released late in the year 1999, made headlines across the nation, with its astounding assertion that 44,000 to 98,000 Americans each year died in US hospitals as a result of errors in their care. Lucian, of course, served on and helped to guide that Committee.

No one but Lucian Leape could have written the book that follows this Foreword. He, and he alone, was present at almost every single step of the 40-year journey between the Harvard Medical Practice study and today. To boot, I know from years of delightful personal collaboration with Lucian, that his memory is astounding, and that he can recall, and has herein set down for all time, otherwise lost details about the people, events, and lessons along the way. This book will be a delight for those who, having seen or heard about part of the patient safety movement, want to experience it vicariously in its entirety.

It is, of course, important to acknowledge that giants, like Lucian, stand always on the shoulders of others before them. There are too many names to summon here, but take note that Ernest Amory Codman, Florence Nightingale, Ellison C. ("Jeep") Pierce, David Gaba, and Richard Cook, for example, are just a few of the medical pioneers of the nineteenth and twentieth century who courageously began to ring alarms about the harm that well-meaning health care can do, and, equally important, to offer ideas about how transparency, systems science, standards, and good leadership can save lives by making care delivery safer just as care itself can save lives by using biomedical breakthroughs. Lucian, of course, gives them their proper due, and acknowledges both his debt and ours.

Note, too, that the journey to patient safety has, in actuality, barely begun. Lucian and his colleagues advocating for safer care, I among them, are all too aware of how incomplete the victory is. To our chagrin, and to the disadvantage millions of patients and families, improving safety still lacks the strategic centering it ought to have in the health care organizations both public and private. Governments around the world still generally lack agencies and individuals responsible for assuring and nurturing safety systems and safety results. Professional training still barely mentions the topic, and the scientific armamentarium for safe systems is almost nowhere taught to the physicians, nurses, and health care managers of tomorrow. No one escapes medical school without studying the Krebs cycle and hearing about the discovery of insulin; but almost all will graduate without 1 minute of learning about human error or a single encounter with the work of James Reason.

As a result, the toll of error and injury to patients continues to be massive. In 2018, three important reports on defects in quality in global health care were published, one ("Crossing the Global Quality Chasm") from the National Academies of Sciences, Engineering, and Medicine in the USA, one from The Lancet Commission on High-Quality Health Systems in the Sustainable Development Goals Era, and one ("Delivering Quality Health Services: A Global Imperative for Universal Health Coverage") from the World Health Organization, OECD, and the World Bank. Though carried out separately, these reports each estimated that over five million deaths a year in the world can be attributed to defects in the quality of health care. Problems in patient safety are high among those causes.

So, the story told in this book, as compelling as it is, will be but Chapter One of the longer term saga of the patient safety movement. The work of safety improvement, indeed, is hardly begun. No one hopes more than does Lucian Leape that the next book will be able to recount vast successes not yet in our hands.

Donald M. Berwick,
Institute for Healthcare Improvement
Boston, MA, USA

Preface

In late1999, Americans were shocked to learn that the number of patients dying in hospitals from medical errors was the equivalent of the crash of a jumbo jet each day. Some experts even said it was twice that many. The response was immediate. Government, hospitals, professional organizations, regulators, and researchers mobilized in a massive effort to reduce medical injury. This is the story of what happened.

It is a remarkable story, full of heroes and villains, awesome successes and discouraging failures. We had much to learn, and we still have a long way to go to make health care safe, but in the past two decades we have made great progress. Health care workers have truly saved millions of lives. Most importantly, we are now poised to dramatically accelerate progress to achieving zero harm.

All histories fall short one way or another. They have more than you want to know about some things, less than you want to know about others, and invariably neglect important events. They suffer from the bias of the writer. This is no exception. It is to some extent a personal history, shaped by my point of view.

I have been privileged to be part of many of the efforts in the journey to make health care safe, sometimes as a participant, other times as an instigator. As a result, I have a wealth of stories to share that illuminate and provide insights into what happened. I think they add interest to the history. Hopefully, you will agree.

More important, having "been there" – and kept notes – I am also able to provide a reasonably accurate account of what actually happened. The desire to provide an accurate account is what motivated me to write this book. I repeatedly heard people telling stories in good faith about how something came about that just weren't true. But they were becoming part of the myth that was growing about how patient safety started. So, I am trying to set the record straight.

But a more important objective is to enable people to understand what patient safety is all about. To help health care professionals, students, administrators, and policymakers understand the basic concepts of error prevention, the key issues that need to be wrestled with, and how to create a culture of safety, and to provide information about the impressive array of safety programs carried out by organizations devoted to keeping us safe.

I also want to enable people working in safety to be more effective by providing them information on what works and what doesn't, and why. How do you change systems? How do you create a supportive, safe, and respectful workplace? How do you engage patients in their care? How do you talk with and support patients after they have been injured? How do you create a culture of safety?

This is not a collection of anecdotes, however. It is a history. Of the ideas, the data, and the theories that drove the patient safety movement. And of the actions of the key players and institutions that made it happen. Of the energy, imagination, and devotion of these leaders, of the strategies they used, and the incredible amount of work they did to make health care safe.

For these stories, I relied not just on my own experience and analysis of published information but on firsthand accounts by the leaders of the organizations who made it happen. In every instance – without exception – these true "movers and shakers" were incredibly generous in sharing information, not just in helping me get the details straight, but also in sharing "back stories."

The process was iterative. For each subject, I interviewed several leaders, usually more than once, and then wrote the story. That account was sent to them for review and editing. It was then revised and sent back once again for a final check on its accuracy. Thus, while the presentations reflect my point of view, to the best of our combined recollections these are the facts.

It is a history of patient safety in the USA. Although there are chapters on developments in the UK and the international safety efforts of the World Health Organization, other important work done elsewhere is not included. Hopefully, however, overseas readers will find useful information and insights throughout the book. The last six chapters on key issues should be of universal interest.

This book is also not a history of everything that happened in patient safety during those early years. Significant advances took place in technology (especially simulation and monitoring), research, training, and education. Leaders in nursing and pharmacy, the frontline professionals who provide patient care, as well as risk managers and others, made important advances to improve safety. A number of health care organizations implemented safety programs. Federal agencies other than the ones described here, such as HHS and DOD, contributed, as did many professional organizations and advocacy groups.

These efforts were important, but they were not the essential drivers of the patient safety movement. An example: 15 years before the legendary IOM report, "To Err is Human," the Anesthesia Patient Safety Foundation pioneered in using human factors principles to make dramatic reductions in the mortality of anesthesia. While the rest of health care took notice, it did not follow suit. This important and successful initiative did not start the patient safety movement. That required the shock from the IOM and the intensive work of the organizations described in the following chapters.

The story runs roughly from 1987 to 2015. It is structured in four parts: Part I, In the Beginning, describes the research and theory that defined patient safety and the early initiatives to deal with it. Part II, Institutional Responses, tells the stories of the efforts of the major organizations that began to apply the new concepts and make patient safety a reality. Most of these stories have not been previously told, so this account becomes their histories as well. Part III, Getting to Work, provides in-depth analyses of four key issues that cut across disciplinary lines and required special attention. Part IV, Creating a Culture of Safety, looks to the future, marshalling the best thinking about what it will take to achieve the safe care we all deserve.

It is an inspiring story, and a hopeful one. I hope you will enjoy it.

Boston, MA, USA   Lucian L. Leape

Acknowledgments

This book tells the story of the efforts of a large number of people who grasped the seriousness of the problem of medical errors and decided to apply their knowledge, skills, and imagination to its solution. The willingness of those individuals to share their experiences and insights made it possible for me to tell their stories. I am forever grateful for their generosity and the privilege of their friendships.

First, I want to express my gratitude to the mentors who inspired me to take on the safety journey. Howard Hiatt, former dean of the Harvard School of Public Health, got me started. Mentor to so many and supporter of numerous worthwhile causes, he conceived of the Medical Practice Study that revealed the extent of medical injury. By including me on the team, he gave me the opportunity to discover the enormity of medical error. His friendship and support have been constant and invaluable ever since, and I am eternally grateful.

Jim Reason taught me most of what I know about errors and their causes. First, through his magnificent book, *Human Error*, still the universally respected "Bible" on the subject 30 years after it was written, and subsequently through our friendship and collaboration over the years on finding ways to apply theory to practice.

Charles Vincent opened my eyes to the psychological impact on patients of our mistakes and the failure to effectively communicate and support them in their hour of need. These perceptions formed the basis for his later work on disclosure and restitution. His method for investigating adverse events provides insights far beyond the usual root cause analysis; I taught it to generations of students over the years. We have become close friends and collaborators on many projects.

Don Berwick, the father of quality improvement, was quick to recognize the importance of patient safety and the applicability of QI principles to its solution. His leadership of IHI and his persuasive powers have inspired thousands. As the reader will discover, his insights and imagination were behind many important safety initiatives. We have partnered on many of these and become good friends. I am honored and delighted to have him write the foreword.

I am grateful to Bob Blendon and Arnie Epstein, department chairs of Health Policy and Management, who provided support at the Harvard School of Public Health for a professor of surgery who had some interesting ideas but few academic health policy credentials. Their encouragement over the years, as well as the welcoming climate in our department, gave joy to my daily work. And I am indebted to my colleague David Bates, with whom I originally conceived the idea of writing the definitive story of the patient safety movement. Our early conversations about the shape of the story, and the importance of telling it, convinced me that this was a task worth undertaking.

Second, I wish to recognize and give heartfelt thanks to the experts and leaders in each topic who graciously helped me write the stories of their institutions. Most of them friends from our years working together, they told me what really happened, turned my general perceptions into specifics, corrected misunderstandings, and helped me get the details straight. They shared the "back stories" that give texture to the narrative. Most importantly, they made sure there were no factual errors. I am very grateful for their generosity in sharing their time, their interest, and their insights. I literally could not have written this history without them:

Ron Arky	Allan Frankel	Patricia McGaffigan
David Bates	John Fromson	Don Melnick
Don Berwick	Tom Gallagher	Gregg Meyer
Rick Boothman	Tejal Gandhi	Julie Morath
Hal Bressler	Atul Gawande	Tom Nasca
Helen Burstin	Paul Gluck	Dennis O'Leary
Carolyn Clancy	Paula Griswold	Diane Pinakiewicz
Jim Conway	Frank Hartman	Peter Pronovost
Jeff Cooper	Marty Hatlie	Edgar Schein
Janet Corrigan	Howard Hiatt	Paul Schyve

Rick Croteau
Connie Crowley-Ganser
Jennifer Daley
Jules Dienstag
Liam Donaldson
Susan Edgman-Levitan
Arnie Epstein
Frank Federico

Jerry Hickson
Gary Kaplan
Leslie Kirle
Ken Kizer
Uma Kotagal
Chris Landrigan
David Lawrence
George Lundberg

Ken Shine
Jim Thompson
Charles Vincent
Bob Wachter
Saul Weingart
Kevin Weiss
Alan Woodward

I wish to thank the hospital patient safety officers and staff who reviewed chapters for clarity and relevance: Susan Abookire, Eric Alper, Janet Barnes, Yvonne Cheung, Pat Folcarelli, Carol Jones, Terry Sievers, and Burt A. Thurlo Walsh. They represent the primary audience for this book, those who do the everyday work of making health care safe. Their contributions helped make it not just authentic, but useful.

I am also grateful to Ariya Kraik, graduate student in health policy and management at HSPH, who provided invaluable assistance in finding articles, inserting references in the manuscript, and constructing the index. She made the whole process much less burdensome and was a joy to work with.

I want to express my appreciation for my editors. As the book was being conceived, Jane Roessner, former editor at IHI, reviewed several of the early chapters and helped me navigate the world of book publishing. Her advice and encouragement were invaluable and deeply appreciated.

At Springer Nature, Richard Lansing provided support and encouragement; his editorial "light hand" corrected errors while preserving the tone and idiosyncrasies of my prose. Margaret Moore put the pieces together and was incredibly helpful in managing the photographs and the production process.

Finally, I wish to thank the Department of Health Policy and Management at the Harvard Chan School of Public Health and the Institute for Healthcare Improvement for funding of open access that makes the book available to all.

The contributions of all those mentioned above made a potentially onerous project one of continuing joy and satisfaction. They were the village that raised this child.

Contents

About the Author

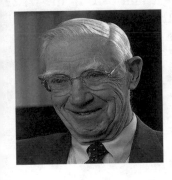

Lucian L. Leape has had two careers, the first as an academic pediatric surgeon. After graduating from Cornell and serving in the U.S. Navy for 3 years, he graduated from Harvard Medical School, cum laude, and trained in general and thoracic surgery at the Massachusetts General Hospital and in pediatric surgery at Boston Children's Hospital. He joined the faculty of the University of Kansas and led the founding of the American Pediatric Surgical Association. He then served as Professor of Surgery and Chief of Pediatric Surgery at Tufts University Medical Center for 13 years. He published over 100 papers and book chapters and a textbook of pediatric surgery.

In 1986, he began a new career in health policy. After a Pew fellowship at RAND, he joined the Harvard Medical Practice Study (MPS) of medical injury and was stunned by the extent of medical errors. In 1994, he published his seminal paper "Error in Medicine" in *JAMA* that called for the application of systems theory to prevent medical errors. He helped found the National Patient Safety Foundation and participated in the Institute of Medicine's committee that published "To Err is Human" in 1999.

Honors include the Distinguished Service Award of the American Pediatric Surgical Association, the Donabedian Award from the American Public Health Association, the duPont Award for Excellence in Children's Health Care, and the John Eisenberg Patient Safety Award from the JCAHO and National Quality Forum. In 2006, *Modern Healthcare* named him as one of the 30 people who had the most impact on health care in the past 30 years. In 2013, he was named a Distinguished Eagle Scout.

Part I
In the Beginning

Chapter 1
The Hidden Epidemic: The Harvard Medical Practice Study

Malpractice! The word strikes terror in doctors' hearts—and with good reason. All doctors are at risk of being sued when things go wrong, and most doctors are in fact sued at some time in their career, whether or not they did anything wrong. For some high-risk special-ties, including neurosurgery, vascular surgery, and cardiology, the percentage sued is very high, and multiple suits are not uncommon. For all doctors, the cost of malpractice insurance is substantial.

So it was not surprising that a sharp rise in medical malpractice insurance premiums in 1985 was viewed by the profession as a "cri-sis." Such "crises" occurred periodically and were not necessarily associated with either an increase in malpractice claims or in payouts. In this case, the rise had several causes. Because of several years of substantial gains from their investments in the stock market, liability insurance carriers had not raised premiums very much for nearly a decade, but annual payouts (claims settlements) had continued their steady increase.

The need to "catch up," coupled with rising reinsurance rates imposed by overseas reinsurers because of strengthening of the dollar, led companies to raise premiums 40–100% or more. On Long Island, malpractice premiums for obstetricians jumped from $68,000 per year to $100,000 [1]. Doctors perceived a crisis.

How big a problem was actual malpractice? No one really knew. No one knew how many people were hurt by negligent care—that is, substandard care. No one knew how many of those patients filed a malpractice suit. Some suspected the number was quite small, but no

© The Author(s) 2021
L. L. Leape, *Making Healthcare Safe*,
https://doi.org/10.1007/978-3-030-71123-8_1

one knew. Doctors seemed to complain about being sued all the time, but no one knew the facts. No one knew what percentage of malpractice suits were successful. Or how many people suffered from injuries that were caused by medical treatment that was not negligent. No one knew.

And no one had any idea of the costs of medical injury—financial, physical, and emotional: not just the costs of continuing medical treatment, but of lost wages, childcare, home assistance, and long-term disability.

Reflecting on all of this, Howard Hiatt, dean of the Harvard School of Public Health (HSPH), and his good friend, James Vorenberg, dean of the Harvard Law School, conceived of the idea of doing a study to answer these questions. What were the costs of medical injury? How much of it was due to negligence? How successfully did the liability insurance system meet its purported objectives of compensating the injured and deterring bad practice? Did the risk of being sued make doctors more careful and thus reduce the likelihood of patients being harmed? Did the system fairly compensate those who were harmed?

Some experts had expressed interest in no-fault insurance that would pay for all the costs of injury for all patients, irrespective of negligence. Would such a scheme be an economically feasible alternative to litigation? Surely among the faculty of their two schools, they reasoned, there should be enough brainpower to answer these questions and perhaps even develop a better solution.

The place to start, they thought, was with the facts. How many people were harmed by medical treatment in hospitals? What percentage was caused by errors? By negligence? Of those harmed by negligent care, how many sued? What were the costs of medical injury—not just for those harmed by bad care, but for all patients, including those who suffered nonpreventable injuries? How were these costs paid for? All was unknown. All was potentially knowable.

With colleagues, they designed a study to get this information. They used as a model a 1978 study by Don Harper Mills of "potentially compensable events" (PCEs): medical injuries for which a jury might award malpractice money damages. Mills and his team had analyzed 20,684 patient charts of patients discharged from 23 California hospitals in 1974. They found that 4.65% of the patients experienced PCEs of varying severity [2].

Like the California study, the Harvard study would also be a review of medical records. However, Hiatt and Vorenberg believed that to influence policy-makers it needed to be designed as a *population-based* study, i.e., based on a scientifically designed sample of patients from all types of acute care hospitals serving all patients in a defined geographic area. Only that way would the information be likely to be used for public planning.

Howard's first thought was to seek the approval of the Massachusetts Medical Society, so he approached the president of the society, whom he knew. She thought it was a very bad idea! As we will see with the AMA later, anything that might possibly make doctors look bad was unacceptable. Similarly, Howard found no "takers" among the various private foundations or governmental authorities in Massachusetts.

But, suddenly, there was interest in New York. Howard described the plan to his friend Alfred Gellhorn, who introduced him to the Commissioner of Health in New York State, David Axelrod, whose response was quite positive. Axelrod took him to meet Governor Mario Cuomo, who said, "We've been looking for you! When can you get started?"

Cuomo was struggling with state spending for medical liability claims that was substantial and increasing. Would the Harvard team be willing to do it in New York State? They were delighted to do so—New York's large size and diversity would make the results more credible. When told how much it would cost, Cuomo commented that he expected it to be several times that amount, and he readily authorized an appropriation of $3.2 million for the study. The Robert Wood Johnson Foundation contributed an additional $250,000.

Hiatt led the research team. Troy Brennan and Nan Laird led the study design. Troy was just finishing his chief residency in medicine at the Massachusetts General Hospital, but he was uniquely qualified for this study. A Rhodes scholar, he was an honors MD and MPH graduate of Yale Medical School, while simultaneously receiving his JD from Yale Law School. Nan Laird was a professor of statistics, later department chair, at the Harvard School of Public Health, and was a national leader in survey design methodology.

In addition to Brennan, three other physicians were members of this planning group: Benjamin (Bunny) Barnes, a surgeon from Tufts; Howard Frazier, a nephrologist and health services researcher at

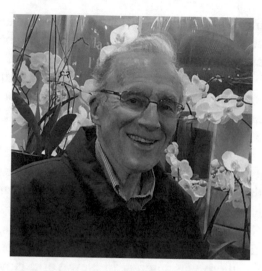

Howard Hiatt.

HSPH; and Lynn Peterson, a Brigham and Women's Hospital internist. Harvard's William Hsiao (later replaced by Joe Newhouse) and Bill Johnson from Arizona State University were the economists on the team. Paul Weiler, professor at the Harvard Law School, oversaw legal issues. Russell Localio served as project manager, and Ann Lawthers oversaw data management.

The team was about 6 months into the study when, in the spring of 1987, Howard Hiatt approached me to determine my interest in joining them. After 20 years in academic pediatric surgery, I wanted to work in health policy and was finishing a year as a fellow at RAND studying epidemiology, statistics, and health policy in preparation for my new career. At RAND I had become involved in several studies of overuse of healthcare services and was leading a study of underuse. I was returning to Boston and looking for additional opportunities in my new career.

Bunny Barnes, an old friend of mine and surgical colleague from my days as a resident at the MGH and on the staff at Tufts, had recommended me to Howard as someone who could contribute to the study because of my newly acquired analytic skills and substantial clinical experience.

I remember the interview well. In my usual blunt manner, I told Howard that I had no interest in working on malpractice! I had not made a career change and spent a year of my life learning how to do health policy research just to waste it on an issue that was so polarizing and for which I saw no reasonable prospect for change. I was cool to the whole idea.

But Howard explained that the scope of the study was much bigger than malpractice in that it would collect interesting and previously undeveloped data about the substance behind malpractice, medical injury, and also measure its costs to patients. That piqued my interest. I wanted to work on quality improvement; injury and costs were clearly quality issues. At the time, I had not thought much about medical errors. Like most of my colleagues, I considered minor errors unavoidable and serious errors malpractice, the result of incompetence or carelessness. Howard offered me a half-time position, which fit nicely with my commitments to continuing research work at RAND. I accepted his offer, not suspecting it would change my life.

I joined the team just after they had completed the study design. The next major effort was to agree on our definitions, particularly the term for medical injury. Many different terms had been used: "unplanned event," "unanticipated outcome," "unexpected result," "adverse outcome," and, of course, just plain "complication." A common thread was that the injury was beyond the control of the caregivers—and therefore not blameworthy.

Measurement of harm at the time was haphazard, even casual, with little analysis and few records. Even surgical departments, which traditionally had weekly mortality and morbidity ("M&M") conferences, classified deaths from complications as due to errors in judgment, management or technique, or "patient's disease." Remedies recommended were better education for residents and admonishing all to try harder.

This lack of consistent terminology, as well as physicians' concerns about culpability, led to substantial underreporting of iatrogenic injuries. Physicians had few incentives to report. Reporting mechanisms were underdeveloped and largely voluntary. States required hospitals to report deaths but rarely investigated their causes. The Joint Commission asked hospitals to report "sentinel events" (serious injuries), but few hospitals did. Surgical departments had M&M meetings, but neither other departments nor the hospitals kept tabulations or continuing records of iatrogenic injuries. Medical injury was largely invisible, and hospitals and doctors liked it that way.

We sought a neutral term that captured all events and to which we could apply a judgment of negligence when indicated. We finally settled on "adverse event." We spent many hours debating its exact definition and ultimately agreed on "an unintended injury that was caused by medical management rather than the patient's underlying disease." The important point was to distinguish harm caused by treatment from harm caused by disease, independent of whether there was an error or negligence. We knew that making this judgment would be difficult for doctors, as it indeed proved to be.

Physicians are very sensitive to any implication that their performance is deficient in any way. Complications were considered either "preventable," which meant someone was to blame, or unpreventable. Most were put in the latter category, which included certain types of complications that everyone knew occasionally happened and were thought to be unavoidable and therefore no one's fault, as well as the occasional unanticipated outcome that seemed to come out of the blue. Our hope was that reviewers could view "adverse event" as a neutral term.

The most common source of injury caused by treatment in the hospital, of course, is a surgical operation, so it was necessary to distinguish this form of planned harm from that due to errors or other failures. Use of the word "unintended" resolved that problem.

We struggled unsuccessfully to devise a reliable way to measure psychological harm, despite its obvious importance, so we restricted our study to physical harm. For "error," we used Reason's definition: "The failure of a planned action to be completed as intended or the use of a wrong plan to achieve an aim." For "negligence," we used the standard accepted legal definition: "Failure to meet the standard of care."

The plan was to obtain data by reviewing medical records of hospitalized patients. We would focus on adverse events that could potentially trigger a malpractice suit. These were injuries that resulted in some degree of disability, temporary or permanent, including death, or were sufficiently severe to prolong the hospital stay. Concurrently, we developed the instruments for data collection and the training materials for record reviewers, both nurses and doctors.

By early 1988, we had settled on our definitions, developed our screening criteria and record review instruments, and constructed instruction manuals for nurse and physician reviews. We designed a two-step review process: First, registered nurses who were trained in record review for quality assurance would read each randomly selected hospital record in search of one or more of 18 screening criteria (such as post-op fever or transfer to an ICU) that suggested the *possibility* of an adverse event. Second, records that met one or more of the screening criteria would then be independently reviewed by two board-certified physicians to determine if, in fact, there had been an adverse event.

Physicians were asked to rate suspected adverse events on a six-point scale based on their confidence—from the information provided in the medical record—that an adverse event had in fact occurred. We used a six-point scale (1 = little or no confidence, 2 = some confidence, 3 = less likely than not, 4 = more likely than not, 5 = highly probable, 6 = virtually certain) to mimic the legal system, which requires a predominance of the evidence with no room for equivocation (50-50).

Reviewers categorized adverse events (AEs) by type (drug reaction, fall, wound infection, etc.) and rated the disability caused by the AE by severity and by duration (temporary or permanent). If an error was found, it was classified as one of five types: diagnostic, prevention, performance, drug treatment, and system. For each type there were additional questions as to the nature of the failure.

Physician reviewers then made a judgment of whether the adverse event constituted negligence, also rated on a six-point scale of confidence. Finally, the AE was rated as to severity (slight, moderate, grave). Except for the well-established definition of negligence, we developed all these definitions and classifications anew, since we found few in the literature and no consensus among physicians or researchers.

The initial screening review of the hospital records was to be performed by a cadre of nurse record reviewers who were skilled at this type of review and were employed by the Hospital Association of New York State (HANYS) which did record reviews as a business. Part of the funding agreement with New York was that HANYS would perform this function for us.

Unfortunately, our project manager had been unable to get agreement on a contract with them, despite many months of negotiations. Time was running out. We were ready to begin the study, but had no one to review the records! Howard turned to me and asked me to see if I could negotiate a contract. I arranged to meet with the head of the HANYS program and flew to Albany on a Saturday morning to meet her over coffee at her home.

Since I had never negotiated a contract in my life, the night before our meeting, I read Roger Fisher's *Getting to Yes*. It was just the ticket. I asked her what they wanted and told her what we wanted, and within an hour we had agreed on the contract and departed friends. At last, the study could begin. We could begin to train these nurses in the use of the record survey instrument.

Finding and training physicians to review the records was more difficult. With help from the NY Department of Health and strong support from the NY State Medical Society, we identified and recruited board-certified internists and surgeons in each of the 51 towns where our study hospitals were. To minimize conflicts of interest, we required that these physicians not be on the staff or have admitting privileges at the hospital whose records were being studied. They were paid the going rate for physician record review.

We met with each group of physicians (typically 4–8 for a hospital) to instruct them in the review process and make sure they understood the definitions. This was a crucial task, since "adverse event" was a new concept for many, and distinguishing treatment-caused injuries from complications of the disease was not something any had ever done.

We also made clear that the term "adverse event" did not mean there had been an error in care. They would find that some were caused by errors and others were not. Part of the purpose of the study was to find out how many there were of each. Despite this caution, we discovered later that many of them considered error the equivalent of negligence, that is, they resulted from the physician not being careful enough. In truth, at that time most of us more or less shared that point of view.

The final design included a random sample of over 31,000 patients who were selected from 51 randomly selected acute care New York hospitals. Government hospitals and mental institutions were excluded. Study hospitals were asked to provide a list of all patients discharged in calendar year 1984. From those lists, patients were randomly selected to reach the appropriate number for each hospital. The hospitals were then asked to make their medical records available for our review.

We were about to launch this enterprise when the leader of data collection, Bunny Barnes, informed Howard that he was leaving the study to go on a round-the-world cruise with his new wife! Howard turned to me to take over. Suddenly, my involvement and time commitment to the study expanded considerably.

We divided the study hospitals into five geographic regions with a similar number of hospitals (10) in each. No one wanted to do the traveling required to supervise data collection in upstate New York, so I volunteered to take it on. From my undergraduate days at Cornell, I knew how beautiful upstate New York was. I looked forward to spending the spring and summer driving around from city to city. By the end of the study, those who chose NYC because it was so easy to get to found that it was rough at times and were envious of my less-stressful experiences.

Data collection began late in the spring of 1988, after training sessions of the physicians at each hospital in each region. We made periodic visits back to oversee the process and personally review a sample of records to make sure they were being reviewed correctly. We later did a formal review of ten charts at each hospital to check reliability of the physician reviews.

Hospitals were very cooperative and retrieved almost all of the records we requested. It is worth noting that at the time we were not required to obtain permission from the patients to review their medical records, something later required by HIPAA rules. This constraint makes it difficult to perform a similar study today.

By mid-1989, we had the results of our initial analysis of the data from the record review in the New York hospitals. In our sample of 30,121 records, we found that 1133 patients had suffered an adverse event, which computed to a serious injury rate of 3.7%, a bit lower than what the Mills study found. Twenty-seven percent of AEs were judged to be due to negligent care. From these data we estimated that in 1984 there were 98,689 adverse events in New York hospitals, of which 13,451 (13.6%) were fatal [3].

There were no differences in rates by sex, but older patients had higher rates. Adverse event rates were substantially higher in some specialties (such as vascular surgery, thoracic surgery, and neurosurgery) than in others. Adverse event rates were higher in large academic medical centers than in community hospitals, but the fraction due to negligence was much lower. Higher negligence rates were found in hospitals with high minority populations.

But the surprising finding was that more than two-thirds of the injuries seemed to be potentially preventable. Reviewers were able to identify specific errors from information in the medical records for 58% of the AEs [4]; subsequent analysis revealed that an additional 11% of AEs resulted from failure to follow accepted practices, raising the total fraction of potentially preventable AEs to 69% [5].

Complications of the use of medications was the most common type of AE, accounting for 19.4% of the total, followed by wound infections (13.6%) and technical complications of surgery (12.9%). Surgical complications accounted for 48% of all adverse events [4] (Table 1.1).

We were very much aware of the limitations of our study—how far it could fall short of our goal of identifying every adverse event and only adverse events. The likelihood is that our numbers *underestimated* the number of AEs. There were opportunities at each stage for missing an adverse event. At the first step, where nurses identified whether the patient met any of the 18 screening criteria, they undoubtedly overlooked a few. Since our screening criteria were not perfect, some injuries almost certainly occurred that did not trigger one of the criteria. And, since all of our information came from the medical record, if the caregiver chose not to record a symptom or event in the medical record, then we could not measure it. We suspected this was not a small problem, but had no way to quantify it.

At the review stage, physicians also undoubtedly failed to find some AEs that were present. Although some of those would be simply

Table 1.1 Major types of adverse events

Type of AE	% of total
Medication errors	19.4
Wound infections	13.6
Technical complications of surgery	12.9
Late surgical complications	10.6
Diagnostic mishaps	8.1
Therapeutic mishaps	7.5
Procedure-related	7.0

Adapted from Ref. [4]

overlooked, others likely resulted from inadequate documentation, ambiguous statements, handwriting problems, and the like. These documentation issues were more common in small private hospitals, where records were less standardized and notes were sparse because only the patient's physician writes progress notes. In teaching hospitals, by contrast, there are multiple notes by residents, medical students, and nurses as well.

Bias also probably played a role, leading physician reviewers to under-identify adverse events and over-label negligence. We defined an adverse event as any injury caused by treatment, whether or not there was an error and whether or not it was preventable. This included common and well-accepted complications. While this seems clear on the surface, it was a new concept to our reviewing physicians.

At this time—remember it was 1988—most physicians considered errors blameworthy; they were thought to result from failure to be careful enough and, therefore, negligent. Some physicians had trouble understanding the term "adverse event" as a neutral descriptor, to be applied to all treatment-related injuries, whether or not they were caused by an error.

Thus, despite extensive training and reviews, some physicians still equated "adverse" with error and accordingly might not call an injury an adverse event if there was no error. Some complications were inevitable, the thinking went; they should not be "held against" the physician. Evidence of this kind of thinking is the fact that several types of adverse events that later studies showed to be quite common, such as hospital-acquired infections, falls, and pressure ulcers, were infrequent in our study.

It is unlikely that we were overcounting. Reviewers would not "see" events that hadn't happened! On balance, we believed that our rates, shocking as they were, *underestimated* the true extent of harm. In fact, later studies would bear this out.

The implications of our findings were profound. If our rates were representative, i.e., if adverse event rates in hospitals across the country were similar to what we found in New York State, then nationwide 1.3 million patients were injured by medical care in American acute care hospitals that year, and 180,000 died from these injuries! These numbers were an order of magnitude higher than had ever been suggested. Medical injury was truly a hidden epidemic.

But I was struck with something else: more than two-thirds of the AE were caused by errors and systems failures that we could detect in the medical record. This meant that of the projected 180,000 deaths each year, more than 120,000 were potentially preventable. I was surprised that no one else in the study group found this particularly alarming or of interest. The focus of the study was on malpractice—the costs of injuries and who paid. But it was the fact that two-thirds were potentially preventable that captured my attention. Surely, we should be able to eliminate those—or at least some of them. Preventing these errors and failures could be a huge agenda for improvement. My colleagues disagreed and warned, "Don't go there. The doctors will hate you."

The results of the study were published in two papers in the *New England Journal of Medicine* in February 1991 [3, 4]. It got substantial local coverage in the New York media and some national notice. The New York State Medical Society was not pleased, but made the best of it by claiming that the 1% negligence rate (27% of 3.7% injury rate) was quite low and showed that doctors were performing at a 99% perfect level! [6] But interest in the study faded quickly. No one knew what to do about it, so after a few commentaries from assorted parties, everyone, lay and professional, pretty much quit talking about it.

The Medical Practice Study did one other thing: it determined the feasibility of no-fault insurance as an alternative to the tort system to compensate patients for medical injury. Malpractice suits only compensate patients whose injuries were caused by negligence and who succeed in winning a malpractice suit. Most people don't sue, and most of those who do don't win. The net result is that very few injured patients are compensated by the tort system.

In a no-fault plan, all patients who suffer a treatment-caused injury are compensated for all of its subsequent costs, irrespective of whether the injury was caused by error or negligence. Importantly, these costs also include lost wages, home care, and long-term disability care.

To determine the feasibility of no-fault compensation, we did a follow-up study of the economic consequences of the adverse events. We interviewed the patients from our study who had been injured—or their next of kin if they had died—to determine the long-term effects of the injuries on the victims (such as permanent disability and inability to work), and we estimated their total costs, medical care, lost wages, disability care, etc., over their lifetimes.

From our analysis, we estimated that the total lifetime cost of adverse events in New York State in 1984 was $3.8 billion in 1989 dollars. Over three-fourths of that cost was paid for by medical insurance or programs such as Medicaid, disability income insurance, and workman's compensation. But the rest was paid by patients.

The cost of a no-fault compensation scheme to compensate for that remainder would be $878 million per year. In that same year, hospitals and doctors in New York paid $1.1 billion for malpractice insurance premiums. The obvious conclusion was that we could compensate *everyone* who was seriously injured for *all* of their expenses for less than the amount that doctors and hospitals were already paying for liability insurance that compensated only the small percentage of patients who received a settlement for malpractice [7].

We called for implementation of no-fault insurance. The potential benefits seemed overwhelming. Only 4% of our patients with significant adverse events ever filed a malpractice claim. Multiple studies have shown that fewer than half of malpractice claims ever result in a payment to the patient. Thus, fewer than 2% of the 98,689 patients who were injured in New York in 1984 were likely to receive compensation. By contrast, a no-fault insurance plan would compensate *all* patients who had significant disability.

Our plea fell on receptive ears. David Axelrod, New York's Health Commissioner who commissioned the study, was in full agreement. He got the governor to propose enabling legislation for statewide no-fault insurance. It was not to be. Axelrod was tragically disabled by a stroke a few months later, and the state fell onto hard fiscal times. Without his leadership and drive, the legislation perished. An unprecedented opportunity for enlightened government and fairness for victims of medical harm evaporated.

Nonetheless, the Medical Practice Study had a profound impact. Although it was designed to address malpractice, its far greater significance came from the revelation of the horrendous extent of harm that resulted from routine medical care. Here for the first time was indisputable evidence that hundreds of thousands of people were being harmed every year by care intended to help them. And, for the first time, evidence that many of those injuries were potentially preventable. Patient safety was a much greater problem than any of us realized. But it would take some time for this to sink in for the medical profession and its leaders.

References

1. Posner J. Trends in malpractice insurance, 1970–85. Law Contemp Probl. 1986;49:37–56.
2. Mills DH. Medical insurance feasibility study. A technical study. West J Med. 1978;128:360–5.
3. Brennan TA, Leape LL, Laird N, et al. Incidence of adverse events and negligence in hospitalized patients: results from the Harvard medical practice study I. NEJM. 1991;324:370–6.
4. Leape LL, Brennan TA, Laird NM, et al. The nature of adverse events in hospitalized patients: results from the Harvard Medical Practice Study II. N Eng J Med. 1991;324:377–84.
5. Leape LL, Lawthers AG, Brennan TA, Johnson WG. Preventing medical injury. Qual Rev Bull. 1993;19:144–9.
6. Zinman D. Study finds hospitals 'harm' some. Newsday 1990 March 1, 1990;Sect. 17A.
7. Johnson WG, Brennan TA, Newhouse JP, et al. The economic consequences of medical injuries: implications for a no-fault insurance plan. JAMA. 1992;267:2487–92.

Chapter 2
It's Not Bad People: Error in Medicine

"Don't go there." Howard Hiatt and Troy Brennan were emphatic: investigating medical error and writing about it would bring the wrath of the medical profession down on my head. But how could we not go there? How could we not go there, now that we knew from the Medical Practice Study (MPS) that 120,000 people were dying from medical errors every year? How could we *not* act?

The Harvard Medical Practice Study confirmed what smaller studies had shown earlier—that nearly 4% of patients in acute care hospitals suffered a significant injury from their medical treatment. What was shocking, and previously totally unrecognized, was that two-thirds of those injuries resulted from errors. Surely we should be able to do something about that.

What was known about how to prevent errors? I knew very little. So, in typical academic fashion, I started my education with a literature search. I clearly remember the day in September 1989 when I went to the Countway Library at Harvard Medical School to carry out a search of the medical literature to find out what was known about preventing medical errors. I came up empty-handed! There were case reports and a few commentaries, reports of surgical complications, and the like, but little about errors or how to prevent them other than to try harder and be more careful. But healthcare professionals—especially doctors, nurses, and pharmacists—are some of the best trained

© The Author(s) 2021
L. L. Leape, *Making Healthcare Safe*,
https://doi.org/10.1007/978-3-030-71123-8_2

and most conscientious workers there are. They were already trying hard and being careful. So why were there no descriptions of error prevention?

I took my search strategy to the librarian and asked for help. She thought the strategy was fine but asked if I had looked in the social sciences or engineering literature. It hadn't occurred to me. When she did, hundreds of references came up. It turned out that many people, in several disciplines—particularly cognitive psychology and human factors engineering—knew a great deal about why people make mistakes as well as how to prevent them. Thus began my education on the mental processes that lead to errors and on the methods of preventing them. I had a lot of reading to do. I dug in.

By early 1990, I had decided to work on a paper to bring these lessons from human factors engineering and cognitive psychology to my profession of medicine. My reading had introduced me to the insights of a host of experts, but three had the greatest influence: James Reason (*Human Error*) [1], the true father of error research, later to become a good friend; Don Norman (*The Design of Everyday Things*) [2]; and Charles Perrow (*Normal Accidents*) [3].

The Causes of Errors

James Reason, of the University of Manchester, UK, is without doubt the person who has contributed the most to the understanding of the causes and prevention of errors. His book, *Human Error* (1990), is the "Bible" of error theory. While Reason had many insights, his most original and useful contribution was to differentiate between active and latent failures. Active failures (or errors) are the individual unsafe acts that cause an injury (such as a nurse's miscalculation of a drug dose). Latent failures (or latent errors) are contributory factors that are "built in" to the system—defects in design—that lay dormant and "set up" the individual to make a mistake. One reason a nurse may make

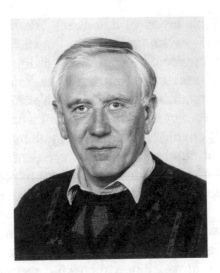

Jim Reason.

an error in calculating the dose of a medication, for example, is the latent failure of a work environment full of interruptions and distractions. Latent errors create "accidents waiting to happen." Latent errors result from poor system design [1, 4].

From this distinction between active and latent errors came the fundamental principle that underlies essentially all safety efforts: errors are not fundamentally due to faulty people but to faulty systems. To prevent errors, you have to fix the systems. As Reason put it so pungently: "Rather than being the main instigators of an accident, operators tend to be the inheritors of system defects. . . . Their part is that of adding the final garnish to a lethal brew whose ingredients have already been long in the cooking" [1].

After studying many industrial accidents, Reason further developed a general theory that accidents result from failures in one or more of four domains: organization, supervision, preconditions (such as fatigue from long hours of work), and specific acts. He is best known for his "Swiss cheese" model that depicts the organizational defenses (systems) as a series of slices of cheese. Each defense has defects, represented by the holes, which vary in size, timing, and position.

Normally the multiple layers of defenses work, but when the defects temporally coincide—when the holes in the slices align—the potential for an "accident trajectory" is created, leading to the failure.

Charles Perrow, professor of sociology at Yale, studied risks and accidents in large organizations. His book, *Normal Accidents: Living with High-Risk Technologies*, advanced the theory that accidents are inevitable in highly coupled and complex systems and hard to predict. From analysis of a number of famous accidents, he described the latent failures and what could have been done to prevent the catastrophes. He has been a consistent and effective promoter of systems theory.

Donald Norman, director of The Design Lab at the University of California, San Diego, is the author of the delightful book, *The Design of Everyday Things*, in which he laments the everyday annoyances— and the error potential—posed by poor design, such as door openers for which it is not obvious whether to push or pull. Though that design failure results only in trivial annoyance, others, such as confusing instructions for programing navigation systems in aircraft, can result in crashes. Norman introduced me to "affordances"—designs that make function obvious, such as door handles that show by their position or design which way to push or pull, and "forcing functions"— designing a process to make it impossible to do it wrong, such as design of a car's ignition switch so that the engine cannot be started unless the gear is set in "park."

This was fascinating stuff. It was all new to me despite my excellent undergraduate and medical education at fine universities. I knew nothing about the extensive knowledge that psychologists and human factors engineers had developed about why we make mistakes, nor about the ideas they had for preventing them. The light bulbs went off: this is what we need! This is something we can use. It was clearly applicable to healthcare: we had to redesign our systems.

The more I read, the more excited I got about the relevance of this knowledge to what we needed to do to reduce iatrogenic harm. I assumed that, like me, very few doctors, nurses, or other healthcare workers had any knowledge of this body of thought. It seemed inescapably clear that healthcare needed to take a systems approach to medical errors. We needed to stop punishing individuals for their errors since almost all of them were beyond their control, and we had to begin to change the faulty systems that "set them up" to make mistakes. We needed to design errors out of the system. I had no doubt we could do that.

Application of Systems Thinking to Healthcare

Healthcare lacked effective systems at many levels. At the most obvious level, there was no fail-safe system for identifying the patient to make sure that a test or medication was being given to the right person. We lacked a system for guaranteeing that a medication dose was correctly calculated and measured out or given to the right patient. The only system for preventing a patient from getting the wrong dose or a substantial overdose of any drug was double-checking by another nurse, but this was required only for certain medications such as narcotics. Nothing prevented a nurse from inadvertently confusing two vials with similar labels, such as solutions of sodium chloride and concentrated potassium chloride, and accidentally giving the patient a lethal infusion of potassium—which, in fact, was not all that rare.

Although the evidence was clear that disinfecting your hands reduced hospital-acquired infections, there was no system to ensure that doctors and nurses did it for every encounter. And, of course, the hospital environment was notorious for distractions and interruptions of nurses and resident physicians, who were also overworked and sleep-deprived—all "preconditions" that are well-known to cause errors.

As noted, my colleagues—particularly Howard Hiatt and Troy Brennan from the MPS—tried to dissuade me from writing about this. They said that "error" was a "third rail" issue that doctors—including my friends and associates—would be very upset if I brought this to public attention, since it would make them look bad; the medical establishment, i.e., the AMA, would line up against me.

I understood that risk but saw no choice. Here was an answer to the problem of medical errors. How could we not pursue it? We needed to make a fundamental change in how we practiced. There was no way to make that happen unless we talked about error. We needed to change physicians' (and nurses' and everyone's) mindset away from thinking of an error as a moral failing to recognizing that it resulted from a systems failure. I was very excited about the possibility of doing this.

Error in Medicine

By mid-1992, I had finally finished the paper. I decided to call it "Error in Medicine" [5]. It was a comprehensive look at the problem. It began by referencing the findings of the MPS, which found that nearly 4 percent of hospitalized patients suffered a serious injury, of which 14% were fatal and 69% were due to errors and were thus preventable.

From these findings we had estimated that nationwide more than a million patients were harmed annually, and 180,000 died from these injuries. I noted that this was the equivalent of three jumbo-jet crashes every 2 days, an analogy that was later picked up by others and became popular after the IOM report came out in 1999. Two-thirds of the deaths, or about 120,000, were due to errors. What could be done about the high rate of preventable injury?

The paper set out to do four things. It first explored why the error rate in medicine is so high. It noted that some of the lack of response comes from lack of awareness—errors are not part of a doctor's everyday experience—and the fact that most errors are, fortunately, not harmful. But a more important factor is that doctors and nurses have a great deal of difficulty dealing with errors. They are taught to believe that they should make no mistakes; when they inevitably do make a mistake, they view it as a character failing.

The second section explored the institutional approach to errors in medicine, which is based on this "perfectability" model: the expectation of faultless performance. This leads to blame when individuals fail, followed by punishment or more training. Since all humans err, any system that relies on error-free performance is destined to fail. I called for a fundamental change in the way we think about errors.

The third section summarized the lessons from the extensive research about the cognitive mechanisms of error in the field of cognitive psychology and the research on latent error (poor system design) and the effectiveness of system design in reducing errors in the field of human factors engineering.

The aviation experience provided a useful model: physicians and pilots are highly trained professionals committed to maintaining high standards while performing complex tasks in challenging environments. But aircraft designers assume that errors are inevitable and design systems to prevent them or, if that fails, "absorb" them with buffers, automation, and redundancy to prevent accidents. Procedures are standardized and pilots use checklists. Training is extensive, both in technical aspects and communication; pilots must take proficiency examinations every 6 months. The other major difference from healthcare is that adherence to standards is monitored and enforced by the Federal Aviation Administration, and accidents are investigated by the National Transportation Safety Board.

The impressive improvement in safety from application of this system-design approach in aviation (where there has been no fatality in the USA from a commercial air flight in more than 10 years!) contrasts dramatically with the medical model that focuses on the individual. There was one exception: the specialty of anesthesia, where application of systems changes had already resulted in dramatic improvements in mortality.

Starting in 1978, Jeff Cooper and his colleagues published a series of pioneering studies of critical incidents in anesthesia [6, 7] in which they identified specific systems failures and recommended system solutions (such as alarms for airway disconnections, procedures and practices for handovers, and greater preparation of residents before their care of patients). That led Ellison Pierce, the president of the American Society of Anesthesiologists, to partner with Cooper and others in 1984 to found the Anesthesia Patient Safety Foundation (APSF), with the mission "To ensure that no patient is harmed by anesthesia." Under Cooper's direction, APSF distributed a newsletter to all anesthesia providers highlighting patient safety issues and established a program to fund grants for research in anesthesia safety.

These efforts were dramatically successful: they reduced the mortality of anesthesia 90%, from 1 in 20,000 to 1 in 200,000, within a decade [8]. In the first years of the APSF grant program, David Gaba's group at Stanford was funded to develop and study the use of simulation to train anesthesia providers to effectively work in teams to manage critical events. The use of simulators was later expanded throughout all of healthcare and in medical schools.

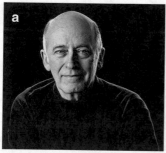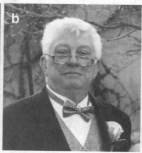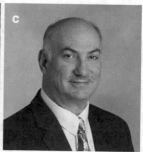

(a) Jeff Cooper, (b) Jeep Pierce, (c) David Gaba.

In the final section, I urged hospitals to implement a systems approach by creating systems for error reporting, changing processes to reduce reliance on memory, standardizing routine procedures, and reducing error-inducing conditions such as long hours and high workloads.

I ended the paper with a summary that was more prophetic than I realized at the time: "But it is apparent that the most fundamental change that will be needed if hospitals are to make meaningful progress in error reduction is a cultural one. Physicians and nurses need to accept the notion that error is an inevitable accompaniment of the human condition, even among conscientious professionals with high standards. Errors must be accepted as evidence of systems flaws not character flaws. Until and unless that happens, it is unlikely that any substantial progress will be made in reducing medical errors" [5].

I knew this was important stuff. I thought it would be a paradigm-shifting paper—as in fact it turned out to be. So I was stunned when *The New England Journal of Medicine* rejected it without even sending it out for reviews! I knew the editor, Jerry Kassirer, from our days together at Tufts, so I called him and asked him to tell me why they had rejected it so I could revise it. I will never forget his answer: "It just didn't meet our standards." I was so stunned that I didn't know what to say, so I said nothing, thanked him, and said goodbye.

Not long after, I happened to see George Lundberg, editor in chief of JAMA, in the hallway at HSPH. He was there that day teaching. I asked him if he would take an informal look at my paper. He did, immediately recognized its "huge importance" (his words), and asked me to submit it to JAMA. I was delighted and greatly relieved. George handled itself at JAMA and accepted it shortly after. It would be months before it was published, however. Such delays—a year sometimes—between acceptance and publication are not unusual with high-impact medical journals, but there was something else going on here.

Response to Error in Medicine

George realized that my paper would be a red flag for many doctors, who were very sensitive to anything that might make them look bad. Their institutional arm was the AMA, which saw its primary responsibility as the defense of physicians' pride and privilege. Naively, I thought the paper offered so much in the way of opportunity to reduce harm to patients that it would be rapidly embraced by doctors. Here

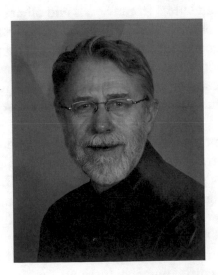

George Lundberg.

was the way they could reduce harm to their patients and decrease the risk of malpractice suits. Why wouldn't doctors be excited about that?

George had the better political sense. He deliberately published the paper just before Christmas, on December 21, 1994, knowing that holiday issues are the least read by the press; hopefully, it would not attract a lot of media attention. It almost worked. Only NPR picked it up: David Baron (later of "Spotlight" fame) recognized its importance and gave it public notice. A month later *The Washington Post* wrote about it and then the reaction began. Lundberg began to receive hate mail, and a lobbying campaign to get rid of him began. James Todd, the executive vice president of the AMA stood by him, however, and the furor subsided.

Curiously, I don't recall receiving any "hate" mail—although I may have just put it out of my mind. I certainly did not get a lot. But he did, and this proved to be an early episode in a series of courageous publishing decisions that ultimately cost him the JAMA editorship. I am forever indebted to George Lundberg, who had the courage to do the right thing.

On the other hand, within days of the publication of *Error in Medicine*, I received letters from friends and others congratulating me and thanking me for the paper. I even received a speaking engagement request. JAMA received a deluge of letters to the editor disagreeing with one or another of the points I had made. It ignored most of them but asked me to respond to nine—a huge number for a single paper. I did so, and the letters and my responses were subsequently published in JAMA [9, 10].

Amazingly, almost as if on cue, suddenly a series of highly publicized events occurred in early 1995 that drew public and professional attention to the paper. In January, *The Boston Globe* reported that Betsy Lehman, a beloved health reporter for the paper, had died from a massive overdose of chemotherapy at the prestigious Dana-Farber Cancer Institute (DFCI). The community was shocked; *Globe* reporters relentlessly pursued the story, with a litany of frontpage articles week after week castigating the Institute for its mistakes and poor systems.

As a leading cancer research organization, DFCI always had a number of new drug trials going on simultaneously. Sometimes these included tests of high doses of toxic chemotherapeutic drugs, and

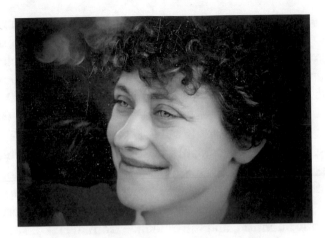

Betsy Lehman.

treatment protocols varied substantially by dose, time of dosage, etc. Study protocols were complicated and many pages long. It was difficult for nurses and doctors to keep it all straight. So, when the physician mistakenly wrote an order for Lehman for a dose that was four times the usual amount, neither the nurses nor the pharmacy questioned it. The system failed.

In April, I was asked to meet with the DFCI staff to talk with them about our new thinking about systems causes of errors in an effort to help the devastated staff deal with the crisis. They were visibly shaken. Years later people commented to me about our session, so I think it helped. The Lehman case was a life-changing event for DFCI, which underwent a major reorganization under the leadership of Jim Conway to dramatically improve its safety and ultimately achieve the lowest medication error rate in the nation.

The Massachusetts Board of Registration in Nursing was not so moved. Four years later (!) it censured 18 nurses for their role in the Betsy Lehman case. I wrote a scathing op-ed for the *Globe* [11].

The Betsy Lehman tragedy, plus several other egregious errors that got national coverage that spring, the amputation of the wrong leg of a patient in Florida, removal of the wrong breast of a patient in Michigan, death from accidental disconnection of a ventilator in Florida, and an operation on the wrong side of the brain of a patient in Chicago, stimulated reporters and others to inquire deeper into why these things happen. They discovered my recently published *Error in Medicine* paper. It undoubtedly got much more early attention because of the coincidence of these tragic accidents.

The combination of the paper and these highly visible preventable deaths also created the climate for a favorable reception of the results of our adverse drug event (ADE) study at the Massachusetts General Hospital and the Brigham and Women's Hospital that David Bates and I published just a few months later in JAMA in July 1995 [12, 13]. Not only did we find high rates of ADEs, further evidence of the seriousness of the error problem, but we were also able to show that underlying systems failures could be identified. (See next chapter.)

It is hazardous to ascribe causation, but it is not unreasonable to conclude that the "one-two-three punch"—the error paper, which raised the issue and recommended a system solution, the serious cases that got public attention, and the evidence from the ADE study that we could identify systems causes underlying medical errors—was instrumental in beginning to get patient safety and systems change on the national agenda.

The paper also influenced the thinking of future leaders in patient safety. Within a year, Jerod Loeb, from the Joint Commission, and Mark Eppinger of the Annenberg Center decided to convene a conference on medical error. Despite the displeasure with Lundberg at the AMA, its legal counsel, Marty Hatlie, convinced the leadership to shift its efforts from tort reform to error prevention. That ultimately led the AMA to found the National Patient Safety Foundation. (See Chap. 5.)

Most importantly, however, the paper influenced Ken Shine, president of the Institute of Medicine (IOM) and its Quality of Care Committee, to make safety a focus of its work in quality of care. (See Chap. 9.) The Committee's later report *To Err is Human* [14] was in many ways a detailed explication of the information in *Error in Medicine*, amplified with patient examples and specific recommendations for policy changes. It brought to public attention what the paper brought to the profession.

Error in Medicine called for a paradigm shift. It challenged everyone in healthcare to change their approach to its most sensitive and most taboo failing: medical errors. It called for replacing a stale, failed policy of blame and retribution after a mistake with a radically new approach to prevent future mistakes. It looked forward, not backward; it replaced fear with hope. It gave medicine a way to deal with our national shame of preventable deaths. "It's not bad people, it's bad systems." would be the guiding principle for the work to follow. Things would never be the same.

References

1. Reason J. Human error. Cambridge: Cambridge University Press; 1990.
2. Norman DA. The design of everyday things. 1st Doubleday/Currency ed. New York: Doubleday; 1990.
3. Perrow C. Normal accidents. Living with high-risk technologies. New York: Basic Books; 1984.
4. Reason JT. Managing the risks of organizational accidents. Aldershot, Hants/ Brookfield: Ashgate; 1997.
5. Leape LL. Error in medicine. JAMA. 1994;272:1851–7.
6. Cooper JB, Newbower RS, Long CD, McPeek B. Preventable anesthesia mishaps - a human factors study. Anesthesiology. 1978;49:399–406.
7. Cooper J, Newbower R, Kitz R. An analysis of major errors and equipment failures in anesthesia management: considerations for prevention and detection. Anesthesiology. 1984;60:34–42.
8. Orkin F. Patient monitoring during anesthesia as an exercise in technology assessment. In: Saidman L, Smith N, editors. Monitoring in anesthesia. Boston: Butterworth-Heinemann; 1993. p. 439–55.
9. Various authors. Letters to the editor. JAMA. 1995;274:457–60.
10. Leape LL. Error in medicine-reply. JAMA. 1995;274:460–1.
11. Leape LL. Faulty systems, not faulty people. The Boston Globe 1999 January 12, 1999;Sect. A15.
12. Bates DW, Cullen DJ, Laird N, et al. Incidence of adverse drug events and potential adverse drug events. JAMA. 1995;274:29–34.
13. Leape LL, Bates DW, Cullen DJ, et al. Systems analysis of adverse drug events. JAMA. 1995;274:35–43.
14. Kohn KT, Corrigan JM, Donaldson MS, editors. To err is human: building a safer health system. Washington, DC: National Academy Press; 1999.

Chapter 3
Changing the System: The Adverse Drug Events Study

It was clear from the beginning of my investigation into the application of systems theory to error prevention in healthcare that however strong the theory and the evidence—and for me it was compelling—the idea of a systems approach to preventing errors would get little acceptance from physicians unless we could demonstrate that it actually worked in healthcare.

Doctors are the ultimate "NIH" (not invented here) thinkers; they have trouble imagining that something that works in another industry would be relevant to healthcare. "Healthcare is different." "Healthcare is special." And, of course, it is, but couldn't we learn from others? Not easily, I knew. It was clear to me that if I wanted to get acceptance of systems theory and motivate doctors—as well as everyone in healthcare—to change, we would have to demonstrate that systems theory could be successfully applied to real-world medical problems.

But it is even more complicated. Any demonstration in healthcare would have to resonate—be applicable—for *all kinds* of physicians. Making a systems change in the operating room, for example, would be of little interest to internists. And a change eliminating errors in the diagnosis of diabetes would not carry much weight with the surgeons. To prove the point, we needed to address a systems failure that affected *all* physicians.

The obvious choice was medication errors. All doctors write prescriptions. Moreover, we knew from the Medical Practice Study that misuse of medications was a serious problem, indeed the most serious

© The Author(s) 2021
L. L. Leape, *Making Healthcare Safe*,
https://doi.org/10.1007/978-3-030-71123-8_3

problem we found, accounting for a fifth of all serious adverse events discovered in the study. Medication errors it would be.

Who knew anything about medication errors? More to the point, who might be interested in collaborating on this type of project? I spoke with Tony Komaroff, professor of medicine at Harvard and editor in chief of the *Harvard Health Letter* and the *Harvard Medical School Family Health Guide.* He knew just the person: David Bates, a young internist-investigator at Brigham and Women's Hospital (BWH).

I first met David on April 12, 1990. We immediately hit it off. He got interested in medication errors when he learned that adverse drug events (ADEs) were the leading type of harm found by the Medical Practice Study. David was also the key person at the Brigham evaluating a computerized physician order entry (CPOE) system being developed by a team led by Jonathan Teich in which physicians were to enter orders on the computer instead of writing them by hand. It seemed obvious that this could be a powerful systems change for reducing errors. Could we demonstrate that it did in fact do that?.

We agreed on a strategy: first, we would do a study to get an accurate measure of the extent of medication errors and the harm they caused. We would categorize them by type and when in the medication process they occurred. And we would see if we could identify the systems failures causing them. Most previous studies of medication errors relied on self-reporting, which was known to be unreliable, and none were comprehensive in the sense of considering all of the stages

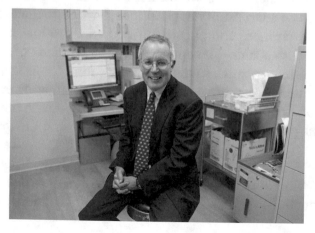

David Bates. (All rights reserved)

in the medication process. Most significantly, none had linked medication errors to harm, and none inquired into underlying causes.

After getting this information, we would implement a systems change, such as CPOE, to see if it reduced the harm. None of this was assured. How to find the errors? How to find the underlying systems failures? All new territory, but very exciting.

Fortunately, the Risk Management Foundation (RMF) of CRICO (the Controlled Risk Insurance Company that provides liability coverage to all the Harvard hospitals and doctors) was intrigued by the Medical Practice Study and was interested in exploring the possibility of *preventing* medical injury, not just paying for its consequences through malpractice suit settlements. They gave us a small grant for a pilot study at BWH. Thus began a long and fruitful relationship with this incredibly enlightened insurer.

We were aware that many complications of the use of medications—such as unpredictable allergic reactions—are not caused by errors, so we decided to focus on drug-related harm, not just errors. Referring to the Medical Practice Study definition of adverse event, we defined "adverse drug event" (ADE) as "an unintended injury caused by use of a medication." To determine those caused by errors, we used the MPS definition: "The failure of a planned action to be completed as intended or the use of a wrong plan to achieve an aim."

Our objective of finding every episode of harm caused by a medication led us to develop a totally new approach to data collection. Rather than rely on reporting of events by the unit nurse, we would have a specially trained nurse visit the study care units in the hospital several times a day to review each patient's record, follow up on laboratory test results, and interview the unit nurses searching for evidence that the patient had experienced an ADE. She would also count the medication errors and find out as much as she could about what caused them. In short, we did everything we could think of to try to find every ADE and every medication error.

The results of the pilot study were encouraging. The intensive data collection enabled us to identify many more ADEs than had been reported in other studies that largely depended on review of medical records [1]. We were also able to determine how many medication errors result in harm. We drew up a proposal for a large multi-institutional study that would have a sample size big enough to have statistical significance. We would also find out if we could identify underlying systems failures. We sought funding from the Agency for Health Care Policy and Research (AHCPR).

Meanwhile, acutely aware of our lack of knowledge and experience in how to train people to find causes of errors, we sought help from a psychologist and were finally steered to Richard Hackman, professor of social and organizational psychology at Harvard. Hackman was an expert on teamwork, having studied airplane crews, sports teams, corporate boards, and even symphony orchestras. He was intrigued by our project, and we enlisted him in our study.

We also recruited David Cullen, a senior anesthesiologist from the Massachusetts General Hospital (MGH) who had research experience and a long-standing interest in patient safety. He had done medication safety research in anesthesia and was very enthusiastic about joining the team. As is often the case in a strong collaboration, we each brought different things to the table. I had clinical experience from my long surgical career to draw on, as well as experience in finding and classifying adverse events from the Medical Practice study. David Bates was an internist at the Brigham with epidemiology training and informatics skills. And David Cullen brought his anesthesia experience and was well positioned to recruit a team at MGH.

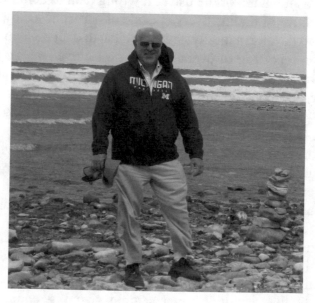

David Cullen.

In 1992 our proposal was funded by AHCPR. We called our coalition the ADE Prevention Study Group and conceived of the project in two phases. In Phase 1 we had two objectives: to identify every ADE and potential ADE (an error that could have but did not result in an ADE) and to identify the systems failure(s) underlying each one. In Phase 2 we would introduce one or more specific systems changes to correct an identified failure and find out whether it prevented ADEs.

The Agency funded Phase 1 but to our disappointment declined to fund Phase 2 until we showed that we had succeeded with Phase 1. Based on our pilot study results, we were confident we would succeed, although we were worried about making the timing work out. We established an investigative team at each hospital and selected 11 nursing units for the study at the 2 hospitals: 5 intensive care units and 6 general, non-obstetric care units. David Bates was the leader of the Brigham team and David Cullen led the MGH team.

As in the pilot study, we identified adverse drug events by having a trained nurse investigator review the charts and laboratory test results of every patient and talk with the nurses in each of the study units daily.

To identify underlying systems failures, something that had not been done before, we developed data forms with questions regarding the what, where, when, and how of each incident. We trained our nurse investigators to use them to assess each ADE they found. We also gathered data about within-team communication, between-team communication, as well as environmental information.

The nurse investigators also inquired about circumstances around the event such as the person's health, job stressors, sleep the previous night, education about the drug, and experience with the drug. In other words, we were looking for all possible explanations for why errors might be made.

To develop and refine our data collection methodology, David Bates and I had multiple meetings with Richard Hackman and his graduate student, Amy Edmondson. Despite this, things almost came unglued at our first training session for the nurse investigators. Through what in retrospect was a major miscommunication, David and I thought Amy was going to do the training. However, when we had the meeting with the nurses, it was immediately obvious that she had no idea that was to be her role. Without revealing our problem to the trainees, I took over and spontaneously ran the program. David and I had thought a lot about our objectives and measures and had spelled them out, so it wasn't starting from scratch, but more planning would have been better. In any case, it had to do. In the end it worked out all right. After a few weeks, the process worked fairly smoothly.

The study team at each hospital conferenced every other week to review every adverse drug event and potential adverse event that had been identified and to classify errors by type. Using the data the nurses had collected about the circumstances surrounding each ADE, we then systematically identified the underlying causes of errors at two levels: the *proximal* (obvious) causes and the *underlying* causes, or *systems failures*. For example, a doctor prescribed the wrong medication (error), because of insufficient knowledge about the drug (proximal cause) due to a failure in the drug knowledge dissemination system (systems failure). Although we were all new at this type of analysis, it proved surprisingly easy to do, which gave us confidence that our findings were valid.

In 1994 we completed the fieldwork and analyzed our data. There had been some pitfalls; partway through the study, a medical unit was switched to a surgical unit, for example. But overall data collection went well. We found 247 adverse drug events in the study population of 4031 admissions, a rate of 6.5 per 100 admissions. Of these, 70 (28%) were preventable [2]. We also found 194 potential ADEs, errors that did not result in harm or were intercepted before the medication was given (Table 3.1).

Errors occurred at every stage of the process. Nearly half (49%) occurred during ordering, followed by nurse administration, 26%; pharmacist dispensing, 14%; and transcription, 11%. Dosing errors were the most common type of medication error, and more than half

Table 3.1 Adverse drug event rates

	No. (%)	Rate/100 admissions
ADEs	247 (100)	6.5
Preventable ADEs	70 (28)	1.8
Nonpreventable ADEs	177 (72)	4.7
Potential ADEs	194 (100)	5.5
Nonintercepted	111 (57)	3.1
Intercepted	83 (43)	2.4

Adapted from Ref. [2]

of these occurred at the physician ordering stage. Fortunately, nearly half of physician errors were intercepted (largely by nurses), but no one backstopped the nurses; only 2% of nursing administration errors were intercepted (Table 3.2).

This rate of ADEs, 6.5 for every 100 patients, was astounding! It was almost ten (10) times higher than had ever been reported. And this was at the two flagship teaching hospitals of Harvard, institutions that considered themselves the best in the country! [2]

To my delight, we were also able to identify systems failures underlying the errors and to categorize them into operationally useful categories. The leading failures were in systems for (1) drug knowledge dissemination (example of an error: failure to reduce dose for elderly patient), (2) dose and identity checking (error: mix-up of two "look-alike" packaged drugs), (3) patient information availability (error: lack of information about reduced kidney function), (4) order transcription (error: handwriting errors), and (5) allergy defense (error: giving medication to a patient known to be allergic to it) [3] (Table 3.3).

We now had evidence that systems failures could be identified in a healthcare environment, the first step in my quest to develop data to convince doctors and hospitals that changing systems would be more effective in reducing harm than punishing people who made mistakes. We still had a long way to go: we needed to show that we could change the systems and that changing them would reduce the harm. But we were on our way. Needless to say, this was pretty exciting.

While we were analyzing our results for publication, we completed planning for Phase 2, the implementation of systems changes in a controlled study to determine if the changes would, in fact,

Table 3.2 Types of medication errors	Type of error	No. (%)
	Wrong dose	95 (28)
	Wrong choice	30 (9)
	Wrong drug	29 (9)
	Known allergy	27 (8)
	Missed dose	24 (7)
	Wrong time	23 (7)
	Wrong frequency	20 (6)
	Wrong technique	20 (6)
	Drug-drug interaction	9 (3)
	Wrong route	6 (2)

Adapted from Ref. [3]

Table 3.3 Major systems failures

System	Attributed errors	
	No.	%
1. Drug knowledge dissemination	98	29
2. Dose and identity checking	40	12
3. Patient information availability	37	11
4. Order transcription	29	9
5. Allergy defense	24	7
6. Medication order tracking	18	5
7. Interservice communication	17	5
8. Device use	12	4
9. Std. doses/frequencies	12	4
10. Std. drug distribution in unit	11	3

Adapted from Ref. [3]

reduce harm. Suddenly the roof fell in! Despite our brilliant results in Phase 1, the rating of our grant proposal to AHCPR fell a fraction of a point below their funding level. We had no funding for the next phase.

We were in deep trouble. We had the team assembled, we had the instruments, and we had the plan all worked out to move ahead. Most importantly, we had a potentially powerful systems change to test— but no money! Into the breach came the Risk Management Foundation, which had funded our original pilot study. They agreed to pay for the project, one more example of their generosity at crucial times that was so helpful for our team. We were profoundly grateful.

The systems change to be tested in Phase 2 at BWH was computerized physician order entry (CPOE) in which all physician orders are written on the computer. This enabled medication orders to be automatically checked for errors such as wrong dose, overlooking a drug allergy, or giving two incompatible drugs, thus preventing the physician from making the error.

This had been our plan from the start. David Bates and colleagues at BWH had been working to get it designed and tested, and it was ready to go. The timing was perfect. This would be a powerful systems change; we anticipated it would have a significant effect in reducing prescribing orders, the most common type of error found in Phase 1.

But what systems change would the MGH implement? They were far from having a computer order entry system, so we needed something else. Fortunately, we were aware that there was some evidence that having a pharmacist present on rounds with clinicians reduced prescribing errors. This made sense, but the practice had not been tested in a controlled trial. We decided to see if implementing this systems change of having a pharmacist make rounds every morning with the physician care team would significantly decrease ADEs.

Morning rounds are when care decisions are made, including what medications to prescribe, so having the pharmacist's input at the time of decision-making might reduce prescribing errors. We would try it in an intensive care unit (ICU) where patients are cared for by a true "team" that meets to make rounds at a predictable time. Another ICU would be the control unit. We began the study.

The big event of 1995 for our research team was the publication of our first two papers from the drug prevention study: the incidence study and the systems analysis study [2, 3]. Prior to submitting the papers to a journal, we ran them by the CEOs of the Mass General and the Brigham, as well as the chair of medicine at the Brigham, Dr. Eugene Braunwald, so they would not be blind-sided by what we anticipated might be extensive publicity when the papers were published.

Despite the fact that the high rates of ADEs could potentially make them look bad, to their credit, neither CEO suggested that we not publish nor, for that matter, change a single word in the papers. They did, however, arrange for and pay for media training for both of us! It proved very helpful. I learned for the first time that when being interviewed, you don't answer the reporter's question but use it to make your points. We were taught some techniques for turning the conversation around to what we wanted to talk about.

George Lundberg welcomed our first two papers, and they were published fairly soon in JAMA in July 1995—just 7 months after my Error in Medicine paper and 5 months after the news about Betsy Lehman's tragic death from an overdose of chemotherapy. The papers got a lot of publicity: all three major television networks covered them on the nightly news, and both David and I had live interviews with them. Ted Koppel even did a special on Nightline about them. Our media training paid off.

But Nancy Dickey, the president of the American Medical Association, was not pleased. In a television interview, she criticized us and said the numbers were exaggerated. Of course, the reverse was true—we knew we missed some, and indeed, later more sophisticated studies showed even higher rates. David Bates was shocked by this. I was not surprised, having previously had a similar experience with her and the Medical Practice Study. To her credit, Dr. Dickey later came around and subsequently became an important advocate for patient safety and led the establishment of the National Patient Safety Foundation.

On the other hand, both of us got favorable letters from other physicians, as well as a number of letters to the editor, most of which were positive. The papers were also well accepted by the general healthcare community. They have since been cited over 2500 times, the most-cited studies of the frequency of harm related to the hospital use of medications.

An interesting sidebar was an episode in the review process after we submitted the papers. As is typically the case, the acceptance was tentative, conditioned on our revising them in response to reviewers' comments. One reviewer wrote a five-page single-spaced review of the systems paper that raised multiple important points, all of which I would have to respond to!

I knew as soon as I read it that it was written by Don Berwick. Don was the founder and CEO of the Institute for Healthcare Improvement (IHI), the pathbreaking organization teaching quality improvement (QI) to healthcare professionals. QI, of course, was about process improvement, or systems change. IHI had applied QI techniques to issues such as overuse and underuse of services, but not to medical errors.

I had met Don some years earlier when I was exploring options for my new career. From talking with him and reading his papers, I immediately recognized that he was the author of the critique. I was reminded of the old saw, "With friends like that, who needs enemies?" But, of course, revising with his points addressed made it a much stronger paper. The paper was also Don's introduction to my work (the review was before my Error in Medicine paper came out) and led him to later involve me in the IHI Breakthrough Collaborative work on adverse drug events and begin our long-term collaboration.

Another interesting wrinkle related to our psychology colleagues. Amy Edmondson became curious about why two of the four seemingly identical nursing units at the MGH had substantially lower rates of ADE than the other two. Were they better managed? Were nurses there more careful? If so, why?

Using the data from our study and further interviews of nurses, she was able to show that the units with the higher rates of reported ADE were those that had more supportive nurse managers. In the units with lower rates, nurses were less likely to report errors because they feared they would be punished or reprimand. In the high-rate units, that wouldn't happen. The high-rate units did not have more ADEs, they just knew about more of them because the environment made it possible for them to be brought to the surface. Edmondson developed this finding into her PhD thesis, and it became the stimulus to her later work. She is now a full professor at Harvard and an internationally recognized expert on teamwork.

Phase 2, studying the effect of our two systems changes—computerized physician order entry (CPOE) at the BWH and pharmacist presence on rounds in the ICU at the MGH—was well underway before the results of the first study came out. Our methods had been worked out and our teams were experienced at finding ADEs. BWH had previously committed to implementing CPOE. At the MGH, the extra cost of including a designated pharmacist as part of the care team for daily rounds in the ICU was funded by the nursing department and pharmacy, who were both keenly interested.

When the results came back from the studies, we were ecstatic. Both systems changes had significant impact. The before-after study at BWH showed that CPOE reduced all medication errors by 83% and ADEs by 17% [4]. The estimated cost saving if the system were implemented hospital-wide was $480,000 per year. The controlled study of pharmacist participation on rounds at the MGH showed a 66% reduction of ADEs caused by errors in prescribing [5]. Finally, we had evidence that systems change worked in healthcare.

Not surprising, our systems change papers received less coverage in the popular media than the studies that had demonstrated the extent of the problem. The media prefer bad news to good. Sadly, evidence of a problem is much more newsworthy than the demonstration of its solution.

However, our colleagues in safety took notice. Here was the proof needed that systems change worked in medicine. The papers were discussed in trade journals, and both systems change papers were part of the evidence cited as part of the Institute of Medicine recommendations in its famous report, *To Err Is Human*, that came out 2 years later. The groundwork was laid. Now began the hard job of getting doctors, nurses, and hospitals to incorporate systems thinking into their work.

BWH Center for Patient Safety Research and Practice

As we concluded our research, I turned my attention to promoting systems change and influencing policy. David kept his focus on research. He wanted to establish a "Center of Excellence," a new vehicle that AHRQ had just announced and was generously funding. Our studies showed how broken the medication delivery system was. Basic research was needed in the epidemiology of medication errors, not just in the hospital, but in all venues. Safe practices needed to be developed for all stages: ordering, dispensing, and administration and for communication and interactions between them. More needed to be known about costs and barriers to improvement.

From his work developing an electronic medical record, David could see the technological explosion that was coming, and he was eager to apply the new technology to medication error problems. There was much to do. AHRQ funded the proposal, and the BWH Center for Patient Safety Research and Practice was born. I was honored to chair its advisory board.

The scope of the Center's work under David's leadership more than lived up to the prospectus. Early on, the group demonstrated the effectiveness of real-time decision support during computer prescribing using alerts to adjust doses for renal impairment and age. Some elderly patients were receiving 10 times the recommended dose of psychoactive drugs! But alerts were not universally regarded as a benefit. If the system provided too many, as it often did, physicians ignored all of them. Center researchers found that if the alert was accompanied by specific advice, e.g., the correct dose, it was readily accepted.

The Center sponsored Rainu Kaushal's first study of medication errors in a pediatric hospital. It found a similar rate of ADE to that found in adult patients, except for newborns, where it was 10 times higher. Potential ADEs—the near-misses—were 3 times as common, testimony to an alert staff and a poor system [6].

The first study of ADE in office patients led by Tejal Gandhi showed that they were even more common than in the hospital. The ADE rate was 21%, of which 36% were preventable [7]. The study was unique and pathbreaking in another way: it demonstrated the value of asking patients about their experiences when assessing harm. We were stunned to find that patients reported 8 times as many ADEs as were noted in the physicians' charts.

From the beginning, a major focus of the Center was on the use and effectiveness of technology to reduce ADE. The early work with computerized ordering helped increase the national will to spread the use of computers into office practice. A pioneering study of bar coding of drugs showed it dramatically reduced errors in pharmacists' dispensing and when nurses give the medication to the patient [8]. Based on this evidence, the NQF endorsed bar coding, and it has since been adopted as standard practice in hospitals nationwide.

Over time David expanded the Center's agenda well beyond the issue of ADEs to patient safety in general. Center researchers studied the costs of adverse events and of adopting information technology in healthcare. They demonstrated that the use of sensors under the mattress to monitor hospitalized patients' vital signs and activity led to improved responses by nurses and a 50% reduction in ICU days. Dr. Patti Dykes, a nurse, developed a fall prevention protocol that decreased its risk by a third. It is now being used at more than 100 hospitals around the country.

David Bates proved to be an incredibly effective leader, who over the years created a leading center—probably *the* leading center—of innovation, research, and development in patient safety. He inspired and mentored a new generation of researchers, attracting postdocs and others from around the world to the center. He has trained more than 100 researchers in patient safety research who have published over 1000 papers on patient safety. His Center exemplifies patient safety research at its best.

References

1. Bates DW, Leape LL, Petrycki S. Incidence and preventability of adverse drug events in hospitalized adults. J Gen Intern Med. 1993;8:289–94.
2. Bates DW, Cullen DJ, Laird N, et al. Incidence of adverse drug events and potential adverse drug events. JAMA. 1995;274:29–34.
3. Leape LL, Bates DW, Cullen DJ, et al. Systems analysis of adverse drug events. JAMA. 1995;274:35–43.
4. Bates DW, Teich JM, Lee J, et al. The impact of computerized physician order entry on medication error prevention. J Am Med Inform Assoc. 1999;6:313–21.
5. Leape LL, Cullen DJ, Clapp MD, et al. Pharmacist participation on physician rounds and adverse drug events in the intensive care unit. JAMA. 1999;282:267–70.
6. Kaushal R, Bates D, Landrigan C, et al. Medication errors and adverse drug events in pediatric inpatients. JAMA. 2001;285:2114–20.
7. Gandhi T, Weingart SN, Borus J, et al. Adverse drug events in ambulatory care. N Engl J Med. 2003;348:1556–64.
8. Poon EG, Keohane CA, Yoon CS, et al. Effect of bar-code technology on the safety of medication administration. N Engl J Med. 2010;362:1698–707.

Chapter 4
Coming Together: The Annenberg Conference

1996 was the year that patient safety began.

One day in the early spring of 1996, Marty Hatlie, a lawyer and lobbyist at the American Medical Association (AMA), called to invite me to participate with the AMA, the Joint Commission on Accreditation of Healthcare Organizations (JCAHO), the American Association for the Advancement of Science (AAAS), and the Annenberg Center for Health Sciences in planning a big meeting on preventing errors.

I didn't know Hatlie, nor was I aware that he had been a diligent opponent of our work on drawing attention to medical error! He was the lead lawyer for the AMA dealing with malpractice issues. When the Medical Practice Study came out in 1991, he coordinated the AMA attack on the study, questioning the methodology and therefore the results. When *Error in Medicine* was published, he coordinated the attack on that as well.

The AMA then, as now, saw its role as advocating for doctors and opposing anything that seemed to be against their best interest. Discussion of errors, or even admitting that they happened, was seen as extremely threatening. The AMA's approach was to deny that doctors made mistakes, to stonewall any investigations, and to push for federal tort reform, the centerpiece of which was a cap on liability payments.

To that end, Hatlie led the AMA's intensive lobbying effort in 1995 in support of federal legislation that would limit the dollar amount of tort settlements in malpractice cases and make it more

© The Author(s) 2021
L. L. Leape, *Making Healthcare Safe*,
https://doi.org/10.1007/978-3-030-71123-8_4

difficult for patients to sue. He was joined in this effort by the American Tort Reform Association and the Healthcare Liability Alliance, a coalition built by Hatlie that included the major hospital associations, liability insurers, and Big Pharma. Together these organizations spent tens of millions of dollars lobbying Congress for the legislation.

Despite these formidable efforts, legislation failed to pass. The timing was bad. 1995 was the year that the public conscience was shocked by stories such as *The Boston Globe* journalist Betsy Lehman's death from an overdose of chemotherapy, the amputation of "the wrong foot" of Willie King in Florida, and a seemingly endless series of mishaps. It was also the year that our research was published that documented that these cases reflected a deeper problem. Although the AMA was successful in the House, the Senate would not cave to the powerful special interests.

With the congressional defeat, Marty and the AMA needed to regroup. Although he later admitted that he began to change his thinking after reading my *Error in Medicine* paper, he was still a skeptical "hired gun." However, he could see that it would help the AMA's somewhat tarnished image if it could show some interest in patient safety.

Jim Todd, executive vice president, and Nancy Dickey, incoming chairman of the AMA Board of Trustees, were easily persuaded to take a new approach. Supporting the Annenberg Conference was just what they needed to improve their image. Todd, a surgeon, had fought,

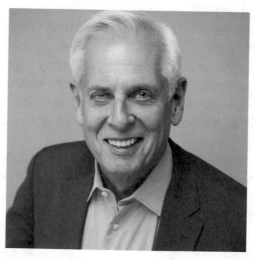

Marty Hatlie.

and lost, a battle to change the tort system from court battles to negotiated claims settlements; after the latest setback at getting tort reform legislation, he was ready for a new approach to the malpractice problem. Hatlie had another prominent ally within the AMA orbit who was a sincere, even passionate, truth teller about patient safety: George Lundberg, editor of JAMA who had published *Error in* Medicine and strongly favored the AMA acknowledging the evidence and changing its position.

The idea for a conference on medical error came from Jerod Loeb, head of research at JCAHO, and Mark Eppinger, the Annenberg Center program director. They approached Deborah Runkle of the American Association for the Advancement of Science (AAAS) in the hope of getting an issue of *Science* magazine dedicated to the topic. The AAAS had a session on medical injury at its annual meeting the year before where Richard Cook, an anesthesiologist and early thinker about patient safety, spoke and I presented the results of the MPS.

Jerod and Mark had developed the proposal for a conference focused on patient safety but had not succeeded in getting funding when Marty approached Jerod about collaborating. Marty convinced the AMA leadership to fund the conference. He also recommended the organizing group invite me, which they agreed to do.

When Marty asked me to join the planning meeting, I accepted without a second thought. Although we had never met, I was sure glad he called me! It was the beginning of a long and productive friendship in the fight for patient safety. Marty remembers that I had one condition: that they invite Jim Reason, the world's leading expert on human error, and pay for his first-class air ticket from Britain, which they did. When Jim accepted, Marty recalls him saying he'd been hoping for such a call for 20 years!

I will never forget the scene as I walked into my first meeting with the planning group at JCAHO headquarters in Chicago in early 1996. When I saw who was there, I suddenly realized that I was not only the sole physician in the group but also the only one who knew anything about medical errors! I was relieved not to have missed it. Clearly, this could be a big deal. They wanted to invite people from numerous industries as well as healthcare, which I thought was a terrific idea. The decision was made that Annenberg would host a program in the fall at the Annenberg Center in Rancho Mirage, CA.

A nationwide call for papers was put out on May 17 for the conference on October 13–15, 1996. To our surprise (and relief), we received an avalanche of proposals for presentation: over 200. To facilitate the review and selection of those we would have on the program, I suggested the committee meet for several days at our vacation home in Newfane, Vermont, in August. That turned out to be great fun and an efficient way to get the job done.

The Conference brochure listed the objectives as:

- Develop an agenda for further research into errors, identify educational or other approaches to their prevention, and target next steps for stakeholders.
- Promote greater understanding of the occurrence of errors and strategies for preventing them.
- Generate candid discussion of accountability in healthcare and explore alternate ways to respond to errors.
- Provide an opportunity for networking in a multidisciplinary setting.

The conference opened on October 13, 1996. Preregistration numbered 274; more than 300 ultimately attended. It was truly a mixed group. Almost 20% of the speakers were scientists and scholars from non-healthcare fields, such as psychology, engineering, and organizational behavior. Another 20% were nonacademic and also not from healthcare, such as lawyers and representatives of patients and families.[1]

The atmosphere from the start was electric. It was the first time that those who were concerned about errors in medicine had ever met together, and to do so with leaders in safety from other industries was exhilarating. I had the privilege of giving the opening keynote address, which I dedicated to the memory of Betsy Lehman. This was followed by a panel presenting different perspectives and an address by Jim Reason on lessons from other sectors. John Nance, pilot and aviation

---

[1] Lead faculty for the conference included, in addition to me and James Reason, Donald Berwick, IHI; Marjorie Beyers, American Organization of Nurse Executives; Victor Cohn, *The Washington Post*; James Conway, Dana-Farber; Nancy Dickey, AMA; Linda Emanuel, AMA; Linda Golodner, Nat'l Consumers League; Brent James, Intermountain Health; John Nance, Alaska Airlines; and Dennis O'Leary, The Joint Commission.

reporter for ABC News, gave his usual stem-winder talk at dinner, telling the riveting story of the crash of the KLM and Pan Am airplanes on the runway in Tenerife in 1977 that killed 538 people.

The second day opened with a presentation of the case of Ben Kolb, a 7-year-old boy who died from a mix-up of medications in the operating room at Martin Memorial Hospital in Stuart, FL. The clinicians involved in the case described the investigation and their despair. What made it memorable was the hospital was transparent from the first conversation with Ben's parents. Driven by the belief that the kind of error that took Ben's life had probably happened many times before in many other hospitals, the hospital CEO, anesthesiologist in the surgery, and risk manager jointly promised Ben's family they would share what they had learned. It was almost unheard of at the time (and, it should be noted, still a challenge 25 years later).

The audience was very moved. It was the part of the conference that most people remember clearly years later. It was also years later that I learned Hatlie had "found" the Ben Kolb case through his contacts at MMI, a liability insurer that wanted to honor the hospital leadership's promise to Ben's family to tell his story so others could be saved. Marty urged it on the program committee because he could see the public interest value of a story where providers communicated openly with the family. That judgment was validated when *USA Today* made it the lead story the next day [1], and the *New York Times Sunday Magazine* featured it as the cover story a few months later [2].

The rest of the meeting consisted of breakout group sessions, where more than 50 presentations were given on issues related to patient safety: education and training, communication, legal issues, organizational processes, human factors, fatigue, drug use, anesthesia, surgery, and medication errors. And, of course, "networking" as attendees found others who shared their interests and concerns.

Dennis O'Leary, president of JCAHO, announced that in an effort to be less punitive, the Commission was changing its response to sentinel events from "Conditional Accreditation" to "Accreditation Watch." The 3-day event concluded with a compelling plenary address by Don Berwick, the founder of the Institute for Healthcare Improvement (IHI).

But the part of the program that would have the most significant long-term impact came on the second day of the conference from something the program committee had not anticipated: a surprise announcement by Nancy Dickey, the incoming chairman of the AMA Board, that the AMA was founding and funding a National Patient Safety Foundation. Modeled on the Anesthesia Patient Safety Foundation, its objective was to fund innovative research projects to move the needle on patient safety and provide a forum for discussion. The JCAHO was a co-sponsor. Patient safety was no longer just a good idea. We would have a gathering, a focus, and a strategy for going forward. It assured that there would be more "Annenbergs."

And indeed there were. The second Annenberg Conference was held in November 1998. The original conveners and the new National Patient Safety Foundation (NPSF) (with Hatlie as its first president) were joined by representatives from the Department of Veterans Affairs. Don Berwick gave the keynote address outlining the components of a safety system. I chaired a panel on Creating a Culture of Safety. The conference focused on the challenges of replacing a culture of blame and punishment with one of cooperation and curiosity that exposes errors as opportunities to change the systems failures that caused them.

Several hospitals reported success in eliminating sanctions for reporting errors. Other presentations included use of information technology to support safe practice, the use of national incident databases as in aviation, and the impact of sleep deprivation on physician performance. There were calls for greater involvement of regulators, legislators, and patients in the dialogue, as the Massachusetts Coalition for the Prevention of Medical Errors was doing.

At the first Annenberg Conference, the memorable event was an uplifting case presentation of hospital transparency after an error. At Annenberg II, it was a depressing story of three nurses who were prosecuted for criminal negligence for their role in a fatal medication error. The audience heard from all parties, including the prosecuting attorney, followed by a presentation on the importance of not punishing individuals for systems failures. It was a stark reminder of how far we had to go to implement the fundamental principle that it isn't bad people, it's bad systems.

The third and final Annenberg Conference, *Let's Talk; Communicating Risk and Safety in Health Care*, was convened in May 2001 in Minneapolis. As the title suggests, speakers and panels addressed the human and legal issues surrounding disclosure. After this meeting, the conferences were sponsored annually by the NPSF and were called Patient Safety Congresses.

"Annenberg," as we all later called the first conference, was the birthplace of patient safety—in the USA and, truly, the world. A number of us on the faculty, Don Berwick, Brent James from Intermountain Health, and I, as well as researchers Richard Cook and David Woods, Jeep Pierce and Jeff Cooper of the Anesthesia Patient Safety Foundation, and Jim Reason and Charles Vincent in the UK, had been speaking out and writing about error prevention for years. Annenberg was the first time we all came together to exchange ideas and make common cause.

For us it was exciting and validating to interact with experts outside of healthcare and reinforce our commitment to the science of safety. It gave weight to our efforts. For others with less experience, some of whom came just out of curiosity, the demonstration of industrial concepts of human factors principles and the efforts to apply them in healthcare by anesthesia, IHI, and others was enabling and energizing. For all, it was a powerful shared emotional experience.

The meeting brought into focus the challenges of the next decade in research, reporting, standardization, changing processes, technology, and culture. It empowered the attendees to continue their work and "carry the word" to a larger audience. The quest for safe healthcare had finally begun.

References

1. Levy D. Medical groups act to curb errors. USA Today 1996 October 14, 1996.
2. Belkin L. How can we save the next victim? The New York Times 1997 June 15, 1997;Sect. 28–33, 44, 50, 63, 6, 70.

Chapter 5
A Home of Our Own: The National Patient Safety Foundation

Prior to the first Annenberg Conference, none of us who were interested in patient safety had given any thought to forming a national organization—except for Marty Hatlie, the AMA's legal counsel. Marty was intrigued by the success of the Anesthesia Patient Safety Foundation (APSF) that Jeep Pierce and Jeff Cooper had founded. He envisioned the formation of a similar national organization as the centerpiece of the refashioning of the AMA's stance on patient safety after its stinging legislative defeat of tort reform.

Hatlie began to internally advocate that the AMA establish a similar organization for all of healthcare, and he ultimately persuaded the executive vice president, Jim Todd, and incoming chair of the Board of Trustees, Nancy Dickey, that they should do this. At Annenberg, Dickey, together with two other AMA trustees, Don Palmisano and Tim Flaherty, decided on the spot to announce that the AMA was founding an independent National Patient Safety Foundation (NPSF).

Some questioned whether the AMA would really permit the Foundation to be independent. Dennis O'Leary, head of the Joint Commission on Accreditation of Healthcare Organizations (JCAHO), was particularly "leery," as was I, having been snookered by the AMA in a previous research program. But we all decided to give it a try, and JCAHO signed on as a sponsor. I thought having a national organization would make a huge difference in improving the visibility of patient safety, which in fact it did.

A few months after Annenberg, in February 1997, the AMA convened a Consensus Conference of a broad group of healthcare leaders

© The Author(s) 2021
L. L. Leape, *Making Healthcare Safe*,
https://doi.org/10.1007/978-3-030-71123-8_5

and safety experts to help it develop the NPSF agenda. Along with several others, I gave a talk to share my vision of what we needed to do for patient safety. Marty Hatlie laid out the objectives of NPSF, his hopes for collaboration across multiple stakeholders, and the details of how it was to be organized.

The group concluded that the first task for NPSF was to establish priorities. The first priority should be to support patient safety research. NPSF could also help by improving taxonomy and making data available on safety to a wide audience. Most importantly, we agreed that, unlike typical medical professional organizations, all stakeholders should be represented.

Unbeknown to most of us at the time, when Dickey and friends announced the formation of the NPSF at Annenberg, it was far from a done deal. It had not been approved by the Board of Trustees of the AMA. It turned out that many Board members were not at all sure that the AMA should be involved in anything to do with medical errors, much less sharing control with other organizations.

It took 7 months and six Board meetings before Dickey and her colleagues convinced them it was the right thing to do. However, once it did so, the AMA was generous in its support, providing $1,000,000 over 3 years, including valuable in-kind support in terms of office space and staff for the foundation in its early years.

Dickey and Hatlie were also very successful in raising money from outside groups. By the time of its official founding in May 1997, funding had been secured from multiple commercial sources, including major grants from 3M ($1m over 3 years), CNA HealthPro ($1m over 3 years), and Schering-Plough (500K over 3 years) as well as substantial contributions from the Physician Insurers Association of America, DuPont, Merck, Hoffman-La Roche, MMI, Kaiser Permanente, and Hoechst Marion Roussel.

The first meeting of the NPSF Board of Directors took place July 28–29, 1997, in Chicago. There were 40 directors in all, representing a wide range of stakeholders. Twelve of us comprised the Executive Committee: Richard Cook, anesthesiologist and safety researcher at the University of Chicago; Nancy Dickey, AMA president; Steve Fountain (Physicians Insurance Association of America); Linda Golodner (National Consumers League); Doni Haas, safety leader at Martin Memorial Hospital; Carol Ley (3M); Jim Macdonald (CNA); Henri Manasse (American Society of Healthcare Pharmacists (ASHP)); Jeep Pierce (Anesthesia Patient Safety Foundation); Diane Pinakiewicz

(Schering-Plough); John Rother (AARP); and myself. Hatlie served as executive director and did all the work of organizing and planning.

The Executive Committee developed a simple mission statement: to assure patient safety in the delivery of healthcare. We would do that by promoting research on error, promoting solutions to prevent patient harm, developing information and educational approaches that advance patient safety, and raising awareness. From the beginning, NPSF funded research through a Research Committee chaired by Jeff Cooper, who held a similar role with the APSA. By the time of the AMA's official announcement of the establishment of the NPSF in October, it was fully functioning.

The first major event the NPSF sponsored was a public briefing in New York on October 9, 1997. Charles Meyers of ASHP issued a public call for bar coding of drugs. But the news hook was the report of a public attitude survey done by Harris Associates of 1513 interviews in August 1997, commissioned by Research!America, and presented by Mary Woolley, its president.

The survey results confirmed the extent of stereotypes about patient safety and highlighted the lack of public awareness of it as a problem, even though safety issues were pervasive. The study found that 42% of respondents had been affected by a medical mistake personally or through a friend or relative, and 84% had heard of a medical mistake situation.

Half of the respondents thought carelessness, improper training, and poor communication were the major causes of mistakes; 75% thought that better training and preventing physicians with bad track records from providing care would be the most effective solution to medical mistakes. A minority believed that lawsuits or government regulation was effective. Healthcare was perceived as moderately safe (5 on a 7-point scale)—and safer than nuclear power (which was far from true), but less safe than airline travel. It was clear we had a long way to go.

The first meeting of the NPSF was held in Chicago December 15–17, 1997, and featured a Workshop on Assembling the Scientific Basis for Patient Safety Research, led by Richard Cook and David Woods, that drew international experts. They made the case for a systems approach and the need to seriously investigate errors. They labeled their session a "Tale of Two Stories," contrasting the usual response to celebrated cases—mostly blame and punishment—with in-depth investigation of a serious adverse event that leads to systems changes.

Meanwhile, at the AMA, all hell was breaking loose. Jim Todd, the CEO who strongly supported founding NPSF had retired and had

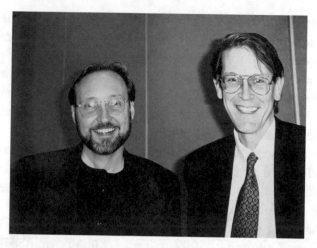

David Woods and Richard Cook.

been replaced by John Seward. One of his first acts was unprecedented and an absolute disaster: he quietly contracted with Sunbeam Products in the summer of 1997 for the AMA to provide, for a fee, an AMA seal of approval of Sunbeam appliances [1].

The AMA membership (and the public) revolted, and there were calls for senior executives, Board chairman Nancy Dickey, and the entire Board of Directors to resign. NPSF funders were outraged and began to grumble about NPSF needing to distance itself from the AMA. AMA management scrambled, fired the CEO, and ultimately paid Sunbeam $9.9 million to break the contract [2]. Things gradually quieted down.

Despite all this, the NPSF rolled ahead. Patient safety was beginning to be talked about widely. In the report of the President's Advisory Commission on Consumer Protection and Quality in the Health Care Industry, led by Don Berwick, head of the Institute for Healthcare Improvement (IHI), reduction of error was one of six recommended national aims, and NPSF was cited. JCAHO revised their sentinel event policy to make reporting voluntary, and the Agency for Healthcare Policy and Research (AHCPR) (later renamed the Agency for Healthcare Research and Quality (AHRQ) identified patient safety as a priority. In November 1998, we held the second Annenberg Conference.

Also in 1998, Ken Kizer, undersecretary for health in the Veterans Administration, established the VA National Patient Safety Partnership and worked with NPSF to explore issues in changing institutional culture. At the urging of George Lundberg, editor of JAMA, Kizer joined me, Steve Schroeder from the Robert Wood Johnson Foundation, Lundberg, and others in issuing a call for action to improve patient safety by a clear focus on medical error [3].

But most importantly, Ken Shine, president of the Institute of Medicine, decided to put quality of care and patient safety on its agenda. Advised by staff who had attended the Annenberg Conference, he convened the IOM Quality of Care Committee. A year later the Committee would issue the legendary IOM report, *To Err Is Human*, that rocked the world (Chap. 9).

Over the next 20 years, the NPSF initiated an impressive array of programs to improve patient safety. In the early years, the focus was on raising awareness and engaging all stakeholders. We viewed NPSF as a catalyst, a force for change, designed to facilitate dialogue and cooperative work on patient safety among diverse stakeholder groups.

To operationalize these goals, NPSF quickly developed activities and initiatives to advance the field. These early years were incredibly productive. From the beginning, NPSF engaged consumer groups and included patients on its Board. The well-funded research grant program facilitated the growth of a cadre of young investigators who focused on this brand new field of patient safety research. The NPSF annual meeting, later named the Patient Safety Congress, provided a forum for presentation of research, education in patient safety, examples of successful practices, and, of course, networking. It attracted an increasing number of attendants each year as the movement took hold.

NPSF also sought to facilitate the *application* of research. To this end, early on it created a comprehensive literature *Clearinghouse*, providing access to literature covering all aspects of medical error and patient safety, as well as a monthly survey of literature, called *Current Awareness* that continues today.

By 2001, the Clearinghouse offered more than 2500 articles, papers, and books on patient safety and healthcare error. A *NPSF website* was created to provide resources, reports, newsletters, and information to practitioners and the public on how to get involved in patient safety initiatives.

For direct help to patient safety practitioners, NPSF established a *Patient Safety ListServ* and a quarterly newsletter. Within a year, the ListServ e-mail discussion group included more than 1300 active subscribers and participants who exchanged patient safety information, strategies, suggestions, and resources.

A newsletter, *Focus on Patient Safety*, gave patient safety professionals up-to-date information on patient safety research and new practices and ideas and monitored the expansion of patient safety initiatives worldwide. All these resources were designed to help those "in the trenches" doing research or redesigning their practices to improve safety.

To advance the role of patients in safety, in 2001 NPSF established a *Patient and Family Advisory Council* (PFAC) to provide input to all Foundation initiatives. The PFAC included the leaders of the major patient advocacy groups. From the beginning of the movement, mothers of children who had died or were seriously harmed by a medical error had spoken out, most notably Sue Sheridan, Helen Haskell, Ilene Corina, and Sorrel King. They were welcomed by the leaders of the movement and contributed to the program at every Congress.

To facilitate training of the next generation of patient safety leaders, NPSF collaborated with the American Hospital Association's Health Research and Educational Trust to establish a *Patient Safety Leadership Fellowship Program*. NPSF also reached out to its corporate and institutional members, creating a *Corporate Council* to educate and involve industry representatives.

In 2002 NPSF initiated *Stand Up for Patient Safety*, a program for hospitals and healthcare systems committed to serious effort to

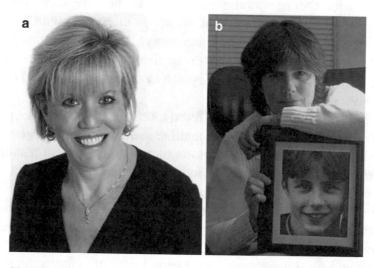

(**a**) Sue Sheridan, (**b**) Helen Haskell and Lewis. (All rights reserved)

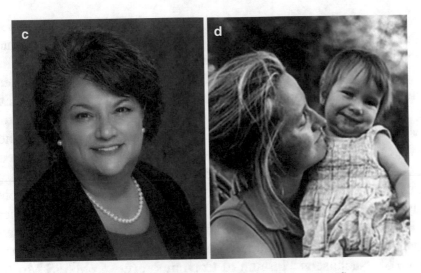

(c) Ilene Corina, (d) Sorrel King and Josie. (All rights reserved)

improve safety. The program offered practical tools to enhance existing patient safety and quality improvement initiatives, educational
programs, information resources, leadership seminars, and online
forums for sharing patient safety innovations and best practices. The
program expanded substantially in 2004 with funding from AIG, the
large insurance company, which brought its hospitals into membership.

At the prompting of patient advocate, Ilene Corina, NPSF initiated
the first annual *Patient Safety Awareness Week*. It is celebrated in
March, coinciding with the date of the death of her son, Michael, from
a medical error. The PFAC published a National Agenda for Action:
*Parents and Families in Patient Safety – Nothing About Me Without
Me*, a white paper outlining how NPSF would lead in education, culture, research, and support of patient engagement. The NPSF website
was generating more than 15,000 hits each week. In 2005, the patient
safety research community's dreams were realized with the launch of
the *Journal of Patient Safety*, with Nancy Dickey as editor in chief.

Despite these awesome early accomplishments of NPSF, there was
turmoil within the organization. Its internal culture was suffering.
Almost from the beginning, turnover of management and chronic staff
unhappiness were the norm. The Board, dominated by the AMA, took
the classic position that it should not interfere with the CEO or

interact with any staff, so these problems remained unresolved. But from the beginning, many other Board members were concerned about NPSF's lack of independence from the AMA.

The AMA's generosity had made the Foundation possible, but the nature of the affiliation with the AMA, including its provision of staffing and office space, represented control. In 2004, the issue came to a head. The Board voted to separate NPSF from the AMA and elected founder and Board member Diane Pinakiewicz to be the president. The AMA was not pleased. It canceled all its funding, including, sadly, the fund for research named for Jim Todd, which had supposedly been endowed in perpetuity.

Pinakiewicz turned things around. She created a new business strategy and moved the headquarters first to distant and inexpensive space at the Massachusetts Museum of Contemporary Art (MASS MoCA) in North Adams, MA, and then to Washington, DC. NPSF began to develop business partnerships across the industry, moving from a contributory revenue model to an earned revenue model. Programs such as Stand Up for Patient Safety and Corporate Council were redefined and grown significantly. The annual Congress grew in number of attendees as well as in the number of commercial exhibitors.

In 2007, in response to a proposal from its chairman, Paul Gluck, and president Pinakiewicz, the NPSF Board decided to establish a think tank to be called the *Lucian Leape Institute*. Over the years,

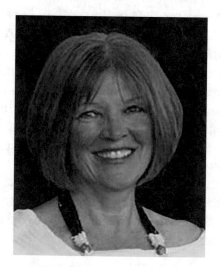

Diane Pinakiewicz. (All rights reserved)

NPSF had created a group of distinguished advisors, leaders in patient safety who were not on the Board but whose support was important to NPSF's mission.

Paul and Diane decided to harness their expertise to provide strategic guidance at the systems level and to identify and tackle the issues that were beyond the capabilities of individual organizations. The Institute was to be the vehicle for doing that. They asked me to chair it. The Board promised adequate financial support for its work.

I liked the idea of an institute for strategic planning but was, to say the least, nonplussed by having it named for me. I wryly observed to them that an "institute" is usually named for someone after they die or contribute a sizeable sum to endow it! I had done neither. But the opportunity to brainstorm with some of my favorite and smartest people was appealing. Further information about the efforts of the Lucian Leape Institute will be found in Chap. 22.

Under Pinakiewicz's leadership, NPSF extended its programs considerably. An important step forward was the formation of the *American Society of Professionals in Patient Safety* (ASPPS) in 2011 to provide caregivers who devoted their efforts to patient safety higher visibility and standing. Membership was open to individuals who were working in formal patient safety roles, as well as clinicians and executives, all in the healthcare workforce, patients, and those working in industry who had a commitment to patient safety.

But more was needed if patient safety was to be recognized as a true discipline. Accordingly, in 2011, NPSF established the *Certification Board for Professionals in Patient Safety*. The Board set appropriate educational and training requirements and developed a qualifying examination for its credential, Certified Professional in Patient Safety (CPPS). In recognition that patient safety must be a team effort with broad responsibility, certification is open to interested parties across multiple disciplines. Within 4 years 1100 individuals were certified. To meet the educational needs of students and professionals, NPSF created a comprehensive online *Patient Safety Curriculum*. By 2018, over 5000 had taken this online course, and 3000 individuals held the CPPS credential.

In 2011, NPSF severed its sponsorship of the *Journal of Patient Safety* which had appointed Charles Denham as editor without consulting NPSF. Denham had already fallen out of favor with NPSF because he had produced a video for the annual Congress and then refused to let NPSF have further use of it, claiming copyright protections. Denham later was forced to leave the National Quality Forum because of undisclosed conflicts of interest and forced to resign as JPS editor (see Chap. 11).

In 2013, Tejal Gandhi, patient safety researcher and head of safety for Partners Healthcare, became president and CEO of NPSF. At the Board's behest, she implemented a new strategic plan to incorporate workforce safety as a critical aspect of patient safety. This was an outgrowth of the LLI white paper on finding joy and meaning in work, *Through the Eyes of the Workforce* [4]. The NPSF vision statement was expanded: "to create a world where patients *and those who care for them* are free from harm".

LLI increased its thought leadership. By 2015, it had published its fifth white paper on transforming concepts. It then convened experts to evaluate best practices for root cause analysis, a core function of safety and risk professionals. The report, *RCA²: Improving Root Cause Analyses and Actions to Prevent Harm* [5], was very well received by the field, and over 7000 persons participated in the initial webcast in 2015 to discuss the report. Since that time, many hospitals

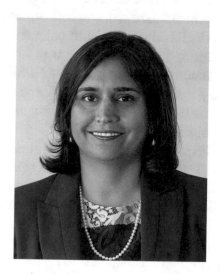

Tejal Gandhi.

and health systems in the USA and abroad have adopted the RCA^2 methodology, and the RCA2 report continues to remain one of the most downloaded reports.

Another high impact report released in 2015 was *Free from Harm: Accelerating Patient Safety Improvement Fifteen Years after To Err Is Human* [6]. The report was the product of a roundtable convened to reflect on what had been accomplished in patient safety since *To Err Is Human* and where the field needed to go. *Free from Harm* has been widely cited, and its eight recommendations have become the basis for safety strategies for a range of health systems as well as for several national safety agencies globally.

Recognizing that leadership is the key to creating a culture of safety, in 2017 LLI partnered with the American College of Healthcare Executives to convene a series of roundtables that examined how leaders can create and sustain a culture of safety. The resulting report, *Leading a Culture of Safety: A Blueprint for Success*, identified practical strategies and tactics to truly advance a safety culture and has had widespread dissemination globally [7]. Many hospitals, health systems, state hospital associations, and countries are using the Blueprint to advance their culture efforts.

But all was not well with the NPSF. While its work continued to expand, it was unable to get adequate, stable, assured funding. At the beginning, a number of generous funders joined with the AMA to get it started. Their support continued for the first few years, but none were willing to commit to long-term annual support. NPSF had come to rely on grants for specific projects and on income from programs such as *Stand Up for Patient Safety*, the *Certification Board for Professionals in Patient Safety*, and the *Patient Safety Curriculum* and fees from commercial exhibitors at the annual Congress. It was not enough.

The problem was resolved in 2017, when NPSF merged with the Institute for Healthcare Improvement. In addition to providing the needed financial support, IHI's global network and forums greatly extended NPSF's reach and provided the means to move thought leadership to action through its collaborative models, expanding safety programs to health systems around the globe. The strategic planning Lucian Leape Institute continued as an active program at IHI.

The impact of NPSF over the years was enormous. From the beginning it was the driving force behind the patient safety movement. Without it, it is unlikely there would have been a national effort; at best, it would have been a slow and stuttering one. AHRQ played a crucial early role in funding patient safety research and advancing training and various programs, but it was NPSF that provided the forum for bringing together the various stakeholders, increasing their awareness, and getting their buy-in. NPSF educated America, and to some extent the world, on what patient safety was all about, and it created the infrastructure that would change a powerful idea into a movement.

Through its support of research, facilitation of communication and education, and dissemination of new safety information, a community that put patient safety "on the map" for many was built. It provided invaluable information, assistance, and identity for individuals who were just beginning to get interested in this new field. It brought together leaders and experts to deepen our understanding of the myriad complex barriers to making healthcare safe and to develop strategies to overcome them.

Its programs stimulated hospitals, educators, and policy-makers to make a commitment to improving safety and provided them with tools to do so. And NPSF embraced diverse groups outside of organized medicine, such as private corporations and patient advocates, giving them a voice and the means to have an impact.

NPSF provided a home for the burgeoning field of patient safety specialists, first with a specialty association, later with specialty certification. The annual Patient Safety Congress conference became the place for safety professionals to come together to learn and share research and experience. The NPSF provided the structure and support for the new patient safety movement. Without it, the movement would have been slow and halting in coming. NPSF was for many years the soul of patient safety.

References

1. Kirk J. Sunbeam, AMA finalize pact: association says consumers will have more data. Chicago Tribune 1997 August 13, 1997; Sect. A3.
2. Japsen B. AMA to pay Sunbeam $10 million. Chicago Tribune 1998 August 1, 1998; Sect. A1, A10.
3. Leape LL, Woods DD, Hatlie MJ, Kizer KW, Schroeder SA, Lundberg GD. Promoting patient safety by preventing medical error. JAMA. 1998;280:1444–7.
4. Institute. LL. Through the eyes of the workforce: creating joy, meaning and safer health care. Boston, MA; 2013.
5. Institute. LL. RCA^2: improving root cause analyses and actions to prevent harm. Boston, MA; 2015.
6. Institute. LL. Free from harm: accelerating patient safety improvement fifteen years after To Err Is Human. Boston, MA; 2015.
7. Institute. INLL. Leading a culture of safety: a blueprint for success; 2017.

Part II
Institutional Responses

Chapter 6
We Can Do This: The Institute for Healthcare Improvement Adverse Drug Events Collaborative

Rewind to 1995, before Annenberg and the NPSF. "Patient safety" was not on many agendas, but methods to change systems to improve quality of care were beginning to be developed. Policy-makers and the healthcare establishment were slow to respond to the new information on the extent of medical error and our calls for a new approach, but one person instantly recognized the challenge: Don Berwick of the Institute for Healthcare Improvement (IHI).

Don Berwick was a pediatrician, an honors' graduate of Harvard and Harvard Medical School, with a MPP from Harvard Kennedy School of Government. "Preparation H" he would call it. He was interested in health policy and quality of care. After joining the Department of Health Policy and Management at the Harvard School of Public Health, he was hired as the vice president for Quality-of-Care Measurement at the Harvard Community Health Plan, where his attempts to motivate physicians and managers by providing them with performance data were not always welcomed. At the advice of the CEO, Tom Pyle, Berwick began to explore approaches to quality in other industries.

Berwick read extensively the literature on quality improvement in industry. He visited and was powerfully influenced by Guy Cohen of NASA and A. Blanton Godfrey, head of quality systems and theory at Bell Labs. At about this time, he had a chance meeting with Paul Batalden, who introduced him to the work of W. Edwards Deming.

© The Author(s) 2021
L. L. Leape, *Making Healthcare Safe*,
https://doi.org/10.1007/978-3-030-71123-8_6

Paul Batalden was also a pediatrician and was COO of Park Nicollet Medical Center when he discovered the work of W. Edwards Deming. Batalden, like Berwick, had been working on improving quality of care for some time, with frustratingly little to show for it. He found Deming's work on quality management in industry fascinating [1].

Deming had been a careful student of approaches to improving industrial and agricultural efficiency during World War II. But in the postwar period, a booming economy and pent-up demand led US manufacturers to focus on production and not worry about quality. Deming was sent instead to Japan, which was struggling to recover from the war, and found his advice eagerly sought—and listened to. The results of his efforts came home to America—literally—in the early 1970s when Japanese cars that were cheaper and better than those produced by the American "big three" entered the market. Deming returned to the USA and found increasing audiences for his courses on quality management.

Batalden took Deming's course and had an epiphany. The approaches Deming was teaching were just what healthcare needed. He persuaded the CEO of the Hospital Corporation of America to fund basic quality improvement courses in their 390 hospitals. Batalden convinced Don Berwick to take Deming's course, which was similarly transforming for him and led to his conversion to quality-focused methods of management and improvement.

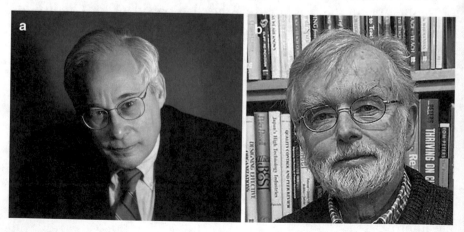

(**a**) Don Berwick and (**b**) Paul Batalden.

At the suggestion of Howard Hiatt, Berwick wrote up his ideas about how these concepts could be applied in healthcare in a NEJM article, *Continuous Improvement as an Ideal in Health Care* [2], launching his career and a new field.

But how to make it happen? Blanton Godfrey had an idea: why not try a demonstration project that paired healthcare organizations that wanted to learn CQI with industrial companies that were actually doing it? Between them and with grant support from the John A. Hartford Foundation, they recruited healthcare organizations and companies to the National Demonstration Project on Quality Improvement in Health Care. Its success led to the founding of IHI in 1991.

Don became familiar with our work on preventing adverse drug events (ADEs) when he was asked by JAMA to review my ADE systems paper in late 1994. IHI was already working on patient safety as a result of Don's introduction to it by Guy Cohen at NASA earlier, and its faculty were engaged in safety designs for several early collaboratives. But Don recognized that it deserved more focused attention. Our ADE systems paper showed what needed to be done. IHI knew how to do it.

IHI was by then the emerging leader in quality improvement in healthcare and had considerable experience in making change. Since its inception, IHI had trained thousands of people from hundreds of healthcare organizations in the fundamentals of improving quality of care through courses on improvement and its annual conference, the National Forum on Quality Improvement in Health Care.

Yet actual change, measurably improved quality of care, was hard to come by. Physicians in particular were often reluctant to participate. They had difficulty reconciling QI concepts with the classical individual performance-centered approach they learned in medical school. The Institute was not having the breadth of impact on quality of care that it desired. IHI needed to try something different to engage organizations in making real, system-level changes that would lead to dramatic improvements in care.

One day, at a meeting of IHI's Group Practice Improvement Network, Don and Paul Batalden were chatting about ways to accelerate improvement in healthcare beyond what IHI had achieved using traditional educational approaches. Batalden sketched a model on a paper placemat and handed it to Don. It contained two new concepts. First, it would pair clinical subject matter experts with quality improvement application experts to help organizations select, test, and implement changes on the front lines of care.

Second, it would bring QI teams from different hospitals together to enhance learning by providing them with instruction on change methods and the opportunity to learn from one another, providing mutual support, reinforcement, and peer pressure. It would build on the work of Tom Nolan, Lloyd Provost, Gerald Langley, and their colleagues in Associates in Process Improvement (API) on rapid cycle change [3]. In a flush of confidence, they decided to name them Breakthrough Series Collaboratives (BTS) [4].

What Is a Collaborative?

A collaborative is a collection of teams of healthcare workers who come together to work on a specific problem. The rationale for the collaborative is that meaningful change requires teamwork and that teams can learn from one another. The collaborative facilitates this interaction by bringing teams together from a number of similar healthcare organizations across the country to work on problems such as overuse of cesarean section or medication errors. The sponsor provides structure, instruction in theory and technique, data collection, and feedback and periodically brings the teams together for reinforcement and learning from one another.

IHI established four aims for a collaborative: to find, describe, and diffuse best practices throughout the collaborating organizations, to improve outcomes in each organization by teaching it to understand its systems of care and change them, to develop expertise in the science of improvement in each topic, and to disseminate the knowledge gained during the collaboratives as broadly as possible to others in the healthcare community.

Participants are educated in the evidence of care process changes that have been proven to be effective for the specific topic, and they are taught to use rapid cycles of change to help test and learn from changes in a short period of time. Teams are challenged to adapt these methods to their own situation to improve care. Early BTS Collaboratives consisted of 20–40 organizations working together for 6–12 months on a specific topic. Over time the model evolved, sometime to incorporate hundreds of organizations in a single collaborative.

How It Works

IHI begins by identifying topics ripe for change. First, a topic has to be a significant quality of care issue. Second, there must be evidence that a different approach is effective, or at least promising. That is, proof that some healthcare organizations had achieved better outcomes by implementing a new system; a gap existed between common practice and what is possible. Third, the problem has to have risen to national, or at least local, attention so there is tension for improvement.

Next, an expert planning group is formed of researchers and specialty practitioners to clarify the nature of the gap and consolidate the scientific knowledge—*what* to do—and the improvement knowledge, *how* to do it. From this review the group identifies "change concepts," which are design ideas (often including human factors concepts such as standardization and reducing reliance on memory) that teams will use to implement the new knowledge. Methods to measure progress are identified, and realistic numerical goals for achievement are created.

Collaborative participants are multidisciplinary teams recruited from hospitals and systems in the wide IHI network. The ideal team varies with the topic but often includes a systems leader "sponsor" who has the authority to get things done, a technical expert who is the improvement leader, a day-to-day leader to make the project go, and at least one clinician champion.

The typical collaborative process starts with a 2-day learning session attended by all participating teams. The planning group instructs participants in improvement methods, the core of which is the "Model for Improvement" first formulated by Associates in Process Improvement. The Model guides teams toward real-world, rapid tests of change: so-called "Plan-Do-Study-Act" or "PDSA" cycles.

The way the Model for Improvement works is that a team identifies a specific aim and plans a small change in process to achieve it. The change is implemented quickly, and just enough data is collected as quickly as possible to see results. If the change fails to yield progress, they start over. If it succeeds, they build on it to improve its success and spread it more widely in the organization. Each test of change informs the rest, as confidence grows in the understanding of what works—a "ramp" of growing knowledge. For any significant aim, a family of changes is required in order to achieve major success. Today, that family of changes is often represented in what IHI calls a "driver diagram."

At the first meetings of the Collaborative, teams decide on their aims, select specific process changes to try out, and plan the initial "tests of change" they are going to carry out when they return home. In subsequent meetings, teams report their progress to the entire group, learn from others, and plan the next changes. (One important rubric of the Breakthrough Series Collaborative model is "All Teach; All Learn.")

During the intervals between the whole-group learning sessions, teams are "supported by conference calls, peer site visits, and Web-based discussions that enable them to share information and learn from national experts and other health care organizations" [4].

A social media network is created for rapid and easy sharing of information. Teams are encouraged to visit other teams. Throughout, the emphasis is on results, not on collecting data. Written progress reports are filed to IHI monthly. Many collaboratives conclude with a National Congress to which all participants as well as other interested healthcare professionals are invited, and the results are reported. Most publish a monograph report or prepare papers for peer-reviewed journals, summarizing the collaborative's experiences.

The Reducing Adverse Drug Events Collaborative

Early in 1995, when the collaboratives were just forming, Don approached me about chairing one of the new breakthrough collaboratives, Reducing Adverse Drug Events. I was delighted to do so. It was exactly what I was looking for: an opportunity to get clinicians to apply what we were talking about regarding changing systems to prevent errors. Unlike the first collaboratives that focused on waiting times and inappropriate care such as high cesarean section rates, the Adverse Drug Event (ADE) Collaborative was IHI's first effort focused solely on the problem of harm resulting from errors in care. It is described in some detail to show how this powerful method of systems change works to actually reduce harm.

In July we began planning the collaborative. We were able to recruit a group of safety noteworthies to advise us, including James Reason, the world's expert on error; Bob Helmreich, developer of aviation crew resource management; Don Norman, psychologist and author of *The Design of Everyday Things*; Earl Weiner, cognitive psychologist and communication specialist; Michael Cohen, founder of the Institute for Safe Medication Practices; Marilyn Bogner, specialist in technology and human error; Charles Meyers, pharmacist leader; David Bates, my research colleague from Brigham and Women's Hospital; and Ken Barker, research pharmacist.

I chaired the planning group of IHI experts, Andrea Kabcenell, Donald Goldmann, Carol Haraden, and Frank Federico, together with Tom Nolan of API and Michael Cohen from ISMP. Ross Baker, psychologist from the University of Toronto, attended as an observer. I think we all had the sense that this could be the entering wedge for getting healthcare to adopt a systems approach to errors.

The initial gathering of teams (called a Change Symposium) for the Breakthrough Series on Reducing Adverse Drug Events and Medical Errors was held January 22–23, 1996. We were delighted that 40 hospitals sent teams. Each consisted of a physician, a nurse, and a

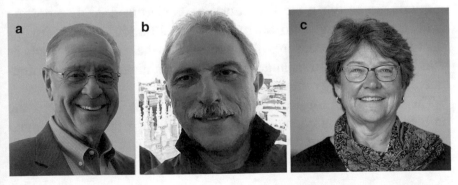

(a) Mike Cohen, (b) Frank Federico, (c) Carol Haraden.

pharmacist. I found it fascinating that for most of these hospitals, it was the first time the participants had ever worked together as a team!

We taught the teams the basic theory of systems redesign and then asked them to identify a specific ADE problem they wanted to work on at home. They were instructed in the use of the API Model for Improvement and PDSA cycles for improvement [3].

Five weeks later, in February, we reconvened the teams for the first learning session. Chuck Kilo from IHI joined Frank Federico as team coaches. Participants were given more specifics of how to use the PDSA cycle, and teams planned their first cycles with faculty coaching. They then went home to carry out their plans. They filed monthly progress reports with IHI, and we had frequent individual and group conference calls.

Early on, we surveyed all participants regarding the extent to which 11 "basic" adverse drug event/medication error preventive measures were already in place in their institutions. These were procedures that were known and had been recommended and talked about for many years. They included unit dosing, standardization of doses, protocols for lethal drugs, pharmacy admixture of IVs, 24-hour pharmacist availability, prohibition of double shifts, etc.

The survey results were sobering. Only 8 of the 41 institutions had as many as 8 of the 11 measures in place; none utilized all. The use of unit dosing, computer drug profiling in pharmacy, and 24-hour availability of the pharmacist was quite high, but for others, such as enforcement of standard protocols, prohibition of double shifts, and use of effective systems to monitor ADEs, the rates were sadly low.

Measuring adverse drug events proved to be a challenge for many hospitals, so early on we developed a standardized ADE reporting form and distributed it to all participants. In addition, participants identified specific measures that applied to their changes, such as blood glucose level for changes in insulin administration and the documentation of allergy information.

The second learning session was held in June. We reviewed the problems in making change, lessons from human factors, and measurement. Teams shared experiences of their successes and failures and interacted with other teams to learn secrets of success. With faculty coaching they refined their projects.

Midway in our Collaborative, in July 1996, IHI held a retreat for the leaders of all six Collaboratives underway to compare notes and learn from one another. All were struggling, with only a modest number of hospital teams notching up major successes in changing their systems. The process seemed straightforward to us; for the hospitals it was anything but.

The third and final learning session was held November 17–19. We focused on lessons learned, how to sustain changes, and strategies for moving forward. Teams presented storyboards of their projects and made presentations of their work and plans. A month later, we presented our experience with the ADE collaborative at the IHI annual forum, and in March 1997 we concluded the collaborative with a National Congress in which all of the groups reported out and presented plans for sustaining the gains.

Results

Of the original 41 teams, 36 completed the collaborative and implemented significant changes. Overall, they implemented 209 ramps, of which 120 were successful. The most common changes were implementing nonpunitive reporting (24 hospitals, 50% success), enforcing standardized prescribing (22 hospitals, 64% success) implementing heparin protocols (18 hospitals, 72% success), and removing KCl from nursing units (15 hospitals, 100% success) (Table 6.1). The change concepts that worked best were reducing reliance on memory, standardization, simplification, use of constraints, forcing functions, and the use of protocols [5, 6].

One of the interesting findings was that success was not related to hospital characteristics such as size, teaching status, ownership, or urban/rural location. It depended instead on the commitment of the team and the support it received from top management.

Table 6.1 Most common changes implemented

Type of change	No. of ramps	No. successful	(%)
Nonpunitive reporting	24	12	(50)
Enforce standardized prescribing	22	14	(64)
Implement heparin protocols	18	13	(72)
Remove KCl from nursing units	15	15	(100)
Ensure documentation of allergy information	12	10	(83)
Standardize medication administration times	12	8	(67)
Implement chemotherapy protocols	9	7	(78)
Implement insulin ordering protocols	7	3	(43)
Totals	119	82	(70)

Lessons Learned

The experience of the ADE collaborative was similar to that of the other IHI collaboratives. Three major factors led to success: strong leadership, effective processes, and appropriate choice of intervention.

Leadership is essential at two levels: the CEO and the team leader. Change of any kind induces resistance. Support from the top is essential to overcome natural and expected objections. At the team level, consistent and persistent leadership was needed to maintain momentum for change and enthusiasm. Teams failed if they had poor leaders or if the leader suddenly left. Although their participation was essential to success, physicians were not necessarily, or usually, the leaders of the teams, which were variously led by representatives from all three professions: nurses, doctors, and pharmacists [7, 8].

Successful teams were also those that were able to define and relentlessly pursue their aims. They had a clear idea of what they wanted to accomplish and were rigorous both about measuring progress and following the PDSA cycle model for improvement. Teams were more likely to succeed when they involved all stakeholders, thus co-opting potential resistors, and if they included a physician.

Successful teams chose practical small-scale interventions that attempted to change processes, not to educate or reform people. The ideal intervention redesigned the work so that it was both difficult to make errors and easy to perform.

Conversely, the most important causes of failure were lack of these features: absence of supportive leadership, failure to clearly define aims, and poor choice of intervention. Failure to involve all stakeholders was almost always a prescription for failure. Resistance by physicians and nurses to change can be profound if they are not involved in the process, especially if the new process requires additional time or effort. Other stumbling blocks were fixating on data collection and focus on the error rather than on the underlying systems failure.

The Breakthrough Collaborative has turned out to be one of the most effective methods for achieving systems change. The limited time frame of the collaborative puts pressure on teams to actually make changes, not just talk about them. The previous experience with many QI efforts was that weeks or months were spent gathering data and talking about and planning elaborate changes. The Collaborative forced action.

The API Model for Improvement and the PDSA method, the use of small tests of change and repeated iterations, is very powerful when used properly. A momentum is developed that energizes the team and facilitates change. But improvement teams often struggle when they are on their own. The collaborative helps them succeed by providing structure, instruction, discipline, and the reinforcement that comes from sharing with others. It is a powerful tool for improving patient safety.

Use of Collaboratives

IHI convened a second collaborative on ADEs that focused on "high-alert" drugs: medications that can be fatal when used improperly. It was one of many collaboratives led by IHI over the ensuing years, teaching hundreds—thousands—of hospital teams the PDSA model. The Massachusetts Coalition for the Prevention of Medical Errors used collaboratives—with the help of IHI—to implement two medication safe practices statewide. (See Chap. 8.)

Some years after IHI introduced the collaborative model, in 2004, Peter Pronovost dramatically demonstrated its effectiveness in reducing central line catheter-associated bloodstream infections (CLABSI) in a statewide collaborative in Michigan [9, 10].

Central lines are plastic infusion tubes inserted into the atrium of the heart via a large vein in the neck. They are typically inserted by a resident physician using sterile technique with the patient in bed. Because they provide reliable access for giving intravenous fluids, blood, and medications, their use is a standard practice for seriously ill patients, who may need them for a long time. But they are risky: infections occurred in 10–20% of patients with long-dwelling catheters; 10% or more of those were fatal. Infection is almost always the result of bacterial contamination at the time of catheter insertion.

Pronovost previously had incredible success in eliminating CLABSI in an intensive care unit at the Johns Hopkins Hospital. He and his team implemented a protocol to ensure that guidelines for the process of inserting the catheter were followed. A key feature was the use of a checklist that specified each step in the process, such as use of a sterile drape, gown, and gloves. (This is the work that introduced the term "checklist" to medicine.)

Johns Hopkins Hospital CLABSI protocol (Adapted from Ref. [9])
1. Implement educational intervention
2. Create a Central Catheter Insertion Cart
3. Asking providers daily whether catheter can be removed
4. Implement a checklist to be completed by the bedside nurse
5. Empower nurse to stop procedures if guidelines are not followed

Checklist for inserting central line (Adapted from Ref. [9])
1. Clean hands
2. Clean the skin with chlorhexidine
3. Drape site
4. Use Hat, mask, sterile gown
5. Use sterile gloves
6. Apply sterile dressing

Pronovost's protocol also introduced a truly radical innovation: if sterile technique was breached, the nurse was empowered to stop the procedure and require the physician to re-prep, re-gown, and re-drape. This was a profound cultural change. It required psychological safety for the nurse, i.e., no fear of speaking up, and physician willingness to accept a role as a true member of a team. As we will see later, these are building blocks of the culture change needed to make healthcare safe.

Pronovost's results were astounding: within months the CLABSI rate was reduced to zero, and the improvement was sustained for more than a year [11]. At last, someone had "gotten to zero"! I considered it then, and still do, a major milestone in the safety journey; it was certainly the most important breakthrough until then.

Building on this success, Pronovost later enlisted the support of the Michigan Hospital and Healthcare Association (MHHA) and secured funding from Michigan Blue Cross-Blue Shield to carry out a state-wide collaborative to implement his protocol. With Christine Goeschel and others, he recruited 127 hospitals to participate in the collaborative run by his team.

Ninety-six hospitals completed the collaborative. They reduced the mean rate of CLABSI/1000 catheter days from 7.7 to 1.4 in 18 months. Even more impressively, over half of the hospitals replicated the Hopkins experience, totally eliminating the infections, getting their infection rates to zero, and keeping them there for 3 years [9].

Dixon-Woods and Bosk subsequently carried out an intensive analysis of how the Michigan collaborative had been so incredibly successful. They concluded that five features were crucial to its success: (1) social pressure among state's ICUs to participate (as the program got underway, ICU leaders didn't want to be left out); (2) creation of a network community by immersion coaching, workshops, and data, as used by IHI; (3) combining grassroots features and inclusion of all stakeholders with a vertically integrated program structure; (4) use of data on infection rates as a disciplinary force by making performance visible and ranking units' performance; and (5) use of "hard edges," coercive measures, by program leaders, such as contacting hospital CEOs to ask for data and asking ICUs to withdraw from the program if the data were not forthcoming (none did) [12].

Motivated by Pronovost's work in Michigan, the World Health Organization launched an international "Match Michigan" program to encourage country organizations to adopt the collaborative method to reduce bloodstream infections. In the UK it was taken up by 215 ICUs. While they were unable to "match" Michigan, they did succeed in reducing the infection rate by more than 50% [13].

In the USA, AHRQ funded Pronovost and JHH faculty to lead a national effort supported by the American Hospital Association and the MHHA. State hospital associations coordinated hospital teams in their states. Following a national campaign, which included promotion by Consumers Union, the Leapfrog Group, the Center for Medicare and Medicaid Services (CMS), and The Joint Commission, 45 states participated. In addition, 22 states instituted required reporting of bloodstream infections [14]. Central line infections in ICU patients have been reduced by 80% [15].

An important result of these successes was that CMS decided that CLABSI was preventable and stopped reimbursing hospitals for the additional costs of bloodstream infections [14].

Thanks to the pioneering work of IHI that developed the Breakthrough Series Collaborative model and the success of Peter Pronovost in applying it on a large scale to get results, the collaborative method has proved to be a highly successful method for changing a system and sustaining the change. Convening collaboratives to address the many other issues in patient safety should be high priority for AHRQ and for state health departments and hospital associations.

Subsequent IHI Initiatives

The Breakthrough Collaboratives added to the influence that IHI was having on quality improvement. By then, the annual National Forum was attracting thousands, and in 1996 IHI teamed with BMJ to host the first European Forum on Quality Improvement in Health Care. At

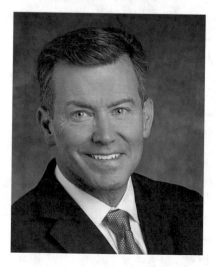

Peter Pronovost. (All rights reserved)

the turn of the century, hundreds of hospitals were engaged with IHI in *Idealized Design* programs for clinical office practices, medication systems, and the ICU. In 2002, IHI launched *IMPACT*, a national network for change.

But the most exciting IHI initiative at this time was *Pursuing Perfection*, a collaboration with the Robert Wood Johnson Foundation to provide $20 million to a small number of hospitals that would make a serious commitment to redesigning processes and building capacity.

The goal was for an organization to show that it could improve not just one or two aspects of care, in one clinic, unit, or department, but could make high levels of performance improvement a way of life for healthcare providers, all the time, in all dimensions of quality, throughout an entire organization or system of care. To undergo *organizational transformation* [16]. The initiative would not only raise expectations among providers, payers, and consumers for higher-quality care; it would demonstrate how to attain this level of achievement.

When the program was launched in 2001, over 220 organizations applied; 12 were selected for Phase 1, the planning process. In 2002, seven US organizations—four hospitals and three outpatient organizations—were awarded Phase II implementation grants of up to $1.9 million each. In addition, six self-funded international sites in Holland, Sweden, and four in the UK joined in this collaborative learning model. (IHI had been working with the National Health Service since 1999.)

The initiative was highly successful, with several hospitals in the USA and overseas achieving transformational change. Cincinnati Children's Hospital attributes its culture change to the Pursuing Perfection initiative.

In 2004, IHI launched its most ambitious project, the *100,000 Lives Campaign*. The design components came from Don Berwick's son, Dan, who had worked on political campaigns. "Some is not a number, soon is not a time," he said—a slogan that resonated as IHI strove for greater and more sustainable impact. They set a date, June 14, 2006, to achieve the goal of saving 100,000 lives—the number the IOM had estimated died every year from medical errors. IHI reached out for support from the AMA, ANA, CMS, and The Joint Commission and found all receptive.

The campaign called on healthcare organizations to reliably—100% of the time—implement six specific interventions: rapid response teams, medication reconciliation, immediate revascularization for myocardial infarction, CLABSI protocol, ventilator-associated pneumonia protocol, and use of perioperative antibiotics.

The campaign was incredibly successful: over 3000 hospitals joined, and by the due date hospital self-reports suggested that the project had saved more than 100,000 lives. This was followed by the five million lives campaign, ending in January 2008, that added six more practices and enlisted additional hospitals. While an accurate count was impossible, the amount of change was substantial. Improving quality and safety was finally becoming ingrained in healthcare.

Of the many other IHI initiatives within the time frame of this book, two deserve brief mention. In 2008, IHI created the IHI *Open School for Health Professions*, with online courses in patient safety and quality improvement provided free to students and at low cost to others. Medical and nursing students rapidly enrolled to make up for their schools' failure to make room for these subjects in their curricula. Within 10 years, 890 voluntary "chapters" of students with faculty advisors had been established in 92 countries, and 4.5 million courses had been completed by 715,000 learners (IHI website). More than 1000 organizations and universities use the courses in their training programs or formal curricula.

The second powerful innovation of this period was the *Triple Aim*, initially crafted by Tom Nolan and another IHI faculty member, Dr. John Whittington. In 2008, recognizing that improving the healthcare system requires simultaneous pursuit of improving the experience of care, improving the health of populations, and reducing per capita costs of healthcare, IHI codified these objectives in a new framework, the Triple Aim. This concept recognized and validated the role of quality improvement in controlling costs and that our responsibilities—and effectiveness—depend on efforts beyond the walls of our healthcare institutions [17].

Conclusion

It is impossible to overstate the impact of IHI on quality of healthcare and patient safety. Under the inspired, skilled, and impassioned leadership of Don Berwick, IHI established a corporate model that has yielded a never-ending stream of innovative and effective methods to improve care and reduce harm. Its influence is global and continually expanding. Its initiatives have both deepened and broadened our understanding of quality of care and the roles of institutions and professionals in providing it. Much of what most people in healthcare understand about quality improvement they learned from IHI.

The merger with the NPSF has led to global expansion of efforts to improve patient safety. IHI support of the Lucian Leape Institute ensures continuing development of innovative strategies to reduce harm. Of all types of quality failure, our inability to prevent harm is the least defensible. Under IHI guidance and inspiration, continued progress is assured.

References

1. Deming WE. Out of the crisis. Cambridge, MA: The MIT Press; 1982.
2. Berwick D. Continuous improvement as an ideal in health care. NEJM. 1989;320:53–6.
3. Langley G, Nolan K, Nolan T, Norman C, Provost L. The Improvement guide: a practical approach to enhancing organizational performance. San Francisco: Jossey-Bass Publishers; 1996.
4. IHI. The breakthrough series: IHI's collaborative model for achieving breakthrough improvement. Boston: Institute for Healthcare Improvement; 2003.
5. Leape LL, Kabcenell AI, Gandhi TK, Carver P, Nolan TW, Berwick DM. Reducing adverse drug events: lessons from a breakthrough series collaborative. Jt Comm J Qual Patient Saf. 2000;26:321–31.
6. Leape L, Kabcenell A, Berwick D, Roessner J. Reducing adverse drug events. Boston: Institute for Healthcare Improvement; 1998.
7. Kilo C. A framework for collaborative improvement: lessons from the Institute for Healthcare Improvement's breakthrough series. Qual Manag Health Care. 1998;6:1–13.
8. Kilo CM. Improving care through collaboration. Pediatrics. 1999;103:384–93.

9. Pronovost P, Needham D, Berenholtz S, et al. An intervention to decrease catheter-related bloodstream infections in the ICU. N Engl J Med. 2006;355:2725–32.
10. Watson SR, George C, Martin M, Bogan B, Goeschel C, Pronovost PJ. Preventing central line-associated bloodstream infections and improving safety culture: a statewide experience. Jt Comm J Qual Patient Saf. 2009;35:593–7.
11. Berenholtz S, Pronovost PJ, Lipsett PA, et al. Eliminating catheter-related bloodstream infections in the intensive care unit. Crit Care Med. 2004;32:2014–20.
12. Dixon-Woods M, Bosk CL, Aveling EL, et al. Explaining Michigan: developing an ex post theory of a quality improvement program. Milbank Qtrly. 2011;89:167–205.
13. Bion J, Richardson A, Hibbert P, et al. 'Matching Michigan': a 2-year stepped interventional programme to minimise central venous catheter-blood stream infections in intensive care units in England. BMJ Qual Saf. 2013;22:110–23.
14. Pronovost PJ, Marsteller JA, Goeschel CA. Preventing bloodstream infections: a measurable national success story in quality improvement. Health Aff. 2011;30:628–34.
15. Wise M, Scott RD, James MB, et al. National estimates of central line–associated bloodstream infections in critical care patients. Infect Control Hosp Epidemiol. 2013;34:547–54.
16. Pursuing perfection: the journey to organizational transformation. An interview with Jim Anderson, President and CEO, Cincinnati Children's Hospital Medical Center. Institute for Healthcare Improvement. Accessed 18 Oct 2020, at http://www.ihi.org/resources/Pages/ImprovementStories/TheJourneytoOrganizationalTransformationAnInterviewwithJimAnderson.aspx.
17. Berwick DM, Nolan TW, Whittington J. The triple aim: care, health, and cost. Health Aff (Millwood). 2008;27:759–69.

Chapter 7
Who Will Lead? The Executive Session

A few weeks after the Annenberg Conference, Saul Weingart called me on the phone, introduced himself and said, "We should do an Executive Session on medical errors." "What is an Executive Session?" I replied. He then told me about the work he had been involved in at the Harvard Kennedy School of Government (HKS) on juvenile justice and community policing. Developed in the late 1970s at HKS, an executive session is a prolonged confidential conversation among leaders in a practice field to solve a complex problem for which there is no evident technical solution.

In contrast to the usual approach to social problem-solving in which ideas are translated from research to practice, the executive session assumes that neither academics nor practitioners have the necessary knowledge, and therefore they must work together to create a solution. Sessions are ideally directed at problems that require changes in policy and management [1]. In a prior session on policing, for example, chiefs of police from major cities developed the concept of community policing.

Saul thought it was a promising model for the infant patient safety movement. I was intrigued from the start. Engaging the leaders of the major healthcare systems was key to getting patient safety moving. If we could get them and leaders of other national organizations to recognize the importance of patient safety, their own role, and the importance of developing meaningful interventions, we might be able to jump-start improvement for safety. This sounded like a good way to do it.

© The Author(s) 2021
L. L. Leape, *Making Healthcare Safe*,
https://doi.org/10.1007/978-3-030-71123-8_7

Saul had come to safety in a roundabout way. After graduating from Cornell, he got a PhD in public policy at the Kennedy School but then decided to go into medicine and graduated from the University of Rochester School of Medicine and Dentistry. During his internal medicine residency at Beth Israel Hospital, he got interested in quality improvement, which he could see as an organizational problem. He came across the announcement of the Annenberg Conference in JAMA and decided to apply. I think he was the only medical resident who attended the conference.

The Harvard politics were a bit sensitive, as the various schools (Medicine, Public Health, and Government) and affiliated teaching hospitals each had an interest and stake in the emerging field of patient safety. To navigate potential territorial conflicts, we sought out Joe Newhouse, the director of the Harvard-wide Division of Health Policy. A nationally known health economist, Joe agreed that his Division's sponsorship would offer the proper auspices for the endeavor.

We formed a planning group that also included Miles Shore, a psychiatrist with long-standing interest in policy and leadership, Joe Newhouse, and the executive director of the Kennedy School Criminal Justice Center, Frank Hartmann, who was an architect of the executive session and a master facilitator.

We identified a diverse group of healthcare movers and shakers—individuals in positions of formal authority and important "influencers." It turned out to be easier than I had expected to recruit key leaders. The people we were after were already aware that medical error was something that they had to deal with. With few exceptions, they readily signed on.

One of those exceptions was David Lawrence, head of Kaiser Permanente, who was initially cool to the idea. I thought that it was absolutely necessary to have him participate since Kaiser Permanente was both a premier provider of healthcare and highly organized, the type of healthcare organization that could more easily implement systems change. Because of its outstanding reputation, having it do so would send a powerful message to the rest of healthcare. So, although we had never met, I shamelessly "twisted his arm" over the phone, telling him he had to do it. Fortunately, he relented and came aboard. I later had the privilege of working with David on the IOM Quality of Care Committee, where his leadership was essential as we fashioned the legendary IOM reports.

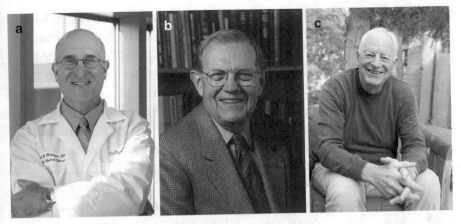

(a) Saul Weingart, (b) Miles Shore, (c) David Lawrence.

We were able to secure financial support from several sources: Agency for Health Research and Quality (AHRQ), Veterans Health Administration, National Patient Safety Foundation, American Society of Health-System Pharmacists, and the WK Kellogg and Robert Wood Johnson Foundations.

Executive sessions follow a loose game plan. The early meetings are designed to draw out the participants by asking members to share personal stories of leadership success and failure. Discussions are topical, prompted by brief presentations and case studies, with the expectation that the discovery of lessons would be an iterative and collective process. Presenters and "reactors" are often drawn from the members. Some of the work of the session is done between meetings. And future agendas are built from the unresolved issues raised at earlier meetings. We would be making it up as we went along—which was the whole idea.

First Meeting, January 22–24, 1998

The first meeting of the Executive Session on Medical Error and Patient Safety convened January 22–24, 1998, at the Kennedy School. We had an unbelievable roster of participants, 30 in all—a "who's who" of leadership in American healthcare delivery—exactly what we had hoped for. As well as leaders from key healthcare organizations, the group included business leaders, editors and news people, and academics. (See Appendix 7.1 for full list of members.)

After dinner, we welcomed everyone and explained what we were up to—the idea behind the executive session—and I gave the basic talk explaining the problem of medical error. The next day in the morning, we had two open discussions in which each member introduced himself and described examples of their leadership success and challenges. This helped create solidarity among the members and began a shared inventory of leadership lessons. Members also discussed the emerging recognition of patient safety as a silent epidemic. We agreed that CEOs are ultimately responsible for the persistence of error and are in the key position to do something about it.

In the afternoon, we had short talks, followed by respondents, followed by discussion. First, Mitch Rabkin, president and CEO of Beth Israel Deaconess Medical Center (BIDMC), talked about barriers, following which members had an extensive discussion about the costs of error and fixing them. (There were little data on this at the time, but they were all keenly aware of it.) Next, Bob Frosch, former director of NASA, described his experience with NASA and other industries, with emphasis on principles of management, management by walking around, and the need for CEOs to think of healthcare as a production process. David Woods, systems engineering professor at Ohio State, spoke about error theory, the Swiss cheese model, and cognitive bias, especially hindsight bias.

Following dinner at the Harvard Faculty Club, John Nance, pilot and ABC News aviation correspondent, gave his exciting talk on aviation safety, emphasizing the value of crew resource management and communication against an authority gradient.

On Saturday, Don Berwick, president of the Institute for Healthcare Improvement (IHI), summarized the previous day's discussions and emphasized the need to adopt in healthcare lessons from human factors research. He then did something quite remarkable that proved to be fundamental to getting the CEOs really engaged: he gave the system CEOs homework. He challenged each of them to personally investigate an incident, including personally interviewing five or six involved participants, and to report back their experiences at the next meeting. He also asked them to invite a human factors specialist to spend a day in their institution and tell them their observations and, finally, to come back to the next meeting with a financial analysis of the cost of one error.

After an extensive discussion on the problems of confidential reporting because of the legal environment—something the group had interest in addressing—we concluded by members identifying a number of tasks for the group:

- Define a working vocabulary for discussions about medical error.
- Identify lessons from other industries.
- Probe aviation for applicable lessons, such as confidential reporting and the value of a NASA-Ames research lab model for medical error.
- Explore the relationship between error reduction and quality of care.
- Identify areas of hazard or vulnerability in medicine.
- Explore the impact of the tort system on reporting and the roles of oversight and regulatory organizations in maintaining accountability.
- Identify constituencies whose voices should be represented at the exec. session.
- Pilot test innovations at home.

The planning group was delighted with how it all went. We clearly had the interest and engagement of key leaders. Our job was to learn with them about how to move the needle on patient safety and to motivate them to take action. We thought we were off to a good start. We planned to have meetings every 6 months for 2–3 years.

Second Meeting: June 25–27, 1998

We had 24 in attendance, including 4 of the 5 who had missed the first meeting. We added a new member to the group: Timothy Johnson, medical editor, ABC News. Mark Moore of HKS gave the after-dinner talk on the role of the executive session and organizational strategy. The idea was to bring everyone, especially the new attendees, up to speed on what we are doing.

On Friday, Miles Shore gave an overview of the first meeting, and new members introduced themselves. I gave a presentation, Medical Error: Working Definitions. We then moved to the CEO's reports on their experiences personally investigating a medical error in their own institutions. For all, it was eye-opening, sobering, and very motivating. Most of them had discovered things they had no idea were going on.

One member investigated an error in which a patient in the emergency department who was having a heart attack had a serious bleed after receiving a clot-busting thrombolytic drug. It turned out that the patient had received the wrong dose of thrombolytic, in part because it was difficult to obtain an accurate weight in the emergency department. On further investigation, it turned out that none of the last six patients with heart attacks had received the correct thrombolytic dose—and none of these cases had been previously identified or reported.

Another investigated a series of infections occurring among the patients of one plastic surgeon. After the second infection, nasal cultures were recommended for the whole operating room team, but the surgeon had refused to have one done. He was later required to have one and it was positive.

All of us learned how pervasive and serious the effects of errors are on the patients and on the staff. The research statistics we had presented earlier were jarring and interesting, but it was the personal stories that compelled these leaders toward resolve to change. Several CEOs were clearly moved by what they found—and that they had been so unaware of what was going on in their own institution. One described how he had reached out to a faculty member with expertise in human factors for advice. To his surprise, the faculty member said, "I've been waiting for your call for 20 years."

Saul Weingart then gave a presentation describing high quality in the service sector, with examples from Taco Bell and the Ritz-Carlton. The goal was to translate promising approaches into concepts that might work in healthcare. We then had a discussion on putting worker safety first: a Harvard case study about Paul O'Neill, the CEO at Alcoa.

O'Neill had initiated a worker safety program at Alcoa in what was already the safest company in his industry. The case study raised for the group the linkage between keeping patients safe and keeping employees safe. Were there common principles? On Saturday, we discussed another fundamental concept in the construction of a safety culture: reporting. We considered confidential error-reporting systems, referring to the Billings work with the ASRS. Don then gave the challenge for the future.

But the big surprise of the meeting was provided by Jim Mongan, CEO of the Massachusetts General Hospital. He had missed the first meeting. After attending this one for 2 days, he announced that he was resigning because "I can't tell my doctors how to practice." We were stunned. Of course, what we were up to was pretty much what he said—not exactly telling doctors how to practice but trying to convince and inspire them to practice differently. That, of course, is what leadership is about. Interestingly, years later (post-IOM and after some good work by members of his own staff), Mongan became a strong advocate for safety. But he wasn't there yet.

Following the meeting, at George Lundberg's urging, six of us wrote an editorial that provided an update on patient safety activities, and he published in JAMA [2]. We discussed the application of human factors concepts to healthcare and described the work being done by NPSF, JCAHO, the Veterans Health Administration, and the Massachusetts Board of Registration in Medicine.

Third Meeting: January 21–23, 1999

Two new members were introduced: Jack Rowe, CEO of Mt. Sinai Hospital in New York, and Troy Brennan, representing Brigham and Women's Hospital.

Our guest was Paul O'Neill, who gave the evening keynote, a compelling description of what he did to reduce harm at Alcoa. Bringing his case study to life, O'Neill emphasized that you cannot provide safe care if you don't provide a safe workplace for your employees. O'Neill told the group that patient safety wasn't a priority—it was a precondition. Paul became an outspoken advocate for patient safety and later joined the Lucian Leape Institute.

In the morning, members gave progress reports. There was no shortage of material! Bob Waller told us about the culture at Mayo, where the long-standing tradition is "the interest of the patient is the only interest." Peter Van Etten described changes at UCSF to hold doctor's accountable. Ken Kizer talked about the considerable changes he and Jim Bagian had made at the VA health system. These included medication bar coding, nonpunitive error reporting, removal of concentrated potassium chloride from floor stock, hazardous drug protocols, nursing upgrades, and assessing pain as the fifth vital sign.

Discussion followed on what needed to be done, and presentations were given on the lack of human factors testing for drug naming and labeling (a recognized contributor to medication errors), nonpunitive reporting, and building a culture of safety, followed by discussions focused on taking action.

Fourth Meeting: June 17–19, 1999

Don Berwick gave the evening keynote on Effective Executive Leadership. In the morning, Saul gave a recap of where we had come during the previous meetings of the executive session, and then we heard progress reports.

David Lawrence told about changes at K-P. He had launched major efforts at all levels—national, regional, and local. He writes a biweekly CEO journal on cases of harm and actions taken and shares best practices system-wide with all 70,000 members. He described his philosophy: no data without stories and no stories without data. But he also offered a cautionary note that effective messages require a relentless drumbeat and that people begin to understand what you mean at about the time when you are tired of saying it. He had stimulated a California statewide ADE initiative and was developing nationwide K-P accountability system. Joyce Clifford talked about nursing innovations at BIDMC.

Gordon Sprenger gave the most complete and inspiring account. He had engrafted patient safety into the governance of Allina, articulated safety as a major organizational goal, and integrated it into the strategic and operational plan. This included designating safety leaders, establishing a safety agenda, establishing the business case, and establishing nonpunitive reporting—including feedback about response. He personally inquired into medical accidents, coached senior managers in nonpunitive reporting, and kept talking with everyone about it.

He supported people who had made errors but had zero tolerance for violation of standards. He has changed the vocabulary from asking "who" to asking "what happened?" They were tapping 3-M engineers to help them with systems change. He disclosed plans to replicate the executive session for all CEO and Board chairs of Minnesota hospitals—which he subsequently did with the help of his safety leader, Julie Morath, and Saul Weingart.

Sprenger, Lawrence, and Robert Waller had spoken out publicly on behalf of patient safety as well as fostering patient safety initiatives within their organizations. Jim Reinertsen, who had moved to become CEO of Boston's CareGroup, made medication reliability one of four corporate priorities. Medication safety teams at each CareGroup hospital attempted to implement 16 best practices in 1 year and demonstrate measurable improvements in the safety of patients on anticoagulants and postoperative pain medications.

We then talked about how doctors and hospitals respond when a patient is harmed. Why are disclosure and apology so difficult? We showed the video from Annenberg of the Martin Memorial case, where the hospital stepped up and took responsibility for a death caused by a mistake. This was followed by a presentation by legal scholar Randy Bovbjerg on alternatives to the tort system and presentations by the executive director of National Alliance for the Mentally Ill, Laurie Flynn, on the consumer's view; Sandy Fleming, executive

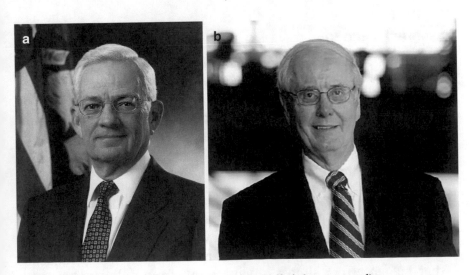

(a) Paul O'Neill and (b) Gordon Sprenger.

director of MA Board of Registration in Medicine; and Dennis
O'Leary, president of The Joint Commission on regulation and over-
sight. We had more discussion of actions that leaders could initiate.
Overall, it was a very feisty meeting, with members fully engaged.

Fifth Meeting: January 27–29, 2000

This was the first meeting after the IOM report came out 2 months
earlier, so we spent a whole session discussing it and its implications
for leadership. We added two new members, Thomas Garthwaite, the
new head of Veterans Health, replacing Ken Kizer, who had stepped
down and Michael Wood, CEO of Mayo, replacing retiring Bob
Waller. Jim Bagian gave the evening talk on his experience as an
astronaut and now director of patient safety for the VA.

An interesting innovation was the presentation of a group of
Harvard Business School-type case studies that Saul Weingart had
commissioned with the goal of capturing the early experience of executive session members' initiatives: creating a safety culture in the VA,
creating a safety program at Allina, and patient safety at Mayo Clinic.
Member reports included David Lawrence's account of many new
activities at Kaiser Permanente.

Lessons Learned

This was the last meeting of the executive session. We discussed how
to spread the message and engage a broader swatch of leaders. We
agreed on our key findings and principles, which in retrospect now
seem remarkably applicable 20 years later. These were later summarized by Saul Weingart in testimony at the AHRQ Patient Safety
Summit later in the year [3]:

1. Medical error is a problem of organizations. Members of the executive session embrace the view that medical error is an attribute of
   the systems and processes by which we deliver care. Scientific evidence and a wealth of experience from other industries demonstrate
   that human errors almost always result from defective systems.

Improvement strategies that punish individual clinicians are mis-guided and do not work. Fixing dysfunctional systems, on the other hand, is the work that needs to be done.

2. Medical error is an executive responsibility. Because managers are responsible for organizing and shaping the systems and processes of care, hospital and health system executives share an essential and nondelegable responsibility for reducing medical error. Moreover, leadership lessons in patient safety can be learned and disseminated. To make progress, healthcare CEOs must commit their own time to working on behalf of patient safety. They must communicate its importance relentlessly. They must hold them-selves personally accountable for patient safety in the same way they do for financial performance.

3. Many important lessons about high-reliability performance can be adapted from manufacturing, aviation, and the service sector. Executives should assess their organizations' core processes for safety, inventory their organizations' patient safety activities, report the results, implement best practices, and create a culture of safety.

4. Medical error is an urgent and strategic priority. Members of the executive session were impressed with the magnitude of harm rep-resented by medical error. Ensuring that care is safe is a profes-sional obligation for healthcare professionals and the organizations where they work. It is an urgent problem that requires the kind of immediate, focused, and sustained attention that motivated organi-zations to ensure Year 2000 (Y2K) compliance. Safety also makes good business sense. It builds consumer confidence and market share. Increased efficiencies and decreased rework may contribute to the bottom line.

5. Error reporting systems must be improved. Healthcare organiza-tions must remain accountable to their patients and to the commu-nity by disclosing errors that result in harm, providing fair compensation for injuries, and introducing measures to prevent recurrence. Physicians have an ethical obligation to inform patients when they have been harmed because of an error in care.

6. Gross negligence and unethical behavior should not be shielded. Professional misconduct is a grave threat to patient safety and should be dealt with accordingly. But errors that do not result in harm must be protected from legal discovery, so that we can learn

from them. Fear of discovery and punishment of clinicians' accidents drives information underground and decreases organizational learning. We need to create robust nonpunitive error reporting systems. Sharing information about errors with frontline workers will build a sense of collaboration and shared mission.
7. The federal government should play an active role in patient safety, requiring pharmaceutical and device manufacturers to use human factors principles in naming, packaging, and labeling medications and to participate in post-market surveillance of adverse events.

Conclusion

Was the executive session a success? It did not create a national consensus or a comprehensive strategy for addressing patient safety. In retrospect, that would have been an unreasonable expectation, and it isn't the purpose of executive sessions. Patient safety was in its infancy. Its definitions, methods, and scope were just developing. The major problems had yet to be defined. Patient safety was not ready for a grand strategy. But it was ready for big thinking.

Moreover, we were beginning to appreciate what an incredibly complex field patient safety is, bridging diverse disciplines from research to clinical care to administration, involving a broad range of stakeholders: patients, doctors, nurses, pharmacists, ancillary medical personnel, administrators, risk managers, lawyers, engineers, and government agencies. Achieving safe healthcare would require major changes in a physician-dominated culture that is more conservative and more authoritarian than in any institution in our society.

But the executive session was extraordinarily successful in other ways. While 99% of people working in patient safety have probably never even heard about it, the session educated major healthcare leaders in depth about patient safety and created awareness and understanding of its complexity. A community of concern developed in which leaders of major organizations in healthcare became colleagues in the pursuit of safe care. It motivated them to take action to advance the cause:

- Dennis O'Leary led The Joint Commission to be more aggressive about safety, setting out National Patient Safety Goals and Standards.
- David Lawrence made major changes at Kaiser Permanente that led it to become a model for patient safety among large healthcare systems.
- Gordon Sprenger made Allina an exemplar of safety.
- Steve Schroeder steered the Robert Wood Johnson Foundation to become the largest private funder of patient safety research and training.

An unanticipated effect of the executive session was its influence on observers. Although membership was by invitation, we encouraged participants to bring colleagues as observers. Two are of particular note. Gordon Sprenger brought Julie Morath, who went on to be a leader in patient safety as COO at Minnesota Children's Hospitals and Clinics, and later as chief quality and safety officer at Vanderbilt University Medical Center and then as the president/CEO of the California Hospital Quality Institute, and member of the Lucian Leape Institute.

The other was Atul Gawande, a surgical resident who I had gotten to know during his year at the Harvard School of Public Health. Atul later developed the surgical checklist for WHO and created Ariadne Labs, an influential collaboration of innovators, implementers, and healthcare leaders focused on quality and safety. His books, *Complications* and *Better*, have succeeded more than any other in making safety issues accessible and understandable to the public.

The Harvard Executive Session concluded shortly after the IOM report was released and just as AHRQ and NQF began to play major roles in developing the foundations for the new field of patient safety (see chapters below). The executive session was complementary to these initiatives in that it helped develop the professional foundation: commitment by key leaders in the field. Patient safety is about changing systems of care. Systems leaders have to make that happen. The executive session set a stake in the ground early on, declaring that the most senior leaders in healthcare organizations had both the responsibility and capability to ensure safe care.

The young National Patient Safety Foundation recognized the potential of the executive session as a reproducible model for engaging leadership and motivating change. It subsequently sponsored executive sessions led by Saul Weingart in Minnesota and Indiana that brought together state hospital association leaders, health system CEOs, and (importantly) hospital trustees to navigate the emerging challenges of patient safety in their regions and communities [1]. Fierce economic competitors created a shared commitment to reducing medical errors and agreed to collaborate on patient safety interventions. This created a reservoir of good will and shared purpose among leaders in Minnesota and the regional Minnesota Alliance for Patient Safety that enabled bold interventions such as the 2003 first-in-the-nation Minnesota Adverse Health Events Reporting Law.

Appendix 7.1: Executive Session Members

CEOs of Healthcare Delivery Organizations

- Harris Berman—CEO of Tufts Health Plan
- Kenneth Kizer—VA Undersecretary for Health, CEO of Veterans Health Admin.
- *David Lawrence—CEO of Kaiser Permanente
- *James Mongan—CEO of Mass General Hospital
- Mitchell Rabkin—CEO of CareGroup (BI-Deaconess Medical Center and its affiliates)
- James Reinertson—CEO of Minnesota HealthPartners
- *Gordon Sprenger—CEO of Allina Health System
- Peter Van Etten—CEO of UCSF Stanford Health Care
- Robert Waller—CEO of Mayo Clinic
- *Gail Warden—CEO of Henry Ford Health System

Leaders of Health-Related Organizations

- Donald Berwick—CEO of the Institute for Healthcare Improvement
- Charles Buck—GE VP for Healthcare Quality

- Joyce Clifford—SVP for Nursing at BI-Deaconess Medical Center
- Dan Creasey—CEO of CRICO (Harvard Medical Institutions Liability Insurer)
- Nancy Dickey—President-elect of the AMA
- Alexander Fleming—Exec. Director of MA Board of Registration in Medicine
- *Laurie Flynn—Exec. Director of National Alliance for the Mentally Ill
- Martin Hatlie—Exec. Director of NPSF
- Henri Manasse—CEO of American Society of Health-System Pharmacists
- Dennis O'Leary—President, the Joint Commission on Accreditation of Healthcare Organizations

Others

- Robert Frosch—Former Administrator of NASA
- Francis Hartmann—Exec. Dir. of KSG Malcolm Weiner Ctr for Social Policy
- Lucian Leape—Adj. Prof. of Health Policy, Harvard School of Public Health
- George Lundberg—Editor in Chief, JAMA
- Joseph Newhouse—Prof. of Health Policy and Management, Harvard
- Steven Schroeder—President of the Robert Wood Johnson Foundation
- Miles Shore—Professor of Psychiatry, HMS
- Saul Weingart—Clinical Fellow, General Medicine, BI-Deaconess
- David Woods—Prof. of Industrial and Systems Engineering, Ohio State Univ.

*Unable to attend the first meeting

References

1. Weingart S, Morath J, Ley C. Learning with leaders to create safe health care: the executive session on patient safety. J Clin Outcomes Manag. 2003;10:597–601.
2. Leape LL, Woods DD, Hatlie MJ, Kizer KW, Schroeder SA, Lundberg GD. Promoting patient safety by preventing medical error. JAMA. 1998;280:1444–7.
3. AHRQ Patient Safety Research Summit, 2000. At https://archive.ahrq.gov/quic/summit.

Chapter 8
A Community of Concern: The Massachusetts Coalition for the Prevention of Medical Errors

One day in January 1997, John Noble, an internist from Boston City Hospital who I knew from somewhere—perhaps residency days—walked into my office and said, "We should form a state coalition for the prevention of medical errors." His idea was to bring to the table the key players in health who tended not to talk much with one another—regulators and the regulated, academics and practitioners, etc.

I thought it was a capital idea. John was at that time a regent of the American College of Physicians and a JCAHO Commissioner. We went to see David Mulligan, the Commissioner of Public Health, who was very supportive. Similarly, when approached, we found the leadership of the Mass Medical Society (MMS) was in favor, and Ron Hollander, president of the Mass Hospital Association (MHA), was downright enthusiastic.

The timing was right. Even before the release of the legendary IOM report, interest in medical errors had begun to develop among the public, health providers, the media, and regulatory agencies. This was especially true in Massachusetts because of the Betsy Lehman tragedy. That such a thing could happen at one of our premier institutions made both patients and professionals feel vulnerable. The fact that these events occur in all settings in spite of extensive oversight and quality monitoring mechanisms led healthcare leaders in Massachusetts to begin to rethink how its industry looked at and learned from medical errors.

© The Author(s) 2021
L. L. Leape, *Making Healthcare Safe*,
https://doi.org/10.1007/978-3-030-71123-8_8

With the commissioner, we called a meeting of leaders of the Department of Public Health (DPH), MHA, MMS, MassPro, the federal peer review organization, and several hospitals. We stated that our hope was to drive improvement by sharing information and to restore the public trust by increasing public awareness of what we were doing to prevent errors. The Coalition would make information available to health professionals and healthcare institutions for quality improvement programs. It would be a vehicle for taking action to improve care. Everyone was enthusiastic.

By May a number of additional organizations had signed up, including the state licensing boards, nurses organizations, the Harvard Controlled Risk Insurance Company (CRICO), the American Association of Retired Persons (AARP), state and federal agencies, and professional associations, as well as several hospitals and clinical researchers.

We agreed on a mission statement that our goal was to develop and implement a statewide initiative to improve patient safety and minimize medical errors. The specific goals were:

- To establish and implement best practices to minimize medical error.
- To increase awareness of error prevention strategies through public and professional education.
- To identify areas of mutual interest and minimize duplication of regulatory and The Joint Commission requirements so that efforts are focused on initiatives that can best improve patient care.

The energy at the first meeting was palpable. Virtually everyone in Massachusetts had been touched by the Betsy Lehman story. Most of the participants, however, knew little else about patient safety. Many were not aware of the Medical Practice Study or of the recent Annenberg Conference. But they were eager to learn and anxious to be at the table. From the beginning, a critical element in moving ahead was the strong support of the DPH and the MHA, who provided staff and office space.

The focus of this and the other early meetings was on framing the problem properly and understanding the perspectives of the different stakeholders (providers, regulators, public, and media). We acknowledged the tension existing between providers and the agencies that regulate them. This was the first time that healthcare providers and government agencies in Massachusetts had ever sat down together to talk openly about medical errors and what they could do together to prevent them.

We believed that the strength of the Coalition would come from participation of representatives from all stakeholders. Thus, a concerted effort was made to ensure that the membership reflected all segments of the healthcare industry, regional interests, providers, payers and regulators, as well as all types of practitioners. We enlisted membership from state and federal agencies with responsibility for licensure and oversight; professional associations representing hospitals, physicians, nurses, nursing executives, and long-term-care institutions; individual healthcare providers; malpractice insurance carriers; accrediting bodies; clinical researchers; and consumer organizations.

Four people provided the leadership that made it happen. John Noble was an academic internist at Boston University who brought a practicing physician's concern about safety, as well as the perspective of the chief regulator, the Joint Commission on Accreditation of Healthcare Organizations (JCAHO), where he was a Board member and later chairman. Leslie Kirle was an enthusiastic administrator and public health advocate who represented MHA's strong commitment and support. Connie Crowley-Ganser, a registered nurse and the quality VP at Children's Hospital, brought the perspectives both of nursing and hospitals. Nancy Ridley was an experienced bureaucrat with the DPH who felt a strong obligation to make healthcare safe.

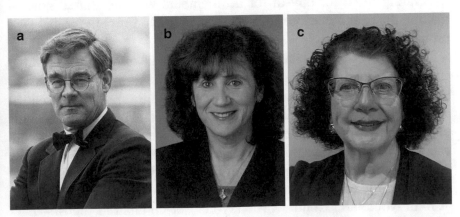

(a) John Noble, (b) Leslie Kirle, and (c) Connie Crowley-Ganser. (All rights reserved)

The energy of these four people, their skills, and their cooperation as a team were crucial to the early success of the Coalition. As noted, members had never all worked together on anything as sensitive as medical errors. These four leaders embodied something quite revolutionary: not just collaboration, but enthusiastic commitment to a cause by a diverse group of key stakeholders.

The Coalition was officially launched on July 31, 1998. The founding members were John Noble (JCAHO), Jim Conway (Dana-Farber Cancer Institute), Connie Crowley-Ganser (Children's Hospital), Harry Greene (MMS), Sheridan Kassirer (Partners Healthcare), Leslie Kirle (MHA), Lucian Leape (Harvard School of Public Health), Randy Peto (MassPro), and Nancy Ridley (DPH).

The mission statement, structure, and process had been developed, and 21 organizations had confirmed their commitment to the Coalition's mission and goals. The Massachusetts Hospital Association took the lead in providing the initial seed money and resources to launch the Coalition and move it forward. DPH and MMS also provided support. The full list of participating organizations is in Appendix 8.1.

We held a press briefing to educate selected print media about the Coalition and its mission. This resulted in several positive stories in key newspapers and journals. It was an important first step in engaging the public in a meaningful dialogue about errors and strategies for prevention.

In a presentation at Annenberg II a few months later, John Noble reflected on the Coalition and its initial success. He noted that the motivating force for buy-in for all members was the shared goal of making the healthcare system as safe as possible for patients and care providers.

From the beginning, the Coalition worked unceasingly to promote communication between key parties. In addition to being a forum for the "heavies" (professional societies and regulators), it also provided a setting that encouraged input from clinicians and consumers as individuals and through their organizations' representatives. The message was clear: patient safety is everyone's responsibility. This emphasis on inclusivity helped enlist broad support for practice and systems changes while building trust and credibility.

John Noble and Connie Crowley-Ganser co-chaired the meetings of the Coalition for the first several years, and they and Leslie Kirle "made things happen." The founding members were the steering committee until a governing Board elected by the members was established in 2002.

Medication Consensus Group

Early on, the Coalition formed a Medication Consensus Group to focus on preventing medication errors. This built on an earlier MHA project that showed poor use of safe medications recommended by the Institute for Safe Medication Practices (ISMP). The group included nurses, physicians, pharmacists, and administrators representing 20 hospitals of different sizes from around the state. They developed short-term (immediate implementation) recommendations, such as unit dosing and removal of concentrated KCl from nursing units, and long-term recommendations such as bar coding, computerized prescriber order entry systems, and electronic medication administration records.

By mid-1999, we had finalized *Best Practice Recommendations to Reduce Medication Errors*. After they were formally endorsed by the Coalition, I made a presentation about it to the MHA Board, assuming their support would be pro forma since the hospital association had been a leader of the medication safety effort even before the Coalition was founded.

To my surprise, some members of the Board, CEOs of hospitals, were dubious. They were concerned about "telling doctors how to practice." Fortunately, others spoke out in its defense, and the Board approved it. The DPH also gave its stamp of approval.

The best practice recommendations were then sent to doctors and hospitals. Again, we got helpful media coverage. In 2001, a survey of Massachusetts hospitals showed that 70% had fully implemented some of the Best Practice Recommendations and 90% had partially implemented some. The recommendations soon spread widely. Within a year they were being used by hospitals in Michigan and Wisconsin in addition to Massachusetts. They were cited in the IOM report.

Looking back 20 years later, it is gratifying to note that while only a few of these practices were in common use at the time, they are now all standard practice. The Coalition was not the only group pushing for standards—ISMP had long advocated most of them—but it was one of the first outside the pharmacy world to do so.

The Medication Consensus Group also developed *Safety First Alerts*. The first three, *Look Alike/Sound Alike Drugs and Packages*, *Transcription and Administration of Medications*, and *Automation*, were published in 2000. The Group also collaborated with the Institute for Family-Centered Care to develop and publish a brochure for patients, *Your Role in Safe Medication Use*. This was distributed to physicians to be given to patients in their offices. It was well received and is still available 20 years later!

Leadership Forum

In July 1999, the Coalition and the Massachusetts Medical Society sponsored another innovation: the first Leadership Forum. We brought experts together with a diverse group of stakeholders to talk for the first time about barriers and solutions to medical errors.

After welcoming remarks by the leaders of the MMS, MHA, and DPH, John Noble gave the history of the development of the Coalition, and I gave the keynote address on creating a culture of safety. Marty Hatlie spoke about the NPSF and Eleanor Vogt presented the new video, *Beyond Blame*. John Nance of ABC News then moderated a star-studded panel of local experts to discuss barriers to talking about errors.

The forum was a great success and became an annual event thereafter, focusing on specific issues, such as reducing restraints and seclusion, communicating unanticipated outcomes and medical errors, and improving safety and quality of ICU care.

Regulatory Consensus Group

A Regulatory Consensus Group was created to align regulatory environments to facilitate adoption of best practices. We had the right people at the table to work on this issue and compare current regulatory requirements. Could we consolidate forms to simplify reporting?

A workshop was held with stakeholders, followed by development of a detailed comparison of requirements levied by the Board of Registration in Medicine (BRM), DPH, the Department of Mental Health (DMH), the Medical Examiner, JCAHO, the Center for Medicare and Medicaid Services (CMS), and the Food and Drug Administration (FDA) for reporting of incidents, time frame, nature of the incident, investigation, corrective measures, definitions, and codes. The group brought awareness in an objective and concrete way to the magnitude of overlapping regulatory requirements and served as the seed for the later work on accountability that the coalition spearheaded.

Restraint Consensus Group

The Restraint and Seclusion Policy and Practice Consensus Group addressed these issues in various venues: psychiatric care, children's care, emergency rooms, and long-term-care facilities. It brought together leaders, staff, administrators, physicians, and nurses from across Massachusetts to review practices, share experiences and techniques that worked, and brainstorm new ideas to minimizing the use of restraints.

The group's report, *Best Practice Recommendations To Improve Patient Safety Related to Restraint & Seclusion Use*, advocated the *appropriate use* of restraints and seclusion by ensuring staff are *well-trained*, implementation of a comprehensive clinical *assessment* before restraints are applied, development of *guidelines* for the need for restraint or seclusion use, routine *monitoring* of the safe use of restraints and seclusion, and *education* of patients and their responsible parties about the organization's restraint and seclusion reduction efforts. The Coalition promoted adoption of these recommendations by developing an improvement workbook and through educational programs and leadership initiatives showcasing restraint-free practices.

Through all the early years, Leslie Kirle of MHA was the person that made the initiatives work. She was the "go to" person who recruited members for consensus groups, organized and convened meetings, and generally made it all work. It was a heady time, with a multitude of projects and intense interest by all members. Many people had good ideas. Leslie turned them into action. But Leslie could only do it part time. She had other duties at MHA. The Board recognized the need for a full-time director. It took more than a year to find the right person, but in the end they succeeded brilliantly.

In 2001, Paula Griswold was appointed as the first executive director. She quickly took over management of the many Coalition activities. In addition to updates on activities of the participants, she built a strong educational component into the monthly Coalition meetings. Coalition members and local or national experts share research and new programs in patient safety. This educational aspect of the monthly meetings has been very helpful to the members and a key reason they attend the meetings regularly.

Also in 2001, Senator Moore succeeded in getting the state legislature to create the Betsy Lehman Center. However, it would be several

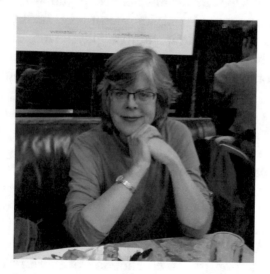

Paula Griswold.

more years before it would be funded and able to carry out its mission of motivating and implementing statewide safety programs. By 2001, coalitions had developed in Michigan, Pittsburgh, and Delmarva (Delaware, Maryland, and Virginia).

DPH Project

But were we actually making patient care safer? By 2002 the Coalition, MHA, and DPH recognized the need for a more aggressive approach to action and research to implement safe practices and to improve reporting. In collaboration with the DPH, we applied for and received a substantial grant from the Agency for Health Research and Quality (AHRQ).

The grant had four aims: to improve the DPH reporting system, to evaluate hospital leadership perceptions of public reporting, to measure perceptions and experience of hospitalized patients concerning adverse events and disclosure, and to develop and implement two safe practices. Eric Schneider, Joel Weisman, and Arnie Epstein of HMS and HSPH and Jack Fowler of the Center for Survey Research led the research team for the first three aims.

The purpose of Aim 1 was to evaluate and improve the DPH mandatory hospital reporting system (MARS), possibly by adopting the National Quality Forum (NQF) list of serious reportable events. After evaluating the content and characteristics of a representative sample of 800 incident reports made by 72 hospitals during 1999–2004, the researchers concluded that if Massachusetts had adopted the NQF standard and accompanying list of reportable events, up to 83% of incidents would not have been reported.

A new system was developed, along with a data abstraction tool to capture key elements from medical records. Use of Internet technology was analyzed to identify where there might be a good fit for the medication error-web-based reporting system, but no solution was identified. In 2003 the project was expanded to include a comparison of MARS to the patient care assessment (PCA) reports required by the Massachusetts Board of Registration in Medicine. However, they were unable to reach the goal of creating a single combined report form.

Surveys

To evaluate leadership perceptions of public reporting, CEOs and COOs were surveyed in six states: two with mandatory reporting and public disclosure (CO and MA), two with mandatory reporting and no public disclosure (FL and PA), and two with no mandatory reporting (GA and TX). The results from the sample of 203 hospitals were surprisingly similar: 69% believed that public disclosure discourages internal (within the hospital) reporting, 79% believed it encourages filing of lawsuits, and only 28% felt it improved patient safety [1]. Although all three groups were strongly opposed to public disclosure, hospitals in states where it was required were less concerned about increased lawsuits, suggesting that familiarity bred less contempt.

Patient perceptions and experience with adverse events in the hospital were evaluated by a patient survey of 2582 randomly selected patients from 16 hospitals in Massachusetts. The results were shocking: 25% of patients reported "negative" events that study physicians identified as adverse events (AEs). Three-fourths of these were significant or serious; 31% were preventable. These rates were 2–3 times those reported by previous record review studies [2].

The study then compared the yield of patient reports to standard record review by examining their medical records using the Medical Practice Study method of nurse screening and two physician independent reviews (Chap. 1). Patients reported AE in 29% of cases, and record review found an additional 11% of patients with AE. But the striking finding was that three-fourths of patient-reported AE were not discovered by record review [3].

Further analysis showed that disclosure of the AE to the patient by the medical team only occurred 40% of the time. Disclosure was more likely if additional treatment was needed and less likely if the AEs were preventable (an error). Patients were twice as likely to rate the quality of care high when there was disclosure [4]. High patient participation in their care was associated with fewer AE (49%) and higher likelihood that patients would rate the quality of their care good or excellent [5].

Implementing Best Practices

The fourth part of AHRQ grant provided support to the Coalition and MHA to develop two voluntary best practice initiatives and get them adopted statewide.

We began by widely soliciting input, calling on clinicians to tell us what "kept you awake at night." To select the practices, we used four criteria: importance, existence of elements of a practice, effectiveness, and feasibility of implementation. From ten widely suggested topics, we chose two: reconciling medications and communicating critical test results. It fell to me and the Coalition staff to make them happen, so I chaired planning groups for each. We made sure to have several change experts from IHI on each committee.

The Reconciling Medications Project

Reconciling medications is the process of making sure that "every hospitalized patient receives all the medications they were taken prior to admission unless they are specifically discontinued by their caregivers and ensuring that they are ordered in the correct dose, route, and frequency." [6] It is a problem because the information may be difficult to obtain, and the responsibility for doing it is unclear. Often, it just isn't done. Reconciling is a classic system problem.

Gina Rogers staffed this project and did a terrific job. We convened a consensus group of physicians, nurses, and pharmacists to develop the best practice, as well as core measurements and an implementation toolkit of suggested strategies for the QI teams to use.

The best practice for reconciling included four steps: (1) establish who (doctor, nurse, pharmacist) has primary responsibility, (2) obtain an accurate preadmission medication list, (3) write accurate admission orders, and (4) reconcile all variances. In addition, the best practice called for providing continuing support and maintenance by adopting clear policies and procedures, adopting a standard form, and providing ongoing education and monitoring.

To implement the practice, we used the IHI Breakthrough Series Collaborative approach in which hospitals use the PDSA (Plan-Do-Study-Act) Model for Improvement. Frank Federico joined us from IHI to help.

The MHA urged all hospital CEOs to participate. Of the 50 hospitals in the state, three-fourths did. Baseline risk assessment in 20 hospitals revealed that 59% of medications were unreconciled. The need for the project was clear.

We brought participating teams together four times in 2003 and 2004 for 2-day learning sessions, coaching on the PDSA method, and to report on progress and share successful strategies. The teams tested implementation strategies and monitored their progress with common measures. They filed monthly reports and communicated with each other over a listserv guided by expert faculty.

Adoption of the safe practice proved challenging. At the conclusion of the collaborative, 64% of hospitals had succeeded in establishing a workable system for reconciliation of medications, but only 20% had succeeded in getting it used hospital-wide at all locations.

A survey of hospital teams after the collaborative ended showed that the factors associated with successful implementation were those common to all collaboratives: strong leadership support, engagement of key stakeholders, use of small tests of change, use of data and examples of errors to motivate change, measuring whether changes are leading to improvement, and attendance at the collaborative learning sessions.

The key lesson specific to reconciliation was that there must be a clear assignment of responsibility—everyone must know whose job reconciliation is, and if it is the admitting nurse, there must be a clear backup assignment of a physician or pharmacist to correct the variances.

The second and even more challenging practice was communicating critical test results.

Communicating Critical Test Results

Communicating critical test results is the process of ensuring that test results are immediately *and reliably* communicated to the responsible physician. For critically ill patients or those with life-threatening conditions, getting the results of blood tests, imaging, EKGs, or biopsies in a timely fashion can make the difference between life and death.

One might assume that would occur without fail. Unfortunately, that is not the case—even in the best of hospitals. Wide variations exist in the definitions of critical test results and how they are communicated to the responsible clinician [7–9]. Each hospital had its own system; there were no uniform standards at the state or national level. Even within a single institution, laboratories, radiology, and cardiology often differed in their practices, and significant delays occur frequently. All shocking, when you think about it. Lives are in the balance—and lives can be lost when treatment is delayed.

The Communicating Critical Test Results collaborative took on these problems. As with the reconciling medications project, a Consensus Group was convened that included the full array of stakeholders: doctors, nurses, pharmacists, and administrators, plus representatives from blood testing laboratories, radiology, cardiology, and pathology.

The process of developing the safe practice recommendations took months, but under the competent leadership of the project director, Doris Hanna, and medication safety expert David Bates, the Consensus Group succeeded in developing a set of Safe Practice Recommendations (Appendix 8.2) and a "starter set" of critical test results.

Recommendations addressed five issues: (1) definition—what tests are critical?, (2) how quickly should they be reported?, (3) to whom?, (4) backup recipient, and (5) how should they be reported?

Definition and timing. The essential first point is that each institution must reach a consensus about which tests are critical. Criteria must be agreed on and applied uniformly in all venues, laboratory, radiology, cardiology, etc., and in all practice areas: inpatient, outpatient, and ED. The typical hospital list is too long, definitions are not clear, and there is no agreed-upon standard for what qualifies as a critical test result (CTR). We recommended a color-code system that is useful and easy to understand:

Red values indicate the patient is in imminent danger of death, significant morbidity, or serious adverse consequences unless treatment is initiated *immediately* (e.g., a blood potassium level of 6 or greater). Results must be reported as soon as possible, at most within an hour.

Orange values are abnormalities that warrant rapid, but not immediate, attention by the responsible clinician (e.g., BUN over 100). The report should be delivered to the responsible party within 6–8 hours.

Yellow values are abnormalities that are not urgent but require diagnosis and treatment in a timely and reliable manner (e.g., a biopsy showing cancer). Maximum time: 3 days.

To whom should the report be given? This must be the person who can take appropriate action. In many institutions the report was delivered to the nurse on the unit, who then had to find the doctor to take action. It was agreed that practice must stop.

Who does the report go to if the ordering provider is not available? This proved to be a difficult problem. If the responsible physician is not in the hospital, finding them quickly can be difficult. If it is a resident, they may no longer be on call. Hospitals must implement call systems that link every patient with a responsible provider at all times.

How should results be reported? For red values, person-to-person verbal communication by phone to the responsible physician was deemed essential. For orange and yellow values, indirect delivery by e-mail or through an intermediary such as a nurse or ward clerk is acceptable. The provider must acknowledge to the sender receipt of the result within the defined time frame (6–8 hours or 3 days), and the system must verify that it happens.

The full set of recommendations can be found in Appendix 8.2, which also includes the implementation context for each recommendation. For example, the recommendation for red results includes the explicit steps of whom to call in addition to the responsible physician; what to do if no response after 15, 30, and 45 minutes; and the failsafe plan at 1 hour.

To facilitate adoption, the consensus group developed a starter set of specific thresholds for red, orange, and yellow values for all laboratory, cardiology, and radiology tests. Hospitals were encouraged to modify these values to make them their own. The starter set is available at http://www.macoalition.org/initiatives.shtml.

As with reconciling medications, the recommendations and starter set of critical test results were disseminated in a statewide collaborative of Massachusetts hospitals where we assisted hospital teams in implementing the system, testing changes, and sharing successful strategies.

A year after the conclusion of the two collaboratives, we commissioned the Center for Survey Research to survey the participating institutions to determine the extent to which they implemented the new practices. How successful were we in actually changing practice?

Of 66 acute care hospitals in Massachusetts, 58 (88%) participated in 1 collaborative and 32 participated in both. For reconciling medications, 50% had some implementation, and 20% had fully implemented them. For communicating critical test results, 65% had some implementation, and 20% fully implemented [10].

These rates were comparable to IHI success rates for collaboratives. It would be another several years before Peter Pronovost demonstrated the power of a more intensive implementation strategy to yield a much higher rate of implementation (75%) of a safe practice for insertion of central lines [11, 12]. (See Chap. 6.)

The major barriers to success were resistance to change, complexity, and competing priorities for staff time. Few teams met as frequently as required, and hospitals sometimes didn't send full teams to collaborative meetings. Despite a lot of advance preparation, getting leaders involved and learning change methods proved difficult for most.

We published the recommendations from each of the initiatives and the results of our experiences in three papers in *The Joint Commission Journal on Quality and Patient Safety* in 2005 and 2006 [6, 13, 14] and an overview paper in Quality and Safety in Health Care in 2006 [10].

Despite the mixed results, these initiatives had considerable impact statewide and on individual participants. They demonstrated that important systems change was possible and that the Coalition was a major force making that happen. A nurse manager at a hospital that implemented both practices commented that the work she did was the most rewarding work she had done during her 25-year career.

But the greatest impact of these initiatives was nationwide when The Joint Commission (whose journal published our results) made them two of their National Patient Safety Goals, signaling to all hospitals not only that these were important, but that hospitals were expected to implement them. By 2006, The Joint Commission reported that 90% of hospitals had improved reporting of CTR and 100% had developed a process for reconciliation.

Impact of the Coalition

The coalition was a powerful force for change in Massachusetts. One reason is clear: from the beginning, the key players—the Department of Public Health, the Massachusetts Hospital Association, and the Massachusetts Medical Society—were enthusiastic participants and provided both leadership and material support. This was several years before the legendary Institute of Medicine report, *To Err Is Human*. The stimulus was much closer to home: the tragic death of Betsy Lehman, which had a powerful impact on our community at every level.

We had another advantage: Several of the national leaders in quality improvement and error prevention were in Boston, and by 1997, thanks to IHI, there was already a cadre of people in the hospitals with first-hand experience in improvement. They welcomed the support of their work and the opportunity to learn from others. The Coalition got the conversation about patient safety into the C-suites and board rooms. Patient safety became a priority.

The support of the Massachusetts Hospital Association was particularly critical. The president, Ron Hollander, strongly supported the coalition and sincerely wanted the effort to succeed, as did his successor, Andy Dreyfus. MHA provided space, staff support, and day-to-day leadership by Leslie Kirle. Likewise, strong support from the Commissioner of Public Health, Howard Koh, and leadership by Nancy Ridley, the DPH representative to the coalition, were critical to getting the coalition going.

Since the coalition came into being, a number of other states and regions have created coalitions: Arkansas, California, Colorado, Florida, Georgia, Iowa, Maryland, Minnesota, Pennsylvania, Tennessee, Texas, Utah, Virginia, and Wisconsin [15].

Under Paula Griswold's leadership, the Coalition expanded its efforts. She made the monthly meetings a "must-do" for members who want to stay current with developments in patient safety. A number of statewide educational programs have been held. The Coalition continued to convene collaboratives, including ones on long-term care and ambulatory care. Keeping up is also facilitated by links to relevant research and notices that the Coalition distributes each month about virtually everything happening in patient safety worldwide. The Coalition website, http://www.macoalition.org, lists initiatives and educational programs.

The Coalition accomplished an incredible amount in the first few years, both in agenda setting and in activities that brought together key stakeholders to produce meaningful deliverables. It was a major force in beginning to change the mindset of its members away from punishment of individuals to changing systems, the paradigm shift that drives patient safety. Its initiatives produced tangible results, driving home human factors lessons about the effectiveness of systems change. It truly changed the conversation and understanding.

Now, more than 20 years after its founding, the Massachusetts Coalition for the Prevention of Medical Errors continues to be a major influence for patient safety in the Commonwealth of Massachusetts.

Appendix 8.1: Initial Coalition Member Organizations

- *American Association of Retired Persons*
- *American College of Physicians*
- *Boston University School of Medicine*
- *Harvard Risk Management Foundation*
- *Health Care Financing Administration*
- *Harvard School of Public Health*
- *Institute for Healthcare Improvement*
- *Joint Commission on Accreditation of Healthcare Organizations*
- *Massachusetts Association of Behavioral Health*
- *Massachusetts Board of Nursing*
- *Massachusetts Board of Pharmacy*
- *Massachusetts Board of Registration in Medicine*
- *Massachusetts Department of Public Health*
- *Massachusetts Extended Care Federation*
- *Massachusetts Hospital Association*
- *Willis Massachusetts Medical Society*
- *Massachusetts Nurses Association*
- *Massachusetts Organization Executives*
- *Massachusetts Peer-Reviewed Organization*
- *Professional Liability Foundation*
- *PRO Mutual Group*

Appendix 8.2: Communicating Critical Test Results

1. Who should receive the results?

   - The results must go to someone who can take action—usually the person who ordered the test or the attending physician. Whoever orders it gets the results and has the responsibility to take action.

2. Who should receive the results when the ordering provider is not available?

   - Have a clear backup system with clear delineation of when to escalate.
   - Link every patient with a responsible provider.
   - Use central call systems with a call schedule for all providers.

3. What results require timely and reliable communication?

   - All parties must agree on which tests require immediate communication; these are the critical test results (CTR).
   - Include all types of tests, all practice areas.
   - Limit the list to those findings that if left untreated could result in harm to the patient. Most of these will require a change in therapy.
   - Recommend three discrete categories according to the maximum amount of time that should elapse before identification of a CTR.
   - Defined by a three-tier system with color labels:
   - Red Zone: Patient is in imminent danger of death, significant morbidity, or serious adverse consequences if treatment is not initiated immediately. Requires immediate clinical response
   - Orange Zone: A significant abnormality that requires rapid, but not immediate, attention. Not a clinical emergency
   - Yellow Zone: Test results that indicate a significant abnormality that my threaten life or cause significant morbidity, complications, or serious adverse consequences unless diagnosis and treatment is initiated in a timely manner. No immediate threat to life

4. When should the results be provided?

   - Red: within 1 hour—requires "stat" page and immediate acknowledgment

- Orange: within the shift (6–8 hours)
- Yellow: within 3 days

5. How is the provider notified?

- Describe explicit steps in notification system; when reporters should initiate and follow up on notifying the ordering provider.
- Use direct person-to-person call to provider, not secretary or other intermediary. (A backup call to a nurse may also be advisable.)
- Develop a fail-safe plan for communicating CTR when ordering or covering provider cannot be contacted within the time frame.
- Ensure 100% acknowledgment for every test result on the list, i.e., that the sender has received confirmation from the responsible recipient that they have received the report. Caller must know that a responsible party has the information—for all three priorities.

6. Establish a shared policy for uniform communication of all types of test results to all recipients:

- Use the same policy regarding definitions and time windows across all domains.
- Encourage and foster shared accountability and teamwork across and between clinical disciplines.
- Decide what information should be included in the report.

7. How to design reliability into the system:

- Use forcing functions at point of ordering to identify the ordering provider.
- Use forcing functions at point of ordering to include a minimum of information to support the interpretation of results.
- Create tracking systems to assure timely and reliable communication.

8. How to support and maintain systems:

- Partner with patients in the communication of test results.
- Provide orientation and ongoing education on procedures for communicating CTR to all health providers.
- Provide ongoing monitoring of the effectiveness of the systems—weekly failure rates, response times, etc.
  Adapted from Ref [13], Table 3

References

1. Weissman JSA, L C, Epstein AM, Schneider EC, Clarridge B, Kirle L, Gatsonis C, Feibelmann S, Ridley N. Error reporting and disclosure systems – views from hospital leaders. JAMA. 2005;293:1359–66.
2. Fowler FJ, Epstein A, Weingart SN, et al. Adverse events during hospitalization: results of a patient survey. Jt Comm J Qual Patient Saf. 2008;34:583–90.
3. Weissman JS, Schneider EC, Weingart SN, et al. Comparing patient-reported hospital adverse events with medical record review: do patients know something that hospitals do not? Ann Intern Med. 2008;149:100–8.
4. Lopez L, Weissman JS, Schneider EC, Weingart SN, Cohen AP, Epstein AM. Disclosure of hospital adverse events and its association with patients' ratings of the quality of care. Arch Intern Med. 2009;169:1888–94.
5. Weingart SN, Zhu J, Chiapetta L, et al. Hospitalized patients' participation and its impact on quality of care and patient safety. Int J Qual Health Care. 2011;23:269–77.
6. Rogers G, Alper E, Brunelle D, et al. Reconciling medications at admission: safe practice recommendations and implementation strategies. Jt Comm J Qual Patient Saf. 2006;32:37–50.
7. Kuperman GJ, Boyle D, Jha A, et al. How promptly are inpatients treated for critical laboratory results? J Am Med Inform Assoc. 1998;5:112–9.
8. Kost GJ. Critical limits for urgent clinician notification at US medical centers. JAMA. 1990;263:704–7.
9. Lundberg GD. Acting on significant laboratory results. JAMA. 1981;245:1762–3.
10. Leape LL, Rogers G, Hanna D, et al. Developing and implementing new safe practices: voluntary adoption through statewide collaboratives. Qual Saf Health Care. 2006;15:289–95.
11. Watson SR, George C, Martin M, Bogan B, Goeschel C, Pronovost PJ. Preventing central line-associated bloodstream infections and improving safety culture: a statewide experience. Jt Comm J Qual Patient Saf. 2009;35:593–7.
12. Dixon-Woods M, Bosk CL, Aveling EL, et al. Explaining Michigan: developing an ex post theory of a quality improvement program. Milbank Qtrly. 2011;89:167–205.
13. Hanna D, Griswold P, Leape L, Bates D. Communicating critical test results: safe practice recommendations 2005. Jt Comm J Qual Patient Saf. 2005;31:68–80.
14. Bates D, Leape LL. Editorial: Doing better with critical test results. Jt Comm J Qual Patient Saf. 2005;31:66–7.
15. Comden SC, Rosenthal J. Statewide patient safety coalitions: A status report. Portland, ME: National Academy for State Health Policy; 2002. Report No.: GNL 44.

Chapter 9
When the IOM Speaks: IOM Quality of Care Committee and Report

On July 7, 1998, I received an invitation from the Institute of Medicine (IOM) to become a member of the Committee on Quality of Health Care in America. The Committee, chaired by Bill Richardson of the Kellogg Foundation, was an outgrowth of an IOM Roundtable on Quality of Care, chaired by Mark Chassin and Robert Galvin.

I was initially reluctant. I had been on several IOM committees by then. Although the quality of their work was impressive, it took a lot of time, and few of the reports seemed to have wide circulation or impact. I called them "shelf research." I wasn't sure I wanted to participate in another.

However, when the staff person calling, Molla Donaldson, told me who else was on the committee—a veritable who's who of quality and policy leadership—I decided to join, if for no other reason than to get to know some people whom I admired. I didn't realize at the time that medical error would be a key focus and that I was a key resource for that. And I certainly had no inkling how much of an impact our work would ultimately have. "Shelf research" indeed!

The IOM Committee on Quality of Health Care in America took its origin from a series of efforts over the previous decade that documented serious problems in healthcare quality. These included a steady stream of research from RAND showing major quality of care shortcomings, the report from the Presidential Advisory Commission on Consumer Protection and Quality in the Health Care Industry [1],

© The Author(s) 2021
L. L. Leape, *Making Healthcare Safe*,
https://doi.org/10.1007/978-3-030-71123-8_9

the findings of the IOM National Roundtable on Health Care Quality [2], and the Milbank Memorial Fund Quarterly Review of evidence of poor quality of healthcare [3].

The Presidential Advisory Commission, appointed by the Clinton administration in 1997 and co-chaired by Donna Shalala, secretary of Health and Human Services, and Alexis Herman, secretary of the Department of Labor, had special weight. The president was concerned about healthcare and especially about the quality implications of "managed care," and he appointed a blue-ribbon committee that included consumers, representatives from business, labor, healthcare providers, health plans, state and local governments, and healthcare quality experts, to insure broad input.

The Advisory Commission's 1998 report, "Quality First: Better Healthcare for All Americans," brought together the evidence for quality problems and the broad consensus for reform [1]. It concluded that quality problems were pervasive and by no means confined to managed care systems. The report was aimed at Congress and policy-makers in Washington and made clear recommendations, including a call for a "Patient Bill of Rights," which the Clinton administration enacted. Otherwise, even though it got a lot of attention, the report resulted in little action.

Enter Steve Schroeder, president of the Robert Wood Johnson Foundation (RWJ). Deeply concerned about the quality of healthcare and anxious to capitalize on the growing pressure for action, Schroeder consulted with Ken Shine, president of the IOM, about moving ahead. Shine was enthusiastic. RWJ gave two million dollars to the IOM to establish the Quality of Care in America Committee. Shine took the unusual step of putting in additional funds from the IOM. Normally, IOM projects were commissioned and funded by Congress or an Executive Branch Agency.

To secure strong leadership, Shine reached out to Bill Richardson, president and CEO of the Kellogg Foundation, to serve as the chair and Janet Corrigan, executive director of the President's Advisory Commission on Consumer Protection and Quality (which was coming to a close), to serve as the project director.

As the project was beginning to take shape, two issues became clear. First, it should "pick up the baton" from the earlier work. Toward

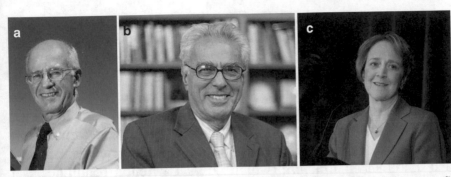

(a) Steve Schroeder, (b) Ken Shine, and (c) Janet Corrigan. (All rights reserved)

this end, the committee was populated with some of the experts who had served on the earlier IOM Roundtable and the President's Advisory Commission.

Second, it would be important to obtain a much deeper understanding of why earlier efforts had fallen on deaf ears and to identify ways to overcome what appeared to be communication barriers.

Accordingly, one of the first activities it undertook was to convene a workshop of people from print and broadcast media and pose the question of how to most effectively get public attention to quality information. Their advice was to keep it simple – things that people can understand – and to frame the issue in terms of a victim and a villain. The obvious candidate: patient safety. Just as plane accidents are understandable, so are medical mishaps. The victims are people just like us; and there was a villain: a defective health care system.

A focus on safety might also enlist the support of the medical profession, which had become defensive about efforts to improve quality. When challenged, doctors would typically counter with "My patients are different." Perhaps shifting the focus to defective systems would bring them aboard.

Safety had another appeal: a movement to do something about it was already underway. The Annenberg Conference had been convened 2 years earlier, sponsored by the AMA, The Joint Commission, and the American Association for the Advancement of Science. The AMA had created the National Patient Safety Foundation, The Joint Commission had strengthened its sentinel events reporting system, and Don Berwick's IHI had conducted a collaborative aimed at reducing medication errors.

The safety problem had been defined, and efforts to change systems had begun. Despite this, most Americans, and most medical professionals, were still unaware and uninvolved. This was a big opportunity to do something about that.

So it was decided that the Quality of Care in America Committee would focus on both quality and safety but lead with safety to get public and political attention. Two subcommittees were formed: one on the *environment* of healthcare (which focused on patient safety) and the other on *structure* (which David Lawrence, head of Kaiser Permanente, had nicknamed the "chassis"). The committees would meet separately and together. I was on the environment subcommittee, chaired by Chris Bisgard, director, Health Services, Delta Air Lines, and Molly Joel Coye of the Lewin Group. Don Berwick chaired the "chassis" one. Don and Dave Lawrence were on both. The first meeting was September 28. Members of the committee are listed in Appendix 9.1.

At the January 1999 meeting of subcommittee on the environment, we focused on reporting of medical errors. Charles Billings, architect of the aviation reporting system, told us that reporting systems don't work unless they are safe, simple, and productive. Safe: the reporter must not be at risk of losing their job or being disciplined for reporting a mistake they have made. Simple: people will not report if the process is too complicated (a long form) or takes too much time. Productive: reporting must lead to a response by the organization to address the issue reported. If nothing happens after people report, they lose interest and stop reporting. We would embrace these concepts in the final report's recommendations for reporting.

At the February meeting of the whole committee, Don Berwick led a discussion of values. He presented six "Aims for Improvement" that he had proposed at an earlier "chassis" committee meeting in Woods Hole: that care should be safe, effective, patient-centered, timely, efficient, and equitable. The aims resonated with all and were quickly embraced. They became the centerpiece of the recommendations in the final report, *Crossing the Quality Chasm.*

Berwick's six aims have proved not only to be most memorable part of the report but also the most powerful. Easily understood, intuitively important, and actionable, they became the framework for thinking about and acting on quality improvement that has motivated practice and research for more than 20 years.

At the March 18 joint meeting of the subcommittees, Berwick presented another organizing concept: the "Chain of Effect" model that shows the relationships among patient and community/microsystem/organization/environment (policy). Don explained the microsystems concept: It is the level—hospital unit or office—where care is given.

Jim Reinertson, CEO of Minnesota HealthPartners, noted that doctors often think they are held accountable as individuals for harm that is actually caused by systems failures. He urged that we not pit professionalism against systems but join them together. All agreed that complexity is a big cause of errors.

We also agreed that we needed better definitions of safety and systems; many are too theoretical. Berwick noted that "standards" can mean three different things: performance standards (desired or expected results), process standards (the agreed way to do things), and measures (such as the "standard kilogram"). All are important, but we needed to explain and distinguish among them.

In April we held a communications workshop. This content-filled meeting was designed both to bring the committee up to date on technological advances and to get advice on how to communicate our findings. Bob Blendon reminded us that the best way to influence the public is to combine a personal case of harm with a villain and a solution.

We agreed that we had to get the public aroused to get the system to change. The definition of poor quality for many people was that your HMO is not letting you get the care you think you need. Some noted that the problem isn't communication, but it is whether the institution responds or doesn't. What is our overall strategy for improving quality? What is our media strategy for making that happen?

Other guest speakers talked about the role of new technologies, such as computerized physician order entry and computerized patient records. I will never forget Joe Scherger's comments. Joe was a primary care doctor who was also associate dean for clinical affairs, at UC Irvine. He made a brief but powerful talk that he summarized by saying that there was one simple thing a physician could do that would simultaneously save time, improve communication, and improve patient satisfaction: "Give your patients your email address."

Reflecting on this as a patient 20 years later, I am struck both with how true it is and how difficult it still seems to be for doctors to do it!

At the April meeting following the communications workshop, we developed the strategy for advancing our recommendations: (1) a broad-based communication strategy involving prominent figures, dissemination of credible data, and gaining access to policy-makers; (2) pressure for public-private-regulatory initiatives, such as quality of care forums, and (3) advocacy for building trust-building actions into healthcare, i.e., open communication when things go wrong.

I made the case for putting less emphasis on mandatory systems for reporting and greater emphasis on developing *response* systems, as recommended by Billings. For example, both USP and ISMP reporting systems identify risks related to naming, packaging, dosing, and use of medications, but the FDA and pharmaceutical industry are slow to respond or don't so at all. State reporting systems are often "black holes."

Don Berwick called for developing illustrative cases—how we do it now, how we should do it using the systems approach, and full root cause analysis. Chris Bisgard noted that the lack of a defibrillator in a single case of cardiac arrest on a Delta flight led airlines to install them on all planes, despite the fact that the cardiac arrest rate was 8 in 50 million!

What policies do we want adopted? One person called for going after the 1% of doctors who are negligent by improving state board functioning. The Committee did not want to do that. We had an extensive discussion about the advisability of having an FAA equivalent for healthcare. I came down strongly on the side of yes, but that proved to be a step too far for the committee. We did agree to press for a federal agency to oversee safety and to change the reimbursement system from pay for volume to pay for quality.

Our discussions were coming to a close. There would be two reports: one on safety and one on quality of care. The safety report would be aimed at a broad audience: both healthcare professionals and the general public. The report on quality (*Crossing the Quality Chasm*) would be targeted to healthcare professionals and would spell out the theoretical concepts and details of what was needed to improve quality of care overall, based on the six aims.

The safety report would be published first since it would grab public and professional attention with its shocking numbers and "victim, villain, solution." Corrigan and her staff were nearing completion; drafts were circulated, and committee members made edits or rewrote substantial segments.

To Err Is Human

The report was titled *To Err Is Human* [4]. It "made the case" for patient safety, explaining the science of error-making and the theoretical and practical evidence for human-factors-based systems changes. In many ways it was an expansion of the ideas set forth in my 1994 paper, *Error in Medicine,* but it provided more detailed descriptions of methods and provided case studies to illustrate the points.

In addition to documenting the need for attention to the issue of patient safety, *To Err Is Human* explained the concept of using a systems approach based on human factors principles and proclaimed that application of this methodology could have a profound effect. It boldly called for a 50% reduction in medical harm in 5 years.

Specific recommendations were made to galvanize the healthcare industry into action to improve safety. The recommendations were nicely summarized in a later report of the Presidential Quality Interagency Task Force [5], excerpts from which I quote here, with my comments in italics:

Establish a Center for Patient Safety at the Agency for Healthcare Research and Quality (AHRQ) with responsibility for promoting the development of knowledge about errors and to encourage the sharing of strategies for reducing errors. The IOM committee recommends substantial budget increases over the next several years. *(This was the most important recommendation. To move ahead in patient safety, we had to have central leadership and funding. Patient safety had to be a national priority.)*

Promote voluntary and mandatory reporting of errors. First, the IOM recommends that *voluntary* reporting systems should focus on errors that result in little or no harm to patients and should be encouraged by AHRQ. Second, a *mandatory* reporting system should be established to allow state governments to collect standardized information on adverse events resulting in death or serious harm. *(Increased reporting was something everyone thought was important. I was not so sure. (See Chap. 17.) But the idea of having a voluntary system to spur improvement and a mandatory system for accountability did make sense.)*

Protect reporting systems from being used in litigation. The IOM urges Congress to pass legislation extending peer review protections to data related to patient safety and quality improvement that are collected and analyzed by healthcare organizations for purposes of improving safety and quality. *(We all agreed this was essential if we were ever to get people to talk about error in the current litigious environment.)*

Make patient safety the focus of performance standards for healthcare organizations and professionals. Regulators and accreditors should require healthcare organizations to have meaningful patient safety programs. Purchasers are also encouraged to provide incentives for patient safety programs. The IOM suggests that professional licensing organizations periodically reexamine and relicense professionals based, in part, on their knowledge of patient safety.

Licensing organizations also need to develop more effective means of identifying unsafe practitioners and taking actions against them. It also suggests that professional societies should promote patient safety education. *(This was our pitch that safety is everyone's business. Healthcare organizations, professional societies, and regulators had to step up.)*

Increase FDA attention to safety in pre- and post-market reviews of drugs. The IOM specifically suggests developing standards for safe packaging and labeling; testing of drug names to prevent sound-alike and look-alike errors; and working with doctors, pharmacists, and patients to identify and rectify problems in the post-marketing phase. *(The failure of the FDA to do this was, we thought, unconscionable. They and the manufacturers knew these were problems and looked the other way. It was time to stop.)*

Encourage healthcare organizations to make a commitment to improving patient safety and to implement safe medication practices. Healthcare organizations should develop a culture of safety and implement nonpunitive systems for reporting and analyzing errors. These organizations should also follow recommendations for safe medication practices as published by professional and collaborative organizations interested in patient safety. (*Of course! The culture had to change. Making that happen would turn out to be the major challenge, still unresolved (Chap. 23)).*

Because the error report was expected to attract public interest and garner attention for the whole quality effort, chairman Richardson and staff director Corrigan decided that it should be released first, and the sooner the better. The report was scheduled to be released on Wednesday, December 1, 1999, so staff made an embargoed copy of the report available to elite media ahead of time and planned for a press conference on the 1st. Then things went awry.

On Monday afternoon, November 29, Don Berwick and I were called by IOM staff and asked to come to Washington immediately. A major television network had decided to break the embargo and go with the story on that night's news. The other networks quickly found out, so all of them were going to be doing the story that evening. The IOM decided to release the report immediately but wanted Don and me to come down for interviews on these national networks that evening.

It was a bit of a circus. I was sent to one network and Don to another, and then we each went to a second. It was hot news, but fortunately the stories were reasonably faithful, and the interviews were on point and not over-sensationalized. What got attention was the estimate that there were up to 98,000 preventable deaths a year due to medical errors. That number also headlined the newspaper stories the next day. In all fairness, the news reports did note that these errors and deaths were due to systems failures, but most viewers and readers were so stunned by 98,000 that it was lost in the uproar.

The 98,000 number was actually a last minute extrapolation that Janet Corrigan made by updating to the present the number of preventable deaths estimated by the Medical Practice Study 9 years earlier, which was over 120,000 [6]. In the interim, thanks to managed care and other cost-cutting measures, the number of patients hospitalized had dropped considerably. One could argue that these were sicker patients, so the number of injuries might not have dropped proportionately, but no matter, 98,000 was shocking enough.

The IOM had never seen anything like it. As I later noted in a NEJM editorial, "The speed and intensity with which the IOM report captured media, public, political, and professional attention surprised everyone. Neither the shocking statistics nor its central message, that errors are caused by faulty systems, was new, but the report forcefully brought them to public awareness." [7] In talks about the report later I would parody a financial house ad, "When researchers speak, no one listens, when the IOM speaks, everyone listens."

In truth, they hadn't listened to the IOM much before, either, of course, but this was different. *To Err Is Human* was by far the most widely disseminated and commented on report ever issued by the IOM, a record that still stands 20 years later. A later survey showed that 51% of Americans were aware of the report, which was unprecedented. Skeptics have argued that we got so much coverage because it was a slow news day. While that may be true, it was also true that the message was powerful and touched everyone. If the timing was good luck, fine. The cause deserved it!

Within days, Congress scheduled hearings, and president Clinton formed the Quality Interagency Task Force—headed, fortunately, by John Eisenberg, administrator of the newly formed Agency for Healthcare Research and Quality (AHRQ)—to analyze the report and make recommendations. The administration—the president, secretary Shalala, and Chris Jennings, the health policy advisor—all wanted to do something, so they acted quickly in response.

The formation of the Task Force was announced by the president at a press conference in the Rose Garden. A number of us were invited to attend. I remember well the tingle that went up my spine, and I gave a silent "Hooray!" when I heard the president of the USA mouth our mantra: "It's not bad people, it's bad systems." Sixty days later, when the Task Force made its recommendations [5], the president called on all federal health agencies to implement the IOM recommendations. The IOM had accomplished an unprecedented act of agenda setting.

The report's shocking numbers and the recognition that errors are caused by faulty systems came from our earlier work, but the IOM report brought them to public and policy-makers attention in a way that those of us devoted to patient safety had been unable to do. Of course I was delighted. As the patient safety expert member of the

IOM committee, it fell to me to be a lead spokesperson for the IOM and an unprecedented opportunity to influence public policy.

The Annenberg Conference in 1996 brought the research and advocacy communities together for the first time to focus on patient safety, but it was the IOM report that brought it to the attention of the public and the medical profession.

The IOM report started the patient safety movement.

Postscript

Fallout from the IOM report was not all positive. Predictably, many physicians took umbrage. They were insulted by what they saw as the implication they were not doing their job properly. A number began to question the numbers. I found this particularly ironic, since none of these objections had been raised 9 years earlier when we published the MPS results. In fact, we were very disappointed at the time with the paucity of reactions!

Over the next year or two, multiple papers were published "proving" our numbers were inflated. We knew, of course, that they were underestimates (see Chap. 1). In fact, ultimately a number of later studies corroborated that, revealing adverse event rates that were 2–4 times what we found [8–11].

Several of the negative papers deserve comment. One from the VA "reanalyzed" our data (without consulting us) and claimed that most of the people who died would have died anyway [12]. Leaving aside the methodologic errors behind this conclusion, its moral repugnancy seemed to have escaped the authors: the implication that it's all right to make fatal mistakes on seriously ill patients!

A more interesting assault came from Clem McDonald and colleagues at the University of Indiana who also "reanalyzed" our data—again without consulting us—using our screening criteria as risk factors to calculate "excess mortality." [13] The fallacy of this approach was so obvious that I was surprised that JAMA would publish it. To its credit, the editor asked me to comment and put the two papers in the "Controversies" section.

I explained why screening criteria cannot be used as risk factors: Risk factors are characteristics that increase the *likelihood* of a future outcome; e.g., the presence of diabetes increases the likelihood of developing a myocardial infarct. Screening criteria are indicators of an outcome that *has already occurred*. A myocardial infarction indicates that a patient could have diabetes, but it does not prove it or cause the diabetes. Risk factors look to the future, and screening factors examine the past [14].

Sadly, their paper also looked at "excess" mortality. I rebutted this directly with the analysis from our study that 86% of the preventable deaths occurred in patients who were not terminal and for whom the error was the major factor leading to their deaths.

An interesting sidebar to this discussion was that Katie Couric of NBC's Today decided to interview the two of us on TV. I told her that I was on vacation in Vermont and could not come to New York. No problem: they sent the TV crew to us and interviewed me in our living room in Newfane, VT!

I took some delight in catching her and McDonald unawares by opening my remarks with praise for his work as a pioneer in the application of computers to medicine. My compliment was sincere: Clem had made significant contributions. The look on Katie's face was priceless. I then went on to say that in this case unfortunately he was wrong and explained the difference between risk factors and screening criteria. I don't remember what Clem said, but I came away feeling we won that one.

But the critique that hurt came from my colleague and co-author of the MPS, Troy Brennan. Troy was not enamored of my work on error, particularly disclosure. He firmly believed that it would lead to more malpractice suits. In a paper in *The New England Journal of Medicine*, he took aim at the IOM report's preventability numbers, which were derived from our study! [15] He debunked our conclusions, asserting that we had not asked about error in the MPS, which was not true [16]. Whether this was intentional or an honest mistake, I don't know. What saddened me, though, was that he never discussed it with me or gave me—his co-author on the study—an opportunity ahead of time to review his paper. I first learned about it when I read my copy of NEJM.

I spoke to the editor, Marcia Angell, about the fact that the paper included a falsehood and asked her to publish my rebuttal. She refused, suggesting instead that I submit a letter to the editor! Before doing so, I consulted with Bill Richardson, chair of the IOM committee, and we agreed that I should write the response, but it would have greater impact coming from the committee. We pointed out the error and also why our estimate of the number of preventable injuries was not an exaggeration [17].

After this flurry of debunking reports in 2000, the academic chatter quieted down, and the serious effort to make healthcare safe began. The problem was, unhappily, worse than our numbers had indicated. But the IOM report got us moving.

Appendix 9.1: Committee on Quality Of Health Care In America

William C. Richardson, Chair, President and CEO, W.K. Kellogg Foundation, Battle Creek, MI.

Donald M. Berwick, President and CEO, Institute for Healthcare Improvement, Boston, MA.

J. Cris Bisgard, Director, Health Services, Delta Air Lines, Inc., Atlanta, GA.

Lonnie R. Bristow, Past President, American Medical Association, Walnut Creek, CA.

Charles R. Buck, Program Leader, Health Care Quality and Strategy Initiatives, General Electric Company, Fairfield, CT.

Christine K. Cassel, Professor and Chairman, Department of Geriatrics and Adult Development, Mount Sinai School of Medicine, New York, NY.

Mark R. Chassin, Professor and Chairman, Department of Health Policy, Mount Sinai School of Medicine, New York, NY.

Molly Joel Coye, Senior Vice President and Director, The Lewin Group, San Francisco, CA.

Don E. Detmer, Dennis Gillings Professor of Health Management, University of Cambridge, UK.

Jerome H. Grossman, Chairman and CEO, Lion Gate Management Corporation, Boston, MA.

Brent James, Executive Director, Intermountain Health Care, Institute for Health Care Delivery Research, Salt Lake City, UT.

David McK. Lawrence, Chairman and CEO, Kaiser Foundation Health Plan, Inc., Oakland, CA.

Lucian Leape, Adj. Professor of Health Policy, Harvard School of Public Health, Boston, MA.

Arthur Levin, Director, Center for Medical Consumers, New York, NY.

Rhonda Robinson-Beale, Executive Medical Director, Managed Care Management and Clinical Programs, Blue Cross Blue Shield of Michigan, Southfield. MI.

Joseph E. Scherger, Associate Dean for Clinical Affairs, University of California, Irvine, CA.

Arthur Southam, Partner, 2C Solutions, Northridge, CA.

Mary Wakefield, Director, Center for Health Policy and Ethics, George Mason University, Washington, D.C.

Gail L. Warden, President and CEO, Henry Ford Health System, Detroit, MI.

References

1. The President's Advisory Commission on Consumer Protection and Quality in the Health Care Industry. Quality first: better health care for all Americans. 1998.
2. Chassin MR, Galvin RW. The urgent need to improve health care quality. Institute of Medicine National Roundtable on Health Care Quality [see comments]. JAMA. 1998;280:1000–5.
3. Schuster MA, McGlynn EA, Brook RH. How good is the quality of health care in the United States? Milbank Q. 1998;76:517–63.
4. Kohn KT, Corrigan JM, Donaldson MS, editors. To err is human: building a safer health system. Washington, DC: National Academy Press; 1999.
5. QuIC. Doing what counts for patient safety. Federal actions to reduce medical errors and their impact. Washington, DC: AHRQ; 2000 February.
6. Leape LL, Lawthers AG, Brennan TA, Johnson WG. Preventing medical injury. Qual Rev Bull. 1993;19:144–9.
7. Leape LL, Epstein AM, Hamel MB. A series on patient safety. NEJM. 2002;347:1272–4.
8. HHS Office of Inspector General. In: Services DoHaH, editor. Adverse events in hospitals: national incidence among Medicare beneficiaries. Washington, D.C: Department of Health and Human Services, Office of Inspector General; 2010:i-iv. p. 1–74.

9. Landrigan CP, Parry GJ, Bones CB, Hackbarth AD, Goldmann DA, Sharek PJ. Temporal trends in rates of patient harm resulting from medical care. NEJM. 2010;363:2124–34.

10. Classen DC, Resar R, Griffin F, et al. 'Global Trigger Tool' shows that adverse events in hospitals may be ten times greater than previously measured. Health Aff. 2011;30:581–9.

11. Makary MA, Daniel M. Medical error—the third leading cause of death in the US. BMJ. 2016;353:i2139.

12. Hayward RA, Hofer TP. Estimating hospital deaths due to medical errors: preventability is in the eye of the reviewer. JAMA. 2001;286:415–20.

13. McDonald CJ, Weiner M, Hui SL. Deaths due to medical errors are exaggerated in Institute of Medicine Report. JAMA. 2000;284:93–5.

14. Leape LL. Institute of Medicine Medical error figures are not exaggerated. JAMA. 2000;284:95–7.

15. Brennan TA. The Institute of Medicine report on medical errors – could it do harm? NEJM. 2000;342:1123–5.

16. Leape LL, Brennan TA, Laird NM, et al. The nature of adverse events in hospitalized patients: results from the Harvard Medical Practice Study II. New Eng J Med. 1991;324:377–84.

17. Richardson WC, Berwick DM, Bisgard JC. Correspondence: The Institute of Medicine report on medical errors. NEJM. 2000;343:663–5.

Chapter 10
The Government Responds: The Agency for Healthcare Research and Quality

When the IOM report started the patient safety movement by converting the safety interest of a few into the concern of the many, those who wished to enter this emerging field had little to work with: few measures, few proven safe practices, and few standards. For the patient safety movement to blossom in the ways envisioned by the IOM, a substantial amount of foundational work would be necessary. Only the government could provide the resources that were needed to accomplish this work.

Fortunately—amazingly, actually—the federal government was ready and willing to provide those resources, thanks to the recent work by John Eisenberg, director of the Agency for Healthcare Policy and Research (AHCPR) and his team. The Agency had been through a tough patch. Commissioned in 1989 to conduct health services research and develop practice guidelines, it did just that under it first director, Jarrett Clinton, a career PHS bureaucrat. But it lost many of its supporters in Congress in 1994 when the Republicans gained control of both the House and the Senate on a pledge to broadly reduce government: the Contract with America. The federal budget for FY 1996 became the focus of an extraordinarily contentious battle between the administration and Congress.

The Agency was caught in the crosshairs. It was linked to the failed Clinton health reform initiative, to which it had supplied data, and its effort to develop practice guidelines was unpopular with many

L. L. Leape, *Making Healthcare Safe*,
https://doi.org/10.1007/978-3-030-71123-8_10

physicians. Worse, its guidelines program had been criticized as being ineffective by the GAO, PPRC, and OTA.

The proverbial "straw" was when the Agency issued a guideline for spine surgery that concluded that there was no evidence to support spinal fusion to treat back pain. Their integrity and pocketbooks challenged, the orthopedists lobbied fiercely to curtail the agency. Enough Congressmen had had back operations or philosophically agreed that the government had no business dictating practice, that they set out to eliminate the agency by reducing its funding to zero.

The House Budget Committee under Rep. John Kasich (R-OH) made AHCPR a symbol of waste and put the agency's name on its "hit list" of 140 discretionary programs to be eliminated [1]. Rep Sam Johnson of Texas mocked it as "the Agency for High Cost Publications and Research." [2] The joint House-Senate committee conference report in June 1996 called for complete elimination of the agency's funding.

By then, Donna Shalala, secretary of Health and Human Services (HHS), had replaced Jarrett Clinton with Cliff Gaus, the highly respected former head of the Association for Health Services Research (AHSR). Gaus went on a campaign to save the Agency. He listened to insurers, hospitals, doctors, and consumers and reframed its agenda to dissemination of guidelines rather than development through a new National Guidelines Clearinghouse to coordinate private sector guidelines.

He partnered with clinical and professional leaders to create the Quality Measures Clearinghouse and enlisted the Health Insurance Association of America (HIAA), the AMA, the Association of American Medical Colleges (AAMC), and the American Association of Health Plans (AAHP) to put their lobbyists to work on Congress for support [3].

The strategy worked, although at a price. In the final appropriations bill, the agency ended up with an appropriation of $125 million, a 21 percent cut from FY 1995. The Agency was directed to stop developing practice guidelines, but it survived. By this time, Gaus had had enough. He believed it was time for a physician to direct the Agency. He recommended John Eisenberg to Shalala, noting that in addition to his superb professional qualifications, he was also her personal physician [3].

Shalala agreed. She was determined to improve quality of care and realized that patient safety could be the wedge. Interest in safety was rising as the result of our research showing the high rate of preventable harm and the efforts of the AAAS and the NPSF. She thought John was just the person to launch a new effort. And, indeed he was.

Eisenberg brought new stature and an impressive set of strengths to the job. He was a nationally known health services researcher who was chairman of the Department of Medicine and physician in chief at Georgetown University, an IOM member, and a former AHSR president. Having chaired the Physician Payment Review Commission (PPRC) for several years, he had developed trusting relationships with key staff on both sides of the aisle. As a physician he brought increased legitimacy to the agency on matters pertaining to clinical care. He was by consensus both brilliant and politically skilled [3].

For John, it was a dream job. It would enable him to leverage his knowledge and skills on the national stage—if he could get Congressional support. Shalala promised to "have his back." He set to work to rebuild the political stature of the Agency on the Hill, shoring up relationships with HHS and members of Congress on both sides of the aisle. He brought in Gregg Meyer to head up the Center for Quality Measurement and Improvement and Nancy Foster as coordinator.

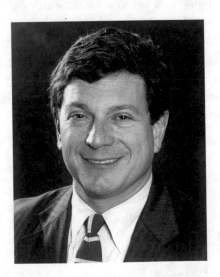

John Eisenberg. (Picture courtesy of the Agency for Healthcare Research and Quality. All rights reserved)

The battle for survival over, the stage was set for moving ahead. In early 1997, the president had established the Advisory Commission on Consumer Protection and Quality in the Health Care Industry and appointed Shalala and labor secretary Herman as co-chairs [4]. In response to its report in 1998, the president established an umbrella organization to coordinate administration efforts to improve quality: the Quality Interagency Coordination Task Force (QuIC), led by Eisenberg and co-chaired by Shalala and Herman. In addition to AHCPR, QuIC included HHS and the Departments of Labor, Veterans Affairs, Defense, and Commerce [5].

In 1998 the tide in Congress turned when Gingrich left the speakership in disgrace. Gaus' efforts had persuaded Congress of the importance of patient safety and the need for its support. The Agency was working with Congress to change its name and mission before the IOM report came out. As a result, a week later, on December 6, 1999, Congress passed the Healthcare Research and Quality Act of 1999 [6] that amended Title IX of the Public Health Service Act to replace AHCPR with the Agency for Healthcare Research and Quality (AHRQ).

Not only did this act get rid of the hated 10-year-old AHCPR, but it greatly expanded the Agency's role in patient safety, calling on it to "conduct and support research and build private-public partnerships to: 1) identify the causes of preventable health care errors and patient injury in health care delivery, 2) develop, demonstrate, and evaluate strategies for reducing errors and improving patient safety; and 3) disseminate such effective strategies throughout the health care industry." [7] It was an incredibly farsighted mandate and a remarkable boon for the cause. In retrospect, it was extraordinary that Congress would designate an agency to focus on patient safety—and fund it.

Response to the IOM Report

The IOM report in late 1999 changed everything. Within days of its release, president Clinton called on QuIC to analyze the report and make recommendations. Thanks to the amount of planning that John and his colleagues had done before the report came out, just 60 days later, in early 2000, the Task Force issued its report, *Doing What*

Counts for Patient Safety: Federal Actions to Reduce Medical Errors and their Impact, which made more than 100 recommendations for federal entities to address safety issues [8].

Doing What Counts was a blueprint for moving ahead in patient safety. Its recommendations were directed at all government departments. It called on AHRQ to take immediate action to establish the Center for Quality Improvement and Patient Safety (CQuIPS)[9] and for AHRQ, the Centers for Disease Control (CDC), the Food and Drug Administration (FDA), and VA to cooperate on research on errors, reporting systems, and applied research on patient safety. CQuIPS was called on to build a national system of errors reporting, promote the development and dissemination of evidence-based patient safety practices, and develop patient safety questions for inclusion in the patient experience survey, Consumer Assessment of Healthcare Providers and Systems (CAHPS).

The National Quality Forum (NQF) was asked to define within 12 months a set of egregious errors that are preventable and should never occur. All federal agencies providing healthcare were directed to develop systems to identify and report and learn from errors. The Health Care Financing Agency (HCFA), which paid for Medicare, was called on to promote the use of error-reduction initiatives by healthcare institutions and to require hospitals participating in the Medicare Program to implement medical error reduction programs.

The FDA was to develop standards for proprietary drug names and for packaging and labels to prevent dosing and drug mix-ups. The VA was asked to invest $47.6 million to increase patient safety training for staff, and the Department of Defense (DoD) was directed to invest $64 million in FY 2001 to implement a new computerized medical record system.

The scope was breathtaking. Healthcare had never seen anything like it.

Shalala asked Eisenberg to brief the president on the report. When he did, he found that Clinton had not only read the entire report but understood it. He asked John whether it was possible, as the IOM report challenged, for healthcare to reduce preventable deaths by 50% in 5 years. John said yes, or even in 2 years or 1 year—because hospitals would manipulate their measures to make it appear that happened.

Such a requirement would divert their attention from improvement to measures. The president saw the wisdom of his answer, publicly approved the report, and called on all federal health agencies to implement the Task Force recommendations.

Congress did its part and appropriated an additional $50 million to the Agency for patient safety research. This single act was crucial to building a cadre of researchers to perform the scientific studies needed to advance the field. It would help establish patient safety as an academic discipline with papers published in the leading journals. It did, in fact, have that effect. Within 2 years, 81 grants were awarded and 100 s of researchers were working on patient safety issues. Without this federal support, research in patient safety would have been slow in coming and spotty at best. It was a foundational initiative.

John Eisenberg was the driving force behind this reinvigorated Agency. His vision of a safer future and how to get there attracted to the Agency an exceptional group of leaders: Gregg Meyer, Carolyn Clancy, and Nancy Foster, among others, who were motivated to get these programs going. Clancy had directed the Outcomes Center at AHCPR prior to the change. They and others who worked at or with AHRQ, or were funded by it, became the first generation of people who made safety their careers. More than any other person, John Eisenberg helped establish patient safety as a science, as a practice, and as an imperative.

Tragically, John could not see the effort through. He died from a brain tumor in early 2002, just as his efforts were beginning to pay off. To honor John's memory, the NQF and The Joint Commission established the John M. Eisenberg annual awards in patient safety that recognize exceptional contributions by individuals and organizations to the advance of patient safety.

Carolyn Clancy took over as director and expanded AHRQ's activities and influence as the major force advancing patient safety. She put emphasis on working strategically with multiple stakeholders—hospitals, health plans, federal and private systems, and patients and families—to actually make changes to make healthcare safer. Patient advocates were added to the National Advisory Council. The CAHPS Hospital Survey (HCAHPS) was launched in collaboration with the Centers for Medicare and Medicaid Services (CMS). Proposals were made to link malpractice reforms with improvement in disclosure, apology, and compensation.

The breadth and depth of AHRQ activities in patient safety are awesome. In addition to funding research, it carries out evaluations of evidence, develops and standardizes safety measures and indicators, develops and maintains surveys, trains patient safety specialists, educates the profession and the public, and provides tools for healthcare organizations to improve safety.

AHRQ has played a critical role in establishing the field of patient safety. A full description of all of AHRQ's programs would require several volumes. What follows is a brief summary of its initial programs in patient safety. Much of this information comes from the AHRQ website, *ahrq.gov*, and AHRQ's 10-year report, *Advancing Patient Safety: A Decade of Evidence, Design and Implementation* [7], also on the AHRQ website.

AHRQ Programs

The Center for Quality Improvement and Patient Safety (CQuIPS)   In 1998, prior to the post-IOM reorganization, AHCPR created a center for quality improvement to bring together agencies within HHS to collaborate on improving quality of care and coordinate support for research. Eisenberg expanded this to include patient safety, renamed it, and brought in Gregg Meyer to organize it. Meyer hired Jim Battles to run the research grants program.

CQuIPS supports investigator-initiated research on patient safety, measurement, and reporting. It "develops and disseminates reports and information on health care quality measurement, reporting, and improvement, collaborates with stakeholders … to implement evidence-based practices, accelerating and amplifying improvements in quality and safety for patients." [9] CQuIPS is also responsible for CAHPS and WebM&M (see below). The Center has been the clearly identifiable part of government devoted to patient safety.

Consumer Assessment of Healthcare Providers and Systems (CAHPS)   This survey initiative began in 1995, before the Agency became involved in patient safety, in response to the recognition that quality of care issues that are important to consumers, such as communication skills of providers and ease of access to healthcare, were often overlooked. The obvious way to find out about them was to ask patients. The Agency began to fund, oversee, and work closely with a consortium of research organizations to conduct research on patient experience and develop the survey.

The survey has since been expanded to ask patients to evaluate their experiences with health plans, providers, and healthcare facilities regarding care coordination, shared decision-making, and patient engagement. The survey is now widely used by healthcare organizations, health plans, purchasers, consumer groups, and accreditation organizations to evaluate providers and improve quality and safety of care. It has been a major factor in teaching clinicians and hospitals to be more aware of patient's concerns and to engage them more meaningfully in their care. It has magnified their voice.

Patient Safety Indicators (PSI)   What everyone wants—CMS, policy-makers, hospitals, and the public—is an *overall* measure of safety. How bad is it? Are we getting better? But there was no such measure, nor even a set of standardized measures that the nation or a healthcare organization could use to identify its safety problems. However, CMS and other payers required hospitals to use ICD-9 billing codes for specific harmful events, such as infections, pressure ulcers, surgical complications, falls, CLABSI rates, etc. Why couldn't hospitals use this "administrative" data to assess and improve their performance?

Under Gregg Meyer's direction, AHRQ created a list of 20 patient safety indicators using billing codes. To develop an overall score, they calculated a weight for each based on national data on risk, reliability of the measure, and extent of harm. The hospital could monitor the rate of each indicator, multiply it by its weight, and sum the values to get an overall measure of safety in the institution. While incomplete—all safety risks were not measured—it was better than nothing and would help hospitals know where to focus their safety efforts.

When the PSIs were released in 2001, AHRQ made it clear that the indicators were designed only for hospitals' internal use for improvement: to "provide information on potentially avoidable safety events …that can be used to help hospitals assess the incidence of adverse events and identify issues that might need further study." [7]

It was not to be. Despite these caveats, CMS and other payers began to use them not only to assess hospitals performance, but to reduce payments if they were deficient. Suddenly PSIs were viewed not as tools for improvement, but as instruments of punishment—a complete inversion of what we were trying to do in patient safety.

The patient safety community was appalled. Hospitals quickly directed their efforts away from improvement to coding of claims, "gaming" the data to minimize penalties. This was exactly what Eisenberg had told the president would happen if hospitals were required to reduce preventable mortality by 50% in 5 years. In the end PSIs may have done more harm than good over the years. Meyer agrees. He considers them "the worst thing I ever did" at AHRQ.

Evidence-Based Practices   Even in these early days, there were a number of established safe practices available. Which should healthcare organizations use? Which safe practices were effective? The newly established standard setter, the National Quality Forum, needed to know, so it turned to AHRQ. The Agency commissioned an Evidence-Based Practices group at the University of California at San Francisco (UCSF), led by Bob Wachter and Kaveh Shojania, to review the evidence and report in 6 months.

Many of us were looking forward to the report, so when it appeared, it was a shocker to find that only a small number of practices were found to have evidence of effectiveness, and most of those with the highest ratings were rarely used or fairly esoteric. These practices received high marks because someone had done a randomized controlled trial (RCT) of their effectiveness. Most of the safe practices in widespread use were not on the list because they had not been subjected to RCTs. The UCSF group had done what they were asked to do: follow the evidence. However, the evidence came from studies that individuals did because of their interest in a specific practice, not because it prevented many errors or was in widespread use [10].

David Bates, Don Berwick, and I were concerned that this would send the wrong message that practices without evidence should be abandoned, so we crafted a critique that was published in JAMA: *What practices will most improve safety? Evidence-based medicine meets patient safety* [11]. JAMA published it together with the authors rebuttal: *Safe but sound: patient safety meets evidence-based medicine* [12] as part of a point-counterpoint analysis to help readers understand the types of evidence needed to support use of a new practice.

Our major point was that the many accepted safe practices in current use should not be abandoned just because they had never been subjected to a controlled trial, as required in the review. (The standing joke about RCTs is that no one had ever done a randomized trial of the effectiveness of parachutes!) Handwashing, read-back, site marking, and unit dosing, for example, were practices without evidence that were clearly of value and should not be abandoned.

The paper was written both to reassure those working on the "front lines" of safety in hospitals and to serve as a resource for the NQF Safe Practices Steering Committee. It seems to have been of some value to both. The Safe Practices criteria were expanded to include experiential evidence of effectiveness. The final NQF list included 34 approved safe practices [13].

WebM&M To engage and inform physicians, AHRQ initiated WebM&M, using the familiar format of mortality and morbidity rounds to make available analysis of real-world medical error cases by experts, monthly. Edited by Bob Wachter, founder of the hospitalist specialty and later chair of the American Board of Internal Medicine, about a third of the cases are also developed as Spotlight Cases that are interactive learning modules for CME. This has proven to be one of the agencies most popular offerings.

Survey on Patient Safety Culture (SOPS) To support the development of a culture of patient safety, AHRQ sponsored the development of patient safety culture assessment tools for hospitals, nursing homes, ambulatory outpatient medical offices, community pharmacies, and ambulatory surgery centers. These surveys enable healthcare organizations to assess staff perceptions of various aspects of patient safety culture. They have played an important role in creating a culture of safety.

National Healthcare Quality and Disparities Report To justify funding, Congress wants to see results. Part of its 1999 mandate was

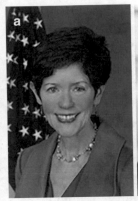
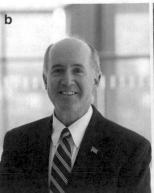
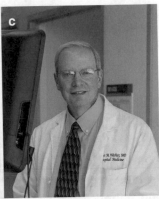

(a) Carolyn Clancy, (b) Gregg Meyer, and (c) Bob Wachter.

that AHRQ produce annual reports on healthcare quality and disparities. The quality reports present trends for access to care, affordable care, care coordination, effective treatment, healthy living, patient safety, and person-centered care. The disparities report provides comparative information according to race and ethnicity, income, and social determinants of health. These reports have helped keep patient safety on the agenda and motivate other agencies to work on safety.

Education and Training AHRQ has developed educational programs for practitioners in several areas. *TeamSTEPPS®* is a training program based on an evidence-based set of ready-to-use materials and curriculum to improve teamwork in healthcare organizations by teaching communication and teamwork skills. The *Patient Safety Improvement Corps (PSIC)* is a partnership with the Department of Veterans Affairs to train midlevel professionals in investigation of medical errors and initiating improvements.

Advancing Pharmacy Health Literacy Practices Through Quality Improvement is a set of modules to help pharmacy faculty integrate health literacy and health literacy quality improvement into the education of pharmacy students and residents.

Central line-associated bloodstream infections (CLABSI) were a serious cause of preventable injury and death. *CLABSI Tools* help care units implement evidence-based practices to eliminate central line-associated bloodstream infections. The *Comprehensive Unit-based*

Safety Program (CUSP) toolkit developed by Peter Pronovost's team includes training tools to make care safer by improving the foundation of how physicians, nurses, and other clinical team members work together [14].

Several of these education and training programs have had substantial impact. CLABSI Tools were used with the CUSP toolkit in a highly successful nationwide initiative led by Pronovost that dramatically reduced CLABSI rates in more than 1000 hospitals across the country [15]. The Patient Safety Improvement Corps (PSIC) has trained teams in every state and has been a major force in disseminating patient safety knowledge throughout the country. TeamSTEPPS has trained 1000 master trainers who in turn train colleagues at their organizations. Almost every hospital now has a patient safety officer; many were trained in this program.

Patient Education   AHRQ has published a number of guides for consumers, such as guides for what to do after leaving the hospital, use of blood thinners, diagnosis and treatment, and questions to ask your doctor.

Health Information Technology   Suddenly, after only 3 years of supporting the full range of patient safety research, in 2003 Congress directed that AHRQ's $50 million annual research funding be devoted to research in information technology. This was a shock because the unrestricted funding had been a powerful incentive for developing new knowledge and attracting new investigators to the field. Research is the coin of the realm in academia, and research gave our new field academic respectability. Our researchers' papers were being published and they were being promoted.

But the need for support of health IT was clear. Hospitals and doctors were being required to implement electronic health records (EHRs) and were having serious problems. The funding resulted in hundreds of projects related to all aspects of implementation of health IT, and the staff made sure other projects were funded as well. In 2004, AHRQ provided $139 million for more than 100 multi-year demonstration grants and contracts to promote the use of health information technology.

Patient Safety Network   To enable healthcare providers and researchers, as well as administrators and patients, to keep up with and easily access the increasing "firehose" of data and patient safety information, AHRQ created a website, psnet.ahrq.gov, with the latest news, research, legislation, and tools for patient safety.

Healthcare-Associated Infections Network   In 2008 Congress directed AHRQ to work with CDC and CMS to develop an action plan to reduce hospital-acquired infections (HAI). Several nonprofit organizations joined what became a major national effort and one of the most successful patient safety campaigns. The reductions in HAI as a result of this program account for a significant share of safety improvement over the past 10 years.

Patient Safety Organizations   From the beginning of the patient safety movement, one of the goals has been to develop national or regional reporting systems so hospitals could share medical error information and learn from each other's mistakes. The IOM called for development of these voluntary systems, but it didn't happen, in part because of hospitals' fear that the information would be legally discoverable and used to sue hospitals and doctors for malpractice.

To eliminate this liability and facilitate sharing of patient error data among hospitals, in 2005 Congress established Patient Safety Organizations (PSOs). Medical error information reported to PSO confidentially is protected from legal discovery. AHRQ also coordinated the development of common definitions and reporting formats to standardize data collection. Since the law was passed, a number of PSOs have developed across the country. Their effectiveness varies, but some have been useful vehicles for sharing lessons learned.

Impact of AHRQ Programs

As is obvious from the above, AHRQ has played an immense role in the development of all aspects of patient safety. It has given substance to "it's not bad people, it's bad systems"—in research, in practice, and in policy. It has been the main funder of patient safety research. It was the prime mover developing a cadre of patient safety researchers and training hundreds of patient safety officers.

It furthered the development of measures and set standards for their use. It developed key surveys and large databases that provide the information upon which public policy and private improvement depend. It motivated other federal agencies, such as CMS and CDC, to become major players supporting patient safety.

To evaluate its national patient safety initiative in September 2002, AHRQ entered into a 4-year contract with the RAND Corporation. In 2005 RAND published the first report [16]. It complimented the agency on "an impressive job in starting the patient safety initiative" that balanced research and translational and practice improvements. It specifically commended AHRQ for its work in support of epidemiology research, development of effective practices and tools, building infrastructure, and achieving broader adoption of effective practices.

Given its crucial role—and incredible success—it is disturbing and puzzling that funding for AHRQ has always been somewhat precarious. The support for research has never been adequate: large numbers of excellent proposals go unfunded each year. The sudden shift of research funding to IT mandated by Congress in the early years has been followed periodically by other requirements to target its efforts to areas of Congressional interest at the time.

As Gray observed, AHRQ's political problems are three-dimensional. Congress is willing to support basic research, as it does with NIH, only if it believes the long-term result will be new ways of preventing or treating disease. AHRQ's results so far have apparently not been sufficiently convincing. Second, when the Agency produces work that affects healthcare practice or policy, it attracts enemies who are vested in the status quo (recall the orthopedists and spine surgery). Third, the agency's work is significant to many parties: policy-makers, decision-makers (providers, purchasers, patients), and researchers. They understandably have competing ideas about how the agency's limited resources should be spent [3].

Thus, despite appeals from many health policy experts over the years to "billionize" the Agency, annual funding has remained in the $300–500 million range. Funding was gradually increased during the Obama years but then cut back by the current administration, which also discontinued several programs.

To health policy experts, it seems obvious that AHRQ should become an institute as part of NIH, with annual funding at $1–2 billion level, which is less than that currently provided for several institutes for conditions that affect far fewer people and cause far fewer deaths. Surely, it is as important to fund research on *how* we deliver care as it is to fund research on *what* care we deliver. NIH has always enjoyed broad bipartisan and public support. If there were a National Institute for Quality and Safety, funding for patient safety would be adequate and secure. A reasonable hope.

References

1. U.S. House Committee on the Budget. Discretionary spending and control act of 1995. Washington, D.C: U.S. G.P.O; 1995. p. 1–64.
2. Sequential votes postponed in committee of the whole. Washington, D.C. Congressional Record; 1995. H8413.
3. Gray BH, Gusmano MK, Collins SR. AHCPR and the changing politics of health services research. Health Affairs. 2003;22:W3–283–307.
4. President clinton announces advisory commission on consumer protection and quality in the health care industry. Washington, D.C.: The White House Office of the Press Secretary; 1997.
5. Clinton WJ. Memorandum on establishment of the quality interagency coordination task force. Washington, D.C: The White House Office of the Press Secretary; 1998.
6. 113 Stat. 1653 – Healthcare Research and Quality Act of 1999. S580, Public Law 106–129. Washington, D.C.: U.S. Government Printing Office; 1999:1653–1676.
7. Agency of Healthcare Research and Quality. Advancing patient safety: a decade of evidence, design and implementation 2009 November 2009.
8. Quality Interagency Coordination Task Force. Doing what counts for patient safety: federal actions to reduce medical errors and their impact 2000 February 2000.
9. Center for Quality Improvement and Patient Safety (CQuIPS). Agency for healthcare research and quality, 2012 at https://www.ahrq.gov/cpi/centers/cquips/index.html.
10. Shojania K, Duncan B, McDonald K, Markowitz A, editors. Making health care safer: a critical analysis of patient safety practices. Rockville: Agency for Healthcare Research and Quality; 2001.
11. Leape LL, Berwick DM, Bates DW. What practices will most improve safety? Evidence-based medicine meets patient safety. JAMA. 2002;288:501–7.

12. Shojania KG, Duncan BW, McDonald KM, Wachter RM. Safe but sound: patient safety meets evidence-based medicine. JAMA. 2002;288:508–13.
13. National Quality Forum. Safe practices for better health care: a consensus report. Washington, DC: NQF; 2003. Report No.: NQFCR-05-03.
14. Pronovost PJ, Marsteller JA, Goeschel CA. Preventing bloodstream infections: a measurable national success story in quality improvement. Health Aff. 2011;30:628–34.
15. Eliminating CLABSI, A national patient safety imperative. Final Report on the National on the CUSP: Stop BSI Project. Agency for Healthcare Research and Quality; October 2012.
16. Farley DO, Morton SC, Damberg CL, et al. Assessment of the national patient safety initiative: context and baseline evaluation report I. RAND Health: Santa Monica; 2005.

Chapter 11
Setting Standards: The National Quality Forum

When AHRQ assumed the responsibility from the Quality Interagency Coordination Task Force (QuIC) report, *Doing What Counts for Patient Safety,* to develop practice changes to reduce harm from medical errors, it faced two problems: there were few proven safe practices, and there was a dearth of standards by which to evaluate them. A standard setter was needed.

Fortuitously, a year earlier, the Advisory Commission on Consumer Protection and Quality in the Health Care Industry had recommended an independent organization be created to standardize performance measures in healthcare by means of a public-private partnership. Under vice president Gore's direction, QuIC advanced the idea of a national standard setter and took steps to establish the National Forum for Health Care Quality Measurement and Reporting, later renamed the "National Quality Forum" (NQF), "a broad-based, widely representative private body that establishes standard quality measurement tools to help all purchasers, providers, and consumers of healthcare better evaluate and ensure the delivery of quality services." [1]

The fledgling National Quality Forum flourished under the leadership of Kenneth W. Kizer, once described by Don Berwick as "…probably the most effective leader in all of American healthcare." Kizer was superbly well-equipped for the task. He was board certified in six medical specialties and had demonstrated his executive skills in several important prior positions. An emergency physician who engineered the statewide EMS system in California and a former US Navy

© The Author(s) 2021
L. L. Leape, *Making Healthcare Safe,*
https://doi.org/10.1007/978-3-030-71123-8_11

diver and diving medical officer, Kizer well understood systems and systems thinking. As an active outdoor sports enthusiast and founding member of the international Wilderness Medical Society, he also had a deep appreciation for safety and planning for the unexpected.

Earlier in his career, as director of the California Department of Health Services and the state's top health official, Kizer orchestrated California's response to the new HIV/AIDS epidemic, led a cigarette tax increase and smoking cessation program that reduced the rate of smoking in California three times faster than the rest of the nation, and pioneered Medicaid-managed care. In 1994, president Clinton appointed him undersecretary for health in the Department of Veterans Affairs (VA) and chief executive officer of the VA healthcare system.

During his 5-year tenure at the helm of the VA healthcare system, Kizer radically transformed it, changing it from a hospital system to a truly integrated healthcare system that was rooted in primary care. He closed hospitals, reduced the total number of acute care hospital beds by some 55% (more than 29,000 beds), opened 300 new community-based outpatient clinics, and hired the first healthcare system chief telehealth officer in the country. All well before the "medical home" concept had taken hold in the rest of healthcare.

He reorganized the whole VA healthcare system into 22 new regional "Veterans Integrated Service Networks" (VISNs) that typically consisted of 8–9 hospitals, 25–30 community-based outpatient clinics, 5–7 long-term care facilities, 10–15 counseling centers, and 1 or 2 residential care facilities. Leaders of hospitals and clinics were proximately responsible to the network chiefs for providing quality care [2–4].

Kizer implemented multiple quality improvement changes that led to decreased death rates, a medication bar code system to check dose timings and reduce prescription errors, and a national formulary that resulted in savings of some $600 million annually. Customer service standards were implemented, and patient satisfaction surveys showed a growing percentage of veterans rated their quality of care as very good to excellent.

As a result of quality assurance measures, illness and death rates from high-volume surgical procedures declined. An observational study published in *The New England Journal of Medicine* found that the VA outscored Medicare's fee for service program for the quality of

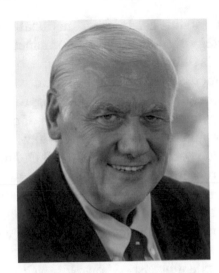

Ken Kizer. (All rights reserved)

preventive, acute, and chronic care [5]. All while the number of veterans served increased by 28% in 4 years.

Despite these truly astonishing improvements in the quality and access to care for veterans that Kizer accomplished in an amazingly short time, political opposition developed, largely as the result of his hospital closings and downsizing. Congressional hearings for his reappointment were repeatedly delayed, although the Congress passed specific legislation extending his tenure at the end of his first term. Finally, after continuing political drama, Kizer had had enough, and motivated in large part by his wife's serious and deteriorating health problems, he decided to leave VA.

After he resigned, *BusinessWeek* reported that the Veterans Affairs system provided "the best medical care in the US." [6] It was a remarkable transformation of a healthcare system that previously had often been regarded with distain by doctors and laymen alike. The *Harvard Business Review* characterized Kizer's work at VA as the largest and most successful healthcare turnaround in US history.

But the Clinton administration was not about to let Kizer go. Vice president Gore's office reached out to Kizer about leading the creation of a new organization that would become the NQF. It would be an independent, consensus-based, financially sustainable organization having equal representation from healthcare's many and diverse stakeholders that would establish a national healthcare quality improvement strategy that included performance measures to track progress toward achieving the strategy.

This was a momentous step. Thanks to the work of Berwick and others, people in healthcare were beginning to talk about quality improvement and patient safety, but standards of care and valid methods for measuring quality and safety were few. Moreover, as later noted by Kizer, "The concept of the National Quality Forum arose in response to the strong American sentiment against government regulation and control of health care quality.... The (Advisory) commission envisioned that...the NQF would devise a national strategy for measuring and reporting health care quality that would advance the identified national aims." [1]

Not everyone was enthusiastic, however. NCQA perceived it as a possible direct threat to what it had been doing for years and its business model. The Joint Commission also had reservations, although they later came around. Kizer recalls that Gail Warden, the inaugural chairman of the NQF board, wondered if the organization would last even 3 years.

The National Forum for Health Care Quality Measurement and Reporting was officially launched on September 1, 1999, with start-up funding from the Robert Wood Johnson Foundation, the California Health Care Foundation, the Horace W. Goldsmith Foundation, and the Commonwealth Fund.

Kizer saw the mission of the Forum as "to improve health care quality; that is, to promote delivery of care known to be effective; to achieve better health outcomes, greater patient functionality, and a higher level of patient safety; and to make health care easier to access and a more satisfying experience. The primary strategy...to accomplish this mission is to standardize the means by which health care quality is measured and reported and to make health care quality data widely available." [1]

Kizer set the context for this enterprise by noting "This strategy is premised on the philosophy that health care quality data are a public good and, therefore, health care quality measurements should be publicly disclosed. It is further based on the belief that making reliable, comparative data on health care quality publicly available will motivate providers to improve the quality of care by providing benchmarks; will facilitate competition on the basis of quality; will promote consumer choice on the basis of quality; and will inform public policy." [1]

Five key strategic goals were initially identified: (1) developing and implementing a national agenda for measuring and reporting healthcare quality, (2) standardizing the measures used to report healthcare quality so that data collection is less arduous for healthcare providers and so that the reported data are of greater value, (3) building consumer competence for making choices based on quality of care data, (4) enhancing the capability of healthcare providers to use quality-related data, and (5) increasing the overall demand for healthcare quality data [1].

From the outset, it has been NQF policy that the organization itself does not develop or test performance measures, but instead uses a multistep consensus process to vet measures created by public and private entities, including, among others, NCQA, CMS, Physician Consortium for Performance Improvement, and medical specialty associations.

NQF endorses only those measures that meet the following criteria: [1] importance to measure and report; [2] scientific acceptability of measure properties, i.e., produces reliable and valid results; [3] feasibility, i.e., require data that are readily available and create as little burden as possible; [4] usability and use, the extent to which they can be used for both accountability and performance improvement; and [5] comparison to related and competing measures to harmonize them or select the best measure [7].

NQF was to be different from any other organization, public or private, in several ways. Indeed, it was broadly viewed as a truly novel experiment in democracy. Membership was open to anyone, organization or individual. Board membership represented a broad and diverse group of stakeholders, including federal agencies (e.g., CMS and AHRQ), state agencies, professional associations (e.g., AHA and AMA), private healthcare purchasers (e.g., GM), labor unions (e.g., AFL-CIO), and consumer groups (e.g., AARP).

Kizer saw the mission of the NQF as blending and balancing consumer, purchaser, payer, and provider perspectives. All Board members had an equal vote. Multiple professional associations initially strongly objected to their vote having the same weight as consumer or purchaser organizations, but Kizer would not budge on this position. The Board's decisions resulted from a consensus process derived from the National Technology Transfer and Advancement Act (NTTAA) and principles formally espoused by the Office of Management and Budget in OMB Circular A-119. [23] A specially convened Strategic Framework Board of experts supported the NQF's nascent efforts by providing an intellectual architecture and principles to help guide measurement and reporting [8].

Kizer believed that ensuring patient safety should be the foundation of healthcare quality. He decided to take advantage of the contemporary surge of interest in patient safety by having the inaugural NQF effort focus on a safety issue: the reporting of serious harmful events. Bolstered by a formal charge from CMS and AHRQ, he asked me and John Colmer, the program officer for the Milbank Fund (which was funding the project), to co-chair a Serious Reportable Events Steering Committee to develop a core set of serious preventable adverse events to enable standardized data collection and reporting nationwide. The primary reason for identifying these measures was to facilitate public accountability through national mandatory reporting of these adverse events—an idea that president Clinton's administration was open to, but which was summarily rejected by the subsequent Bush administration.

Serious Reportable Events

The first charge to the Steering Committee was to develop a definition of "serious, avoidable adverse events." We were then to apply a consensus process to develop a set of these events. The final set would be voted on by the then 110 NQF member organizations and the Board of Directors. If approved, it would then be issued as a nationwide recommendation. In addition, we were to identify potential candidates for additional measures that needed more research, discuss issues relating to implementation, and develop a plan for dissemination of the measures.

The Steering Committee was composed of representatives from a cross section of healthcare providers, experts in quality and safety, public interest groups, regulators, and others. Broad representation of stakeholders was to be a cardinal principle of operation for the NQF, so a serious attempt was made to make sure all stakeholder sectors were well represented for this first effort. (Appendix 11.1)

I could see several pitfalls ahead. Following the release of the IOM report, *To Err Is Human*, the most common reaction from the public and the press was to call for required reporting of adverse events. Many people seemed to think that if people just knew about them, they would be taken care of. Doctors and others would be shamed into doing something. Those of us working in safety knew there was much more to it than that. Reporting does not automatically or necessarily lead to change.

Safety experts and policy-makers identify two kinds of reporting: reporting for improvement and reporting for accountability.

Reporting systems for improvement are voluntary and based on frontline caregivers' desire to prevent harm. As Charles Billings, architect of the aviation safety reporting system, has noted, voluntary reporting only works when it is *safe* (does not result in punishment), *simple* (the act of reporting only takes a few minutes), and *productive* (reporting results in positive changes) [9].

Creating a safe environment for reporting within hospitals has long been challenging. Despite national campaigns, 20 years after the IOM report, nearly half of nurses surveyed say they do not feel safe talking about errors. On the other hand, outside the hospital, national voluntary systems, such as those run by specialty societies, ISMP, and the National Nosocomial Infection Survey, rely on reports from caregivers and have been quite successful.

Reporting systems for accountability rely on reports from *institutions*—in healthcare, primarily hospitals—and are mandatory. They are based on the concept that hospitals have a duty to prevent serious harm that we know how to prevent, such as amputation of the wrong leg or giving a blood transfusion to the wrong person. These events result from major system breakdowns, and it is the institution, not individual caregivers, that is in charge of the systems.

The public expects healthcare providers to ensure that care is safe, and it looks to the government to make sure that providers take the actions necessary to make care safe. The occurrence of a serious preventable adverse event suggests that a flaw exists in the healthcare organization's efforts to safeguard patients. It is reasonable for the public to expect an oversight body to investigate such occurrences.

These serious reportable events are healthcare's equivalent of airplane or other public-transportation crashes. And most people think the public has a right to know about them when they occur [10]. If so, then not only reporting, but making the reports public should be mandatory.

Reporting is of little value if it doesn't lead to improvement. The healthcare organization must also be required to investigate the event to determine the underlying system problems and/or failures (i.e., root cause analysis) and then correct the failures to prevent recurrence of the event. This information should be disseminated to other healthcare organizations so all can benefit from the lessons learned.

In the USA, the only mandatory systems for reporting of serious events are those run by the states. However, in 1999 only 15 states had such programs, and these varied considerably in what hospitals were required to report and what happened when they did. In most cases, nothing happened: no analysis and no feedback to the hospital—and no reporting of results to the public. The programs were typically understaffed, underfunded, and ineffective [10]. Perhaps providing a nationally accepted, industry-endorsed list of serious preventable adverse events would be an incentive for improvement.

My personal feeling was that it was important to focus on clearly defined adverse events, not on errors or vague things like "loss of function," which appeared in some systems. I argued for events that were simple to define and "unfudgeable," i.e., not susceptible to interpretation or debate about whether it is or is not reportable. At the time, hospitals routinely gamed the system, going to great lengths to "prove" that an event was not preventable and therefore didn't need to be reported. However, if certain events were by definition preventable, perhaps this charade could be curtailed.

The Steering Committee met for the first time on December 20, 2000. We defined "serious, avoidable adverse events" as patient harms that hospitals can reasonably be expected to prevent 100% of the time. We had interesting, thoughtful, and sometimes spirited discussions about the purpose of the list, preventive strategies, priorities, verifiability of reporting, and specificity of events. I suggested we eliminate "unanticipated" as being too difficult to define and too easy to weasel. More easily than I had expected, we agreed on the definitions of an adverse event and a serious event, as well as the criteria for inclusion on the list. We did a first pass, discussing a list of 25 candidates for inclusion that the NQF staff had prepared.

Mandatory reporting is a contentious issue. Many have strong feelings about the public's right to know when these events occur, while hospitals are afraid of liability and loss of reputation from going public with a mistake. Although some hospitals had gone public and found their honesty led people to trust them more, most still did not believe in this degree of transparency.

At the Steering Committee's second meeting in February 2001, Kizer announced a special advisory panel of state health professionals to help us ensure our list would be relevant. We agreed on four criteria for selection of events for the list: events must be (1) serious, (2) clearly definable, (3) usually preventable, and (4) quantifiable (i.e., capable of being easily audited). In other words, they should be events that are serious and obvious to all observers when they occur (the "unfudgeable" part).

In April we approved the final report. However, the group did not agree with Ken's interest in calling them "never events," undoubtedly rooted in the firmly held doctrine in medicine that you cannot say that anything "never" happens. So it was decided that the list should be officially titled "Serious Reportable Events." Nevertheless, they quickly began to be referred to as "never events."

In the final version, 27 items were grouped into 6 categories: (1) surgical events (e.g., wrong site, retained foreign body), (2) device or product events (contamination, malfunction), (3) patient protection events (suicide, infant discharged to wrong person), (4) care management events (death or disability from medication error, blood mismatch, kernicterus), (5) environmental events (death or severe disability from electric shock, burn, falls, restraints), and (6) criminal events (sexual assault, impersonation) [11]. The full list is shown in Appendix 11.2. In 3 subsequent updates, the list has been expanded to 29 events.

The Committee's report was readily approved by the NQF Board, with only the American Hospital Association and one state hospital association voting against the report's adoption, and it was published a few months later in early 2002. It was generally well received by the press and the public. It did, in fact, become the model for some state reporting systems. Later, CMS used the list to deny payments for

Medicare patients. This was not our intended use, and the matter was vigorously debated and discouraged during the Committee's deliberations. However, I personally felt it had merit. The best way to get hospitals' attention is to hit them in the pocketbook.

All in all, this was an interesting and important initiative. We established important definitions and expectations. Within 2 years, the number of states with mandatory reporting of serious events increased to 20, and by 2010, 27 states and the District of Columbia had enacted mandatory reporting systems, incorporating all or part of NQF's list.

Safe Practices for Better Healthcare

The reporting initiative got national attention and started the NQF on the way to Kizer's goal of it becoming "the" trusted and respected national standard-setting organization. He then took on the second QuIC challenge, to "identify a set of patient safety practices critical to prevention of medical errors." This initiative was more ambitious than the reporting project and destined to have far greater impact. It was to be a list and description of evidence-based and standardized care processes that promote safety and reduce patient harm. The objective was to stimulate healthcare organizations to adopt a systems approach by providing effective processes that could be used "off the shelf," saving the care team the effort of developing their own new practices and systems de novo.

To begin the initiative, NQF asked AHRQ to commission an independent review of the evidence behind safe practices. As described in the previous chapter on AHRQ, this effort was led by Kaveh Shojania and Bob Wachter of UCSF [12]. But they found only 11 practices that met its criteria! As noted in the previous chapter. David Bates, Don Berwick, and I were concerned that the many accepted safe practices in current use would be suspect just because they had never been subjected to a controlled trial. Our paper and a rebuttal by the authors were published in JAMA as part of a point-counterpoint analysis [13, 14]. The Safe Practices Committee expanded its criteria to include experiential evidence of effectiveness.

Other sources of candidate practices were the Leapfrog Group, NQF member organizations, Steering Committee members themselves, and an open call for candidate practices to more than 100 medical, nursing, and pharmacy specialty societies.

The final criteria for inclusion as a safe practice were:

1. Specificity. The practice must be a clearly and precisely defined process or manner of providing a healthcare service.
2. Benefit. Use of the practice will save lives endangered by healthcare delivery, reduce disability or other morbidity, or reduce the likelihood of a serious reportable event.
3. Evidence of Effectiveness. There must be clear evidence that the practice would be effective in reducing patient safety events. This includes not just research studies, but broad expert agreement or professional consensus that the practice is "obviously beneficial" as well as experience from nonhealthcare industries transferable to healthcare (e.g., repeat-back of verbal orders or standardizing abbreviations).
4. Generalizability. The safe practice must be able to be utilized in a variety of inpatient and/or outpatient settings and/or for multiple types of patients.
5. Readiness. The necessary technology and appropriately skilled staff must be available to most healthcare organizations [15].

The practices were organized into five broad categories for improving patient safety: (1) creates a culture of safety, (2) matches healthcare needs with service-delivery capabilities, (3) facilitates information transfer and clear communication, (4) adopts safe practices in specific clinical settings or for specific processes of care, and (5) increases safe medication use.

The final list of 30 practices included both those with research evidence of effectiveness and those that were already in wide use and well accepted. Some examples of the latter practices included the following: staffing of ICUs with critical care specialists (intensivists); "read-back" of orders; prohibited abbreviations; medication reconciliation; hand hygiene; unit dosing; adoption of computerized patient order entry; the universal protocol for preventing wrong site, procedure, and patient for all invasive procedures; and protocols for prevention of central line-associated bloodstream infections (CLABSI), surgical site infections, MRSA, and catheter-associated urinary tract infections [15]. (For the full list, see Appendix 11.3.) The list was formally approved by the NQF Board in late 2002.

In April 2004, the Leapfrog Group adopted the full list of safe practices as their fourth safety "leap." (Three of the safe practices were based on its first three safety leaps.) Also in 2004 several purchaser coalitions (e.g., Pacific Business Group on Health, The Employer Alliance Health Care Cooperative, Midwest Business Group on Health, among others) endorsed the safe practices.

Individual hospital adoption of the safe practices has varied greatly. Although now widely accepted as the standard toward which to strive, they are not easy to implement. (See Chapters 6 and 8.) Success requires strong support at the executive level, education and training of personnel, a "champion," and teamwork. Physician buy-in is critical. Outside pressure, as from The Joint Commission, has helped.

NQF has periodically updated the safe practices in response to the development of new practices as patient safety matured. In the first update, in 2006, safe practices were added that addressed leadership and staffing, and the practices were harmonized with safety initiatives from other national groups such as the CMS, AHRQ, and The Joint Commission. In 2009, practices were added to address pediatric imaging, organ donation, caring for caregivers, glycemic control, and prevention of falls.

Performance Measures

While the serious reportable events and safe practices were highly visible projects, multiple other projects were concomitantly undertaken by NQF during its formative years. For example, performance measures were endorsed for, among other things, adult diabetes care, home healthcare, cardiac surgery, child healthcare, medication safety, hospital care, substance use disorders, and nursing care.

Likewise, a consensus framework for hospital care performance evaluation was developed, approved by the Board, and published, as were position papers or guidance documents on the role of hospital governing boards in promoting quality care, health information technology and electronic health records, health literacy, pay for performance, and improving healthcare quality for minority populations.

The NQF also closely worked with the eHealth Initiative, CMS, AHRQ, and other groups to facilitate the adoption of health information technology and new payment models that supported quality improvement. Kizer strongly lobbied HHS secretary Tommy Thompson to promote the adoption of electronic health records, and he worked closely with CMS administrator Scully to promote adoption of public reporting of performance measurement data.

Throughout this time, a problem that plagued the NQF's efforts was the lack of stable financing and especially not having funds to undertake projects that were "for the public good"—i.e., projects that were not linked to a specific healthcare constituency and its interests. Kizer spent a large amount of time finding and cobbling together funds to finance the many projects that NQF undertook in these early years.

New Leadership

At the end of 2005, Kizer stepped down, and Janet Corrigan took over as president of the National Quality Forum. Corrigan was ideally suited to the role. An expert in health policy and management, she was highly respected for leading the staff at the Institute of Medicine that produced the legendary *To Err Is Human*. But most notably, Corrigan was the executive director of president Clinton's Advisory Commission on Consumer Protection and Quality, which recommended the creation of NQF.

Corrigan faced several challenges. Despite generous support from several foundations, the financial situation was precarious. Other reliable sources were needed. In addition, the endorsement process had become unruly. It needed to be put on more rigorous scientific foundation. It needed to continue expanding the membership base, but more importantly it needs expanded public support. Corrigan brought in Helen Burstin from AHRQ to straighten it out.

Corrigan envisioned new opportunities for NQF. She believed that the NQF would be more effective if it focused more on measures needed to achieve national safety and quality goals. But what were the national priorities; what were the goals? And who set them? Well, it wasn't clear. AHRQ had its priorities, as did CMS, IHI, and others, but there was no uniformity, no consistency, and no single voice.

With support from the Robert Wood Johnson Foundation, in 2007 Corrigan persuaded HHS to ask NQF to establish the National Priorities Partnership (NPP) to provide input to the secretary for consideration as it developed priorities. Under the leadership of Helen Burstin, NPP was developed as a public-private partnership of 51 partner organizations that represent the diverse perspectives of consumers, purchasers, healthcare providers and professionals, community alliances, health plans, accreditation and certification bodies, and government agencies. NPP identified six national priorities that were embraced by many national organizations and health systems.

As the debate around health reform heated up in 2009, NQF helped organize a coalition of quality leaders known as Stand for Quality to encourage legislators to provide stable and adequate support for the core measure activities recognizing that they are fundamental building blocks for virtually all approaches to payment and delivery system reform and for recognition of the important role of having a public-private partnership to carry out this work.

The passage of the Affordable Care Act (ACA) in 2010 permitted the realization of these goals. Federal support of NQF's work increased. ACA directed HHS to obtain multi-stakeholder input on setting priorities and selecting measures for use in various federal

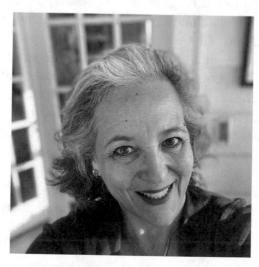

Helen Burstin. (All rights reserved)

programs. Significant support was provided for HHS to contract with a "voluntary consensus standard setting body" (aka NQF) to conduct much of this work.

In response and to complement its priority-setting NPP, NQF developed the Measure Applications Partnership (MAP) to advise the federal government and private sector payers on the optimal measures for use in payment and accountability programs. This closed the loop linking the endorsement process to measures needed to advance the goals established by the NPP. Under the leadership of Helen Burstin, the MAP built on the earlier efforts of the various "quality alliances" but provided for a more patient-centered, coordinated approach to measure selection across various providers, settings, and programs.

MAP has two overarching objectives: to *focus* accountability programs on achieving the NQS priorities and goals and to *align* measurement across the public and private sectors and across settings and populations served. The MAP Coordinating Committee and workgroups are composed of representatives from more than 60 private sector stakeholder organizations, 9 federal agencies, and 40 individual technical experts.

CMS found the recommendations of the MAP essential in 2012 when it adopted value-based purchasing for Medicare and Medicaid services that linked hospitals' payments to their success in achieving reductions in specific measured bad outcomes, such as catheter-associated urinary tract infections and central line infections. Suddenly, the incentive for hospitals to implement safe practices increased dramatically. CMS contracted with the MAP for further measures to use in this program.

Through the MAP the NQF has advised the government on the selection of measures for use in more than 20 federal public reporting and pay-for-performance programs. About 300 NQF-endorsed measures are currently in use in federal, state, and private sector programs. Over 90 percent of all Medicare payments are now performance-based.

The ACA placed responsibility for setting national priorities within CMS. NQF's National Priorities Partnership provides input to CMS for this function and also plays a role in convening stakeholders to develop action plans to achieve the national priorities and goals.

ACA also charged HHS with developing a National Quality Strategy (NQS) to improve the delivery of healthcare services, patient outcomes, and population health and required that the NQS be shaped by input from a broad range of stakeholders. HHS requested NQF to convene the NPP to provide input to the secretary for consideration as it developed this national body of work. In 2011 it established six priorities: healthy living, prevention of leading causes of mortality, patient safety, person and family engagement, communication and coordination, and affordable care.

NQF thus manages the "supply chain" for quality and safety priorities, setting standards and applying them: the NPP, which sets priorities and goals; measure stewards, who develop and test measures; the evaluation and endorsement consensus process; the MAP that advises on selection of measures for use in accountability applications; and public and private accountability efforts. It is the neutral convener of multi-stakeholder groups that provide the "bridge" between public and private sectors.

In addition to NPP and MAP, the NQF has a broad array of quality and safety programs. Its health IT initiatives support the complex move toward electronic measurement to facilitate data sharing between healthcare providers and their patients. NQF provides information and tools to help healthcare decision-makers and has programs in person- and family-centered care, effective communication, palliative and end-of-life care, and disparities [16].

Many of these programs have been institutionalized by NQF into multi-stakeholder Standing Committees in topical areas. Standing Committees are charged to review and recommend submitted measures for endorsement to NQF's Consensus Standards Approval Committee that considers all measures recommended for NQF endorsement.

Conflict of Interest Scandal

In 2014, the patient safety movement was rocked by its first major scandal when Charles Denham reached an out-of-court settlement with the US Department of Justice for receiving over $11 million from a medical products company, CareFusion, to promote their products [17, 18]. Denham had served as co-chair of various NQF committees that produced safe practices reports dating back to 2003; he was chair of the Leapfrog Group's Safe Practices Committee and editor of the *Journal of Patient Safety*. Denham's exposure was a blow to the entire patient safety community, but NQF by far suffered the greatest fallout.

The leadership of NQF was taken completely by surprise. Despite NQF's strict conflict of interest policies, Denham had not disclosed his commercial ties. NQF immediately severed its ties to Denham and his foundation TMIT.

Denham had come under suspicion earlier at NQF in 2009 when concerns were raised by both staff and committee members when he lobbied the committee to insert a specific recommendation in Safe Practice 22 (surgical site infection prevention) to use chlorhexidine gluconate 2% and isopropyl alcohol solution as skin antiseptic preparation, i.e., CareFusion's ChloraPrep. After investigation, the recommendation was replaced with a more generic one, and Denham was removed from his co-chairmanship of the Safe Practices Committee, but no one knew he was being paid by CareFusion.

There was another problem. For years, Denham had been providing substantial financial support for NQF. Much of the staff work for the Safe Practices Committee was supplied gratis by Denham's "non-profit" company, Health Care Concepts. Between 2006 and 2009, this organization donated grants totaling $725,000 to NQF.

When the scandal broke, NQF officials said that Denham never reported his conflicts, despite a specific requirement for all members to do so. After his firing, NQF took immediate steps to strengthen its processes to ensure the integrity of quality measures and safe practices, and it reviewed all of the standards set by the committee Denham co-chaired. It also established a policy of not accepting money from funding organizations whose leaders are on its committees. Denham was also relieved of his editorship of the *Journal of Patient Safety* and his leadership of a committee of the Leapfrog Group.

Conclusion

NQF is one of the few healthcare organizations defined as consensus-based by the National Institute of Standards and Technology, part of the Department of Commerce. This status allows the federal government to rely on NQF-defined measures or healthcare practices as the best, evidence-based approaches to improving care. Because they must meet rigorous criteria, NQF's endorsed measures are trusted and used by the federal government, states, and private sector organizations to evaluate performance and share information with patients and their families.

NQF's prompt and transparent response to the Denham affair confirmed its legitimacy as standard setter. It has continued to expand its role as envisioned by Kizer to promote effective care, achieve better outcomes, improve patient safety, and improve access to care through rigorous measures and collection and analysis of data.

Working together, NQF and AHRQ became the institutional foundation that permitted patient safety to advance both as a science and in practice. They represent the ideal of a public-private partnership where collaboration, commitment, leadership, and good will produce powerful and important change.

Appendix 11.1: Serious Reportable Events Steering Committee [11]

John M. Colmers (Co-Chair), Program Officer, Milbank Memorial Fund, New York, NY

Lucian L. Leape, MD (Co-chair), Adj. Professor of Health Policy, Harvard School of Public Health, Boston, MA

Becky Cherney, President and CEO, Central Florida Health Care Coalition, Orlando, FL

Robert M. Crane, Senior Vice President and Director, Kaiser Permanente Institute for Health Policy, Oakland, CA

David M. Gaba, MD, Director, Patient Safety Center of Inquiry, VA Palo Alto Health Care System, Palo Alto, CA

Mark Gibson, Policy Advisor to the Governor of Oregon, Salem, OR

Sr. Mary Jean Ryan, FSM, President and CEO, SSM Healthcare, St. Louis, MO

Paul M. Schyve, MD, Sr. Vice President, Joint Commission on Accreditation of Healthcare Organizations, Oakbrook Terrace, IL

Gerald M. Shea, Assistant to the President for Government Affairs, AFL-CIO, Washington, DC

Drew Smith, JD, Senior Policy Advisor, AARP Public Policy Institute, Washington, DC

Capt. Frances Stewart, MD, USN, Program Director for Patient Advocacy and Medical Ethics, Department of Defense (Health Affairs), Falls Church, VA

Renee Turner-Bailey, Executive Director of Healthcare Quality Consortium, Ford Motor Company, Dearborn, MI

Appendix 11.2: NQF Serious Reportable Events [11]

Event	Additional specifications
1. Surgical events	
A. Surgery performed on the wrong body part	Defined as any surgery performed on a body part that is not consistent with the documented informed consent for that patient Excludes emergent situations that occur in the course of surgery and/or whose exigency precludes obtaining informed consent
B. Surgery performed on the wrong patient	Defined as any surgery on a patient that is not consistent with the documented informed consent for that patient
C. Wrong surgical procedure performed on a patient	Defined as any procedure performed on a patient that is not consistent with the documented informed consent for that patient Excludes emergent situations that occur in the course of surgery and/or whose exigency precludes obtaining informed consent Surgery includes endoscopies and other invasive procedures

Event	Additional specifications
D. Retention of a foreign object in a patient after surgery or other procedure	Excludes objects intentionally implanted as part of a planned intervention and objects present prior to surgery that were intentionally retained
E. Intraoperative or immediately postoperative death in an ASA Class I patient	Includes all ASA Class I patient deaths in situations where anesthesia was administered; the planned surgical procedure may or may not have been carried out. Immediately postoperative means within 24 hours after induction of anesthesia (if surgery not completed), surgery, or other invasive procedure was completed
2. Product or device events	
A. Patient death or serious disability associated with the use of contaminated drugs, devices, or biologics provided by the healthcare facility	Includes generally detectable contaminants in drugs, devices, or biologics regardless of the source of contamination and/or product
B. Patient death or serious disability associated with the use or function of a device in patient care, in which the device is used for functions other than as intended	Includes, but is not limited to, catheters, drains and other specialized tubes, infusion pumps, and ventilators
C. Patient death or serious disability associated with intravascular air embolism that occurs while being cared for in a healthcare facility	Excludes deaths associated with neurosurgical procedures known to be a high risk of intravascular air embolism
3. Patient protection events	
A. Infant discharged to the wrong person	
B. Patient death or serious disability associated with patient elopement (disappearance) for more than 4 hours	Excludes events involving competent adults
C. Patient suicide or attempted suicide resulting in serious disability, while being cared for in a healthcare facility	Defined as events that result from patient actions after admission to a healthcare facility. Excludes deaths resulting from self-inflicted injuries that were the reason for admission to the healthcare facility

Event	Additional specifications
4. Care management events	
A. Patient death or serious disability associated with a medication error (e.g., errors involving the wrong drug, wrong dose, wrong patient, wrong time, wrong rate, wrong preparation, or wrong route of administration)	Excludes reasonable differences in clinical judgment on drug selection and dose
B. Patient death or serious disability associated with a hemolytic reaction due to the administration of ABO-incompatible blood or blood products	
C. Maternal death or serious disability associated with labor or delivery in a low-risk pregnancy while being cared for in a healthcare facility	Includes events that occur within 42 days postdelivery Excludes deaths from pulmonary or amniotic fluid embolism, acute fatty liver of pregnancy, or cardiomyopathy
D. Patient death or serious disability associated with hypoglycemia, the onset of which occurs while the patient is being cared for in a healthcare facility	
E. Death or serious disability (kernicterus) associated with failure to identify and treat hyperbilirubinemia in neonates	Hyperbilirubinemia is defined as bilirubin levels >30 mg/dl Neonates refer to the first 28 days of life
F. Stage 3 or 4 pressure ulcers acquired after admission to a healthcare facility	Excludes progression from Stage 2 to Stage 3 if Stage 2 was recognized upon admission
G. Patient death or serious disability due to spinal manipulative therapy	
5. Environmental event	
A. Patient death or serious disability associated with an electric shock while being cared for in a healthcare facility	Excludes events involving planned treatments such as electric countershock

Event	Additional specifications
B. Any incident in which a line designated for oxygen or other gas to be delivered to a patient contains the wrong gas or is contaminated by toxic substances	
C. Patient death or serious disability associated with a burn incurred from any source while being cared for in a healthcare facility	
D. Patient death associated with a fall while being cared for in a healthcare facility	
E. Patient death or serious disability associated with the use of restraints or bedrails while being cared for in a healthcare facility	
6. *Criminal events*	
A. Any instance of care ordered by or provided by someone impersonating a physician, nurse, pharmacist, or other licensed healthcare provider	
B. Abduction of a patient of any age	
C. Sexual assault on a patient within or on the grounds of the healthcare facility	
D. Death or significant injury of a patient or staff member resulting from a physical assault (i.e., battery) that occurs within or on the grounds of the healthcare facility	

Appendix 11.3: NQF Safe Practices [15]

1. Create a healthcare culture of safety
2. For designated high-risk, elective surgical procedures or other specified care, patients should be clearly informed of the likely reduced risk of an adverse outcome at treatment facilities that have demonstrated superior outcomes and should be referred to such facilities in accordance with the patient's stated preference
3. Specify an explicit protocol to be used to ensure an adequate level of nursing based on the institution's usual patient mix and the experience and training of its nursing staff
4. All patients in general intensive care units (both adult and pediatric) should be managed by physicians having specific training and certification in critical care medicine ("critical care certified")
5. Pharmacists should actively participate in the medication-use process, including—at a minimum—being available for consultation with prescribers on medication ordering, interpretation and review of medication orders, preparation of medications, dispensing of medications, and administration and monitoring of medications
6. Verbal orders should be recorded whenever possible and immediately read back to the prescriber—i.e., a healthcare provider receiving a verbal order should read or repeat back the information that the prescriber conveys in order to verify the accuracy of what was heard
7. Use only standardized abbreviations and dose designations
8. Patient care summaries or other similar records should be prepared with all source documents immediately at hand (i.e., they should not be prepared from memory)
9. Ensure that care information, especially changes in orders and new diagnostic information, is transmitted in a timely and clearly understandable form to all of the patient's current healthcare providers who need that information to provide care
10. Ask each patient or legal surrogate to recount what he or she has been told during the informed consent discussion
11. Ensure that written documentation of the patient's preference for life-sustaining treatment is prominently displayed in his or her chart
12. Implement a computerized physician order entry system
13. Implement a standardized protocol to prevent the mislabeling of radiographs
14. Implement standardized protocols to prevent the occurrence of wrong-site procedures or wrong-patient procedures

15. Evaluate each patient undergoing elective surgery for his or her risk of an acute ischemic cardiac event during surgery, and provide prophylactic treatment of high-risk patients with beta-blockers

16. Evaluate each patient upon admission, and regularly thereafter, for his or her risk of developing pressure ulcers. This evaluation should be repeated at regular intervals during care. Clinically appropriate preventive methods should be implemented consequent to the evaluation

17. Evaluate each patient upon admission, and periodically thereafter, for the risk of developing deep vein thrombosis (DVT)/venous thromboembolism (VTE). Use clinically appropriate methods to prevent DVT/VTE

18. Use dedicated antithrombotic (anticoagulation) services that facilitate coordinated care management

19. Upon admission, and periodically thereafter, evaluate each patient for the risk of aspiration

20. Adhere to effective methods of preventing central venous catheter-associated bloodstream infections

21. Evaluate each preoperative patient in light of his or her planned surgical procedure for his or her risk of surgical site infection (SSI), and implement appropriate antibiotic prophylaxis and other preventive measures based on that evaluation

22. Use validated protocols to evaluate patients who are at risk for contrast media-induced renal failure, and use a clinically appropriate method for reducing risk of renal injury based on the patient's kidney function evaluation

23. Evaluate each patient upon admission, and periodically thereafter, for his or her risk of malnutrition. Employ clinically appropriate strategies to prevent malnutrition

24. Whenever a pneumatic tourniquet is used, evaluate the patient for his or her risk of an ischemic and/or thrombotic complication, and use appropriate prophylactic measures

25. Decontaminate hands with either a hygienic hand rub or by washing with a disinfectant soap prior to and after direct contact with the patient or objects immediately around the patient

26. Vaccinate healthcare workers against influenza to protect both them and patients from influenza

27. Keep workspaces where medications are prepared clean, orderly, well lit, and free of clutter, distraction, and noise

28. Standardize the methods for labeling, packaging, and storing medications

29. Identify all "high-alert" drugs (e.g., intravenous adrenergic agonists and antagonists, chemotherapy agents, anticoagulants and antithrombotics, concentrated parenteral electrolytes, general anesthetics, neuromuscular blockers, insulin and oral hypoglycemics, narcotics, and opiates)

30. Dispense medications in unit dose or, when appropriate, unit-of-use form, whenever possible

References

1. Kizer KW. The National Quality Forum seeks to improve health care. Acad Med. 2000;75:320–1.
2. Kizer KW. Re-engineering the veterans healthcare system. In: Ramsaroop P, et al., editors. Advancing federal sector health care: a model for technology transfer. New York: Springer-Verlag; 2001.
3. Kizer KW. The "new VA": a national laboratory for health care quality management. Am J Med Qual. 1999;14:3–20.
4. Stires D. How the VA Healed Itself. Fortune. 2006;2006:130–2, 4, 6.
5. Jha AK, Perlin JB, Kizer KW, Dudley RA. Effect of the transformation of the veterans affairs health care system on the quality of care. NEJM. 2003;348:2218–27.
6. Arnst C. The best medical care in the U.S. Bloomberg Businessweek July 17, 2006.
7. Measure Evaluation Criteria. National Quality Forum. 2020., at http://www.qualityforum.org/Measuring_Performance/Submitting_Standards/Measure_Evaluation_Criteria.aspx.
8. Kizer KW. Establishing health care performance standards in an era of consumerism. JAMA. 2001;286:1213–7.
9. Billings C. Some hopes and concerns regarding medical event-reporting systems. Arch Pathol Lab Med. 1998;122:214–5.
10. Leape LL. Reporting of adverse events. N Engl J Med. 2002;347:1633–8.
11. Serious Reportable NQF. Events in healthcare. Washington, DC: National Quality Forum; 2002.
12. Shojania K, Duncan B, McDonald K, Markowitz A, editors. Making health care safer: a critical analysis of patient safety practices. Rockville: Agency for Healthcare Research and Quality; 2001.
13. Leape LL, Berwick DM, Bates DW. What practices will most improve safety? Evidence-based medicine meets patient safety. JAMA. 2002;288:501–7.
14. Shojania KG, Duncan BW, McDonald KM, Wachter RM. Safe but sound: patient safety meets evidence-based medicine. JAMA. 2002;288:508–13.
15. National Quality Forum. Safe practices for better health care: a consensus report. Washington, DC: NQF; 2003. Report No.: NQFCR-05-03.
16. The National Quality Forum. 2020 at https://www.qualityforum.org.
17. Wachter B. Patient safety's first scandal: the sad case of chuck Denham, CareFusion, and the NQF. The Hospital Leader: Society of Hospital Medicine (SHM); 2014.
18. CareFusion to pay the government $40.1 million to resolve allegations that include more than $11 million in kickbacks to one doctor. Washington, D.C: Department of Justice Office of Public Affairs. 2014.

Chapter 12
Enforcing Standards: The Joint Commission

On March 30, 1981, Ronald Reagan, president of the USA, was shot in an assassination attempt. During his lifesaving surgery at the George Washington Hospital, the nation was riveted by the clear and calm account of its progress by the hospital's physician spokesman, Dennis O'Leary. Five years later, O'Leary became the head of the Joint Commission on Accreditation of Hospitals.

History of the Joint Commission[1] [1]

The Joint Commission has been for many years the principal driver of healthcare quality in hospitals and, in more recent decades, other types of healthcare organizations. Its roots go back to the early years of the twentieth century when medicine was undergoing rapid changes as the result of scientific advances in understanding the causes of diseases, the use of antisepsis, and the development of x-rays. Over a short period, hospitals move from "pest houses" to essential resources and proliferated. But quality of care varied widely. A few people began to be concerned.

---

[1] Most of what follows of the early history of The Joint Commission comes from its excellent 50-year anniversary report, *Champions of Quality in Health Care*.

© The Author(s) 2021
L. L. Leape, *Making Healthcare Safe*,
https://doi.org/10.1007/978-3-030-71123-8_12

One was Ernest Amory Codman, a surgeon at the MGH in Boston who developed the End Result Idea, a system for following up patients after surgery to determine their outcomes. The Idea was sufficiently unpopular with his colleagues at the MGH that he found it necessary to leave and found his own hospital in 1911. He kept meticulous records and later published his results in *A Study in Hospital Efficiency* [2]. Along the way, however, he went out of his way to publicly accuse surgeons and hospitals of being more interested in making money, for which he was widely ostracized.

At about the same time, in 1912, a prominent Chicago surgeon, Franklin H. Martin, and several others founded the American College of Surgeons (ACS). The purpose was to distinguish those who were trained in surgery from others, to establish the specialty. Their other concern was about the lamentable state of hospitals, which led them to call for "a system of standardization of hospital equipment and hospital work." Ernest Codman was tapped to chair a Hospitalization Standardization Committee.

In 1918 the ACS initiated the standardization program. In its initial foray surveying hospitals of 100 beds or more, only 89 of 692 hospitals surveyed met the minimum standards! Although that number was reported out to the college, the list of the names of the hospitals was burned to keep it from being obtained by the press! The hospital standards approval process was here to stay, however, and by 1950, half of all hospitals, 3290, were on the ACS approval list.

But the ACS was in financial trouble and unable to sustain the program. It approached the American Hospital Association (AHA) about taking it over. The AHA was interested and willing to provide financial support. The American Medical Association (AMA) got wind of this and made a counteroffer. The AMA had an accreditation program for internships and residencies and disliked the idea of a program run by administrators, not doctors. After months of wrangling, the three parties, along with the American College of Physicians (ACP), worked out their differences and in 1951 founded the Joint Commission on Accreditation of Hospitals (JCAH).

In the early years, the JCAH carried on the ACS standards. Surveys focused only on the hospital environment, what Donabedian would later call "structure." They examined physical aspects, such as proper use of autoclaves, function of clinical laboratories, medical staff organization, and patient records. An early effort to include evaluation of clinical care was shot down by the AMA, who consistently claimed this to be the prerogative of physicians. They even threatened to absorb JCAH into the AMA if they did not get their way.

The enactment of Medicare in 1965 was a watershed moment for JCAH. The legislation gave it "deemed" status, meaning that hospitals that were accredited by JCAH were deemed to have met the Medicare *Conditions of Participation*. This may have been of necessity—the federal government had no capacity to inspect hospitals and the states were notoriously poor at it—but it had immense impact and dramatically enhanced the prestige and power of JCAH as a "quasi-public" licensing body. The flip side was that it exposed it to much greater public accountability.

The JCAH board saw the new status as an opportunity to elevate the standards and use the surveys to improve quality of care. By using lessons learned from the surveys, they could move standards from "minimum essential" to "optimum achievable." They undertook a major project to elevate the standards over the next few years.

These were also the years of rising concerns about civil rights, however, and the JCAH soon found itself in the crosshairs of public interest groups that were concerned—justifiably—about poor conditions in municipal hospitals in major cities. The Commission was pushed to deny accreditation to these hospitals in order to stimulate increased funding.

Not only would this be counterproductive, but closing the hospitals would deny care to indigent people, and most of these hospitals would be able to get certification from their state or the Department of Health, Education and Welfare (HEW). The JCAH stuck to provisional accreditation and consulting with hospitals on how to improve.

However, in 1971 the preamble in the new *Accreditation Manual for Hospitals* declared that patients were entitled to "equitable and humane treatment" and that "no person should be denied impartial access to treatment ... on the basis of such considerations as race, color, creed, national origin or the nature of the source of payment for his care." The first patients' bill of rights. It was not just a statement. Observance of patient rights would be a factor in the determination of accreditation.

The tension between the JCAH's concept of its accreditation role as informing and stimulating hospitals to improve quality of care and the public's desire for accountability came to a head a few years later when Congress passed legislation that gave HEW (now Health and Human Services (HHS)) authority to do "validation" studies of accredited hospitals in which they would conduct surveys in response to complaints alleging noncompliance with Medicare standards and to establish standards that exceeded those of the JCAH. The Commission was being pushed to be not just an accreditor, but a certifier, i.e., a regulator. It continued to resist but in some states it did begin to survey hospitals with state licensing teams.

It seemed to work. In 1979, a General Accounting Office (GAO) report endorsed The Joint Commission process as superior to that of HHS and later commended its cooperative relationships with states for licensure and accreditation. The Commission focused on improving its surveys.

The Agenda for Change

In 1986, the course of The Joint Commission changed dramatically when Dennis O'Leary was appointed president. O'Leary was a board-certified internist and hematologist. He grew up in Kansas City, graduated from Harvard and Cornell Medical School, and trained in internal medicine at the University of Minnesota and Strong Memorial Hospital in Rochester, NY. He had been at George Washington University Medical Center since 1971 where he had taken on progressively more administrative duties, including chairing the medical staff executive committee at the hospital and being the dean for clinical affairs at the medical center.

O'Leary had a clear idea of what he wanted to accomplish. He wanted The Joint Commission to change the focus of accreditation to performance improvement.

The time was ripe. In the 1960s, Avedis Donabedian at the University of Michigan had developed his classical definition of quality of care as encompassing three components, structure, process, and outcome, but his teachings had little impact except in academe. The Joint Commission focused on structure, and practicing physicians were too busy in the 1960s and 1970s keeping up with the fast pace of scientific advances that were transforming medicine to give much thought to how their systems worked or to analyzing their results. (Codman redux!)

But costs were increasing almost exponentially. When Medicare was introduced in 1965, it was estimated that it would cost $275–325 million a year [3]. The actual expenditure in 1966 was $1.8 billion, and by 1985 the expenditure was $71 billion and seemingly out of control [4, 5]. Questions began to arise for the first time about the effectiveness of care. What were we getting for our money?

In 1973, John Wennberg, a researcher from the Harvard Center for Community Health and Medical Care, added fuel to the fire when he published the results of his studies of geographic variation that showed two- to fourfold variations in the provision of common surgical procedures, such as tonsillectomy, hemorrhoidectomy, and prostatectomy [6]. Charles Lewis had previously shown three- to fourfold variation in the rates of performance of six surgical procedures in Kansas, including tonsillectomy, appendectomy, and herniorrhaphy [7]. These differences were not trivial, and the conclusion was inescapable: either too many patients were getting the service in one area or too few in the other. Did the doctors know what they were doing? Over the next few years, Wennberg expanded his studies to other regions, but the results were similar.

It took a while for people to take notice, but by the early 1990s, a movement was afoot in medicine to take a different approach to quality of care. Paul Batalden and Don Berwick had studied under Deming and began work on applying industrial continuous quality improvement (CQI) concepts to healthcare [8]. Berwick had founded the Institute for Healthcare Improvement (IHI) (see Chap. 6).

O'Leary and his senior colleagues Jim Roberts and Paul Schyve could see that its applications in healthcare were the future. It was time to get The Joint Commission on board. Schyve was the director of standards at The Joint Commission from 1986 to 1989 and then vice president for research and standards. He would function as The Joint Commission's quality and safety guru for the next two decades, representing it to the NQF and participating in NPSF and LLI initiatives.

There were other pressures as well: by this time The Joint Commission had 2600 standards! Hospitals and doctors wanted relief,

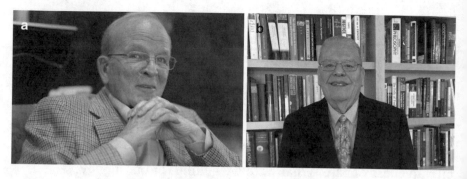

(a) Dennis O'Leary and (b) Paul Schyve.

and they wanted accreditation to be more relevant to their work. Why not focus on quality of care?

Changing Accreditation

O'Leary and his staff proposed that the Commission change the accreditation survey focus from standards for organizational structure to standards important to the provision of quality care. A steering committee of six board members plus Paul Griner, John Wennberg, Steven Shortell, and Lincoln Moses was formed to guide them.

Steven Shortell ended up leading the reorganization of the accreditation manual to a series of chapters on clinical care functions and a series on management support functions. The hospital standards manual shrunk from 2600 standards to less than 500. The Joint Commission was now talking about performance, not structure. The new standards had clearly moved the bar to a higher level.

Meanwhile, work was begun to develop clinical indicators—discrete measures of outcomes and related processes—in selected areas such as the management of heart attack, heart failure, and pneumonia. Indicator data were then gathered from accredited hospitals and analyzed through an Indicator Measurement System. Integrating these data into the accreditation process was a challenge, however, since they were not standards against which to measure compliance, but more like a rifle shot that defined a narrow significant goal.

The Commission also changed its name to the Joint Commission on Accreditation of Healthcare Organizations (JCAHO) to reflect its increasing scope. It was already accrediting long-term care organizations, mental health institutions, and ambulatory surgery centers, among others; it now added home care. Five public members were added to the board. In 1990, JCAHO changed its mission statement to "improve the quality of healthcare provided to the public."

Hospitals resisted the changes. External factors, such as the failed Clinton health plan and continuing increases in healthcare and survey costs, compounded the problem. The combination of anxiety over the new standards and potential public disclosure of performance led the AHA at one point to seek O'Leary's ouster as The Joint Commission president and replace him with a senior AHA staff member who had previously been The Joint Commission surveyor. However, Board leaders, headed by incoming Board chair William Kridelbaugh of the American College of Surgeons, successfully deflected the assault.

In 1994 and 1995, the Commission piloted a new approach to accreditation: the Orion Project. The Orion Project tested several innovations in the survey process: changing surveys from announced to unannounced so hospitals had to be continuously ready, use of an integrated team of surveyors who were all on-site at the same time, use of laptop technology by surveyors, focus on the effectiveness of staffing, and including performance measures in the accreditation process.

After testing in several states and refining them, some of the innovations were rolled out nationwide. These were major changes in the accreditation process, but the new approach was well-received. A survey of hospitals showed that 80% found new process "more interactive, consultative, and valuable" than previous accreditation surveys. By 1995 accreditation included six new functional areas: patient rights and organizational ethics, care of patients, continuum of care, management of the environment of care, management of human resources, and surveillance and prevention of infection.

Focus on Patient Safety: Sentinel Events

Something else was happening in 1995. Starting with the death of Betsy Lehman in Boston from an overdose of chemotherapy, a number of nationally reported cases of major medical mishaps were reported in the press. These led the public and advocacy groups to raise questions about the effectiveness of The Joint Commission accreditation. If it was doing its job, how could these things happen?

O'Leary recalls that some years earlier, in 1990, I had visited The Joint Commission to suggest that, based on our experience with the medical practice study in New York, The Joint Commission should pay more attention to patient safety issues in accrediting hospitals. The discussion was cordial, but The Joint Commission had a substantial development agenda on its plate and was not anxious to add more to its agenda. However, the seed had been planted.

The patient safety shocker that spring for The Joint Commission was when it learned that a surgeon in an accredited hospital had amputated the wrong leg of a diabetic patient with severe peripheral vascular disease. Wrong-site surgery? Who had ever heard of that? Nor were there any identifiable case reports in the medical literature. (It was not so rare, it turned out. In the ensuing years, The Joint Commission would typically learn of 50–75 new cases of wrong-site surgery each year.)

Reacting to this and the other major mishaps, The Joint Commission moved into action. Rick Croteau, a senior surveyor, former aerospace engineer and surgeon, was tasked with creating an entirely new policy framework for addressing what came to be known as sentinel events. His knowledge of systems thinking, analysis, and applications would stand him in good stead.

A sentinel event was defined as "a serious undesirable occurrence that results in the loss of patient life, limb, or function." A new performance improvement standard was added that required "intensive assessment of undesirable variation in performance," i.e., root cause analysis (RCA) for each sentinel event, as well as the creation of a corrective action plan. A monograph describing a thorough RCA and how to perform one was also prepared and released by The Joint Commission. Hospitals experiencing a sentinel event were placed in Conditional Accreditation until they had submitted a thorough RCA and had it approved.

In early 1996, vice president for performance measurement Jerod Loeb conceived of holding a national conference on medical error. He persuaded the American Association for the Advancement of Science (AAAS), the Annenberg Center, and the AMA to be co-conveners (Chap. 4). At the conference in the fall, the Commission announced that in an effort to be less punitive, it was changing its policy regarding sentinel events from "Conditional" Accreditation to "Accreditation Watch."

It didn't work. Although The Joint Commission leaders thought this was making their response to sentinel events less punitive, hospitals saw it as a stigma—less threatening, perhaps, but punitive, nonetheless.

By 1997, antagonism between The Joint Commission and hospitals was again in full flower. Some of this related to the formal initiation of ORYX, a next iteration of efforts to integrate clinical indicators into the accreditation process. ORYX set requirements for the number and types of standardized measures each organization had to collect and report. To ease the burden for hospitals, The Joint Commission approved the use of commercial measurement systems to collect the data, audit its reliability, and transmit it to the Commission. But the process was expensive and labor-intensive.

Adding to the friction was the Commission's decision to improve public transparency by introducing quality check on its website. Quality check was a directory of accredited organizations and their performance reports. The combination of these initiatives with the perceived threat of exposing their patient safety performance was almost too much for the hospital field to tolerate.

Hospitals would agree with doing an RCA in principle (how could they not?), but in practice they regarded this expectation as intrusive. A more collaborative approach was needed. Reporting of sentinel events was made voluntary. Hospitals were "encouraged" to report sentinel events and to do RCAs. "Accreditation Watch" would only be assigned if a hospital failed to do an RCA for review by The Joint Commission or if it did not report a sentinel event that The Joint Commission learned of by other means, such as from a patient complaint or a story in the press.

Although their brief was with The Joint Commission, hospitals had many reasons for not wanting to report sentinel events in addition to resistance to performing RCAs. Their lawyers were concerned that despite all assurances of confidentiality, information might be revealed that would lead to a lawsuit. CEOs worried about damage to the reputation of their hospitals if events became known. In addition, if the internal environment was punitive, as most still were, the CEO might not even know an event had occurred. And, despite all the efforts of patient safety experts, many people clung to the idea that some injuries are not preventable and therefore didn't need to be reported.

Sentinel Event Alerts

Since 1995, The Joint Commission had been steadily amassing details regarding sentinel events and their related RCAs and correction plans into a "Sentinel Event Database." The Database now contained a great deal of useful information about the prevalence of serious hazards. Why not disseminate these "lessons learned" widely? To every hospital. The idea of a Sentinel Event Alert was born.

In 1998, the first "Sentinel Event Alert" was issued, describing patient deaths resulting from accidental infusion of concentrated potassium chloride (KCl). Nurses confused its vial with that of dilute sodium chloride, which was used to "flush" intravenous lines. This rarely occurred, but when it did, it was deadly.

The Alert recommended that concentrated KCl be removed from nursing units and that its use be restricted to the pharmacy, where it could be better controlled. This was a classic example of a "forcing function," a powerful human factors technique for preventing error. It worked. Hospitals complied, and within a few years, deaths from accidental infusion of KCl virtually disappeared. Sentinel Event Alert was one of The Joint Commission's most successful initiatives.

In 1999 O'Leary invited me to speak to the Board at their annual planning retreat. I urged them to take the lead in patient safety and to do three specific things: (1) define and require implementation (i.e., inspect for) of known safe practices, (2) replace scheduled triennial inspections with unannounced inspections, and (3) move their reporting system to a separate entity with confidentiality protection. I have no idea whether my entreaties helped, but unannounced surveys were later implemented, and in 2001 The Joint Commission defined 11 new safe practices that they began inspecting for in January 2003.

The Commission continued to push hospitals to focus on quality improvement, but in 1999, the IOM report, *To Err Is Human*, put the spotlight on safety. In that year, The Joint Commission rolled out a major new chapter on patient safety for its accreditation standards manual and changed its mission statement to ". . . continuously improve the *safety and* quality of care provided to the public." However, it needed to do more. It needed to motivate hospitals to implement safe practices.

Patient Safety Goals

Sentinel Event Alerts gave hospitals an incentive to deal with patient safety issues, but many did not know how. Removing concentrated KCl from nursing units was simple: issue a decree (although it is interesting that some hospitals didn't.) But few hazards could be dealt with that easily; most required changing a process. Thanks to IHI and others, some hospitals were beginning to learn how to do this, but it was difficult work, and most were still not engaged. By this time, however, the National Quality Forum (NQF) was identifying evidence-based safe practices that hospitals could adopt. Hospitals wouldn't have to reinvent the wheel; they would just have to put it on.

The Joint Commission Sentinel Event Database was the treasure trove of information that made the Alerts possible. Why not take the next step and recommend safe practices to address the high-priority problems? In addition to The Joint Commission, the NQF, IHI, and others were developing safe practices.

In 2002, the Commission established a Sentinel Event Alert Advisory Group of nurses, physicians, pharmacists, risk managers, and engineers to formalize the work already being done to identify patient safety issues based on lessons learned from sentinel events—the Alerts—as well as from accreditation surveys and recommendations from the NQF and other safety organizations. The Advisory Group analyzed potential remedies for practicality, cost-effectiveness, and evidence.

From this analysis, Patient Safety Goals were developed. Each goal had one or more specific recommendations—the practice changes to be implemented. Box 12.1 shows one of the early goals, reporting critical test results, that was informed by our work at the Massachusetts Coalition for the Prevention of Medical Error (Chap. 8) (Box 12.1).

Box 12.1 Patient Safety Goal 2

Goal 2	
Improve the effectiveness of communication among caregivers.	
NPSG.02.03.01	
Report critical results of tests and diagnostic procedures on a timely basis.	
--Rationale for NPSG.02.03.01--	
Critical results of tests and diagnostic procedures fall significantly outside the normal range and may indicate a life-threatening situation. The objective is to provide the responsible licensed caregiver these results within an established time frame so that the patient can be promptly treated.	
Elements of Performance for NPSG.02.03.01	
1. Develop written procedures for managing the critical results of tests and diagnostic procedures that address the following:	**R** ⊙
The definition of critical results of tests and diagnostic procedures	
By whom and to whom critical results of tests and diagnostic procedures are reported	
The acceptable length of time between the availability and reporting of critical results of tests and diagnostic procedures	
2. Implement the procedures for managing the critical results of tests and diagnostic procedures.	**R** ☐
3. Evaluate the timeliness of reporting the critical results of tests and diagnostic procedures.	**R** ☐

Note that these were goals, not required practices. In line with the commission's commitment to encourage voluntary improvement, the goals were to be aspirational statements of intent for organizations to pursue. Recommendations, not requirements. A hospital's progress in implementing them would, however, be evaluated during accreditation surveys, and performance expectations that followed each goal were surveyed and scored. Compliance data were aggregated and periodically published in *Joint Commission Perspectives*.

The first set of six Patient Safety Goals was published in January 2003:

1. Improve the accuracy of patient identification.
2. Improve the effectiveness of communication among caregivers.
3. Improve the safety of high-alert medications.
4. Eliminate wrong-site, wrong-patient, and wrong-procedure surgery.
5. Improve the safety of infusion pumps.
6. Improve clinical alarm systems.

Each goal had two or more specific recommendations. More detailed processes for achieving the Goals were available for each safe practice from other sources such as IHI and the Massachusetts Coalition. At the time they were released, Rick Croteau noted: "These six Joint Commission National Patient Safety Goals and recommendations provide a clearly defined, practical, and achievable approach to addressing…the most critical threats to patient safety." [9]

The Advisory Group continually reviews the goals. It adds new goals annually and retires old ones as high compliance rates are achieved. In 2004, Goals 1b (time-outs) and 4 were consolidated into a new "Universal Protocol" for the prevention of wrong-site, wrong-person, wrong-procedure surgery. A seventh goal was added to address healthcare-acquired infections, which included complying with CDC hand hygiene guidelines. By 2008, 16 goals had been issued, including the first call to involve patients in their care: Goal 13, Encourage Patients' Active Involvement in Their Own Care as a Patient Safety Strategy.

The Goals were well accepted by hospitals. Follow-up data from surveys in 2005 showed high rates of implementation for a number of specific recommendations: 95% use of two identifiers for patient identification, 82% use of time-outs, 90% implementation of critical test result procedures, 99% removal of KCl, and 96% use of a wrong-site checklist. They have been an effective mechanism for motivating hospitals to improve patient safety.

Core Measures

By 2000, The Joint Commission, working with expert panels, had expanded its original core measure sets for acute myocardial infarction (AMI), heart failure (HF), and pneumonia to a total of 14 individual measures. Box 12.2 shows the core measures for AMI. Hospitals began collecting measures July 1, 2002. (Box 12.2)

Box 12.2 AMI Core Measures

Aspirin within 24 hours of arrival
Aspirin prescribed at discharge
Beta-blocker within 24 hours of arrival
Beta-blocker prescribed at discharge
ACEI for LVSD prescribed at discharge
Smoking cessation counseling/advice
Thrombolysis within 30 minutes
PCI within 120 minutes

Adapted from Ref. [9]

Responding to the pleas from hospitals to reduce duplication of effort, the Commission worked with the Centers for Medicare and Medicaid Services (CMS) to create one common set known as the Specifications Manual for National Hospital Inpatient Quality Measures to be used by both organizations.

The measures worked. From 2002 to 2005, hospitals adherence improved: AMI 87 to 90%, pneumonia 72 to 81%, and CHF 60 to 76%. Some improvements were dramatic. For example, hospitals provided smoking cessation advice to 92.1 percent of patients in 2005 compared with 66.6 percent in 2002. More importantly, outcomes improved: the inpatient mortality rate for heart attack patients declined from 9.2% in 2002 to 8.5% in 2005, representing thousands of lives saved [10].

Currently, The Joint Commission's ORYX initiative integrates performance measurement data into the accreditation process. The measures are aligned as closely as possible with the Centers for Medicare and Medicaid Services (CMS), and chart-abstracted data are publicly reported on The Joint Commission's *Quality Check*® website.

Public Policy Initiative

In 2001, The Joint Commission launched a set of public policy initiatives to amplify its patient safety and quality improvement messaging. It convened a series of topic-oriented roundtables to frame relevant discussions and develop recommendations. Each roundtable had 30–45 participants and met on 2–3 occasions. The Joint Commission staff used the input to draft a white paper. Each white paper was eventually 35–50 pages long and contained findings, recommendations, and accountabilities for seeing each recommendation through to fruition.

The first paper on the nurse staffing crisis struck a chord in the hospital, nursing, and patient safety communities and was an immediate success, eventually being downloaded from The Joint Commission website almost two million times. The report of a roundtable on patient safety and tort reform was also a hit and was downloaded over 300,000 times. A number of other roundtables were convened in the next few years.

Accreditation Process Improvement

In 2000, The Joint Commission decided it had to do more to improve its accreditation process. The triennial inspections had been a tremendous burden for hospitals. For several weeks beforehand, all work other than patient care stopped as hospital departments got their records in shape for the survey. Everyone dreaded them. Worse, they often failed to identify some serious performance problems.

O'Leary asked Russ Massaro, a seasoned surveyor who knew how the minds of healthcare organization leaders worked, to rethink the process. The result was the Shared Visions-New Pathways initiative that was launched in 2004. It completely changed the accreditation process in three fundamental ways.

First, organizations were asked to periodically do their own in-depth self-assessments and share the results and their plans for improvement with The Joint Commission. From now on, surveys would concentrate on the findings from the self-assessments and hospital-reported data, such as from ORYX and sentinel events.

Second, and this was a biggie, on-site surveys from here on would be unannounced. Gone was the dreaded triannual ritual of stopping work to get ready for The Joint Commission. You would have to be at the top of your game at all times. Unannounced meant finding out that the survey would be tomorrow.

Finally, instead of focusing on records, the on-site reviews would focus on the care actually provided to patients. They would use a tracer methodology in which the care to individual patients in the hospital at the time was evaluated by observing and interviewing the patients and hospital staff in real time. Patient care was reviewed for relevant standards compliance, such as medication management and nurse staffing.

It was a huge change. And it was very successful. The reviews engaged doctors, nurses, and other frontline staff. Suddenly, surveys made sense to them, while also giving them an opportunity to demonstrate their skills. Hospitals welcomed the new accreditation process. This was now continuous engagement with The Joint Commission toward the mutual goal of continuous improvement.

Conclusion

What do we make of all this? First and foremost, The Joint Commission has clearly been a leader in reducing harm in healthcare. Without its influence—and persistence—we would not have made the progress we have made in many areas and likely not made any at all in others. Deciding what to do for patient safety and how to do it has been an incredibly complicated business, and the Commission has navigated that thicket well.

From the beginning, the patient safety movement has had to confront the tension between those who call for the greater accountability and regulation that has worked so well in other hazardous industries such as transportation and nuclear power and those who believe that making real change is voluntary and that our job is to motivate people and provide them with the tools to do it.

Your author has found himself squarely in the middle of this debate, embracing the need to change the culture and helping to teach professionals to change systems, but also of the mind that we need to do much more to hold the leaders of healthcare organizations publicly accountable for failure to prevent harm, particularly serious harm where the methods are known, such as serious reportable events.

The Commission has also found itself in the middle, and over the years it has experimented with one approach and another regarding reporting of sentinel events, collection and reporting of data, and how to respond to failures revealed by accreditation visits. All compounded by the ambiguities and vicissitudes that result from the fact that participation by hospitals is voluntary and from changes in views about whether accreditation suffices for deemed status or state licensing.

Compounded also by pushback on all sides: consumer groups who want tougher oversight, hospitals and doctors who want less, and Congress who doesn't know what it wants or changes what it wants according to external pressures. To say, "You can't please everyone" is an understatement at best.

Despite all this, The Joint Commission has been a well-spring of innovations, a great many of which have measurably reduced harm and improved quality of care. More than any other organization, public or private, it has consistently pursued a data-driven analytic approach to helping hospitals improve care. We can all sleep better knowing that it will continue to be a major force for improving patient safety in the future.

References

1. Brauer CM. Champions of quality in health care: a history of the joint commission on accreditation of healthcare organizations. Lyme: Greenwich Publishing Group, Inc.; 2001.
2. Codman EA. A study in hospital efficiency: as demonstrated by the case report of the first years of a private hospital. Boston: s.n.; 1915.
3. Myers RJ. Table 6: estimated progress of supplementary health insurance benefits trust fund. In: Executive hearings before the committee on ways and means HoR, 89th congress 1st session on H.R. 1 and other proposals

for medical care for the aged: part 2. Washington: U.S. Government Printing Office; 1965.

4. Davis MH, Burner ST. Medicare expenditures, by type of service, selected years, 1966-1993. Health care financing administration, office of the actuary, office of national health statistics; 1995.

5. Waldo DRLK, Lazenby H. National health expenditures, 1985. Health Care Financ Rev. 1986;1985(8):1–21.

6. Wennberg JE, Gittelsohn A. Health care delivery in Maine I: patterns of use of common surgical procedures. J Maine Med Assn. 1975;66:123–49.

7. Lewis CE. Variations in the incidence of surgery. NEJM. 1969;281:880–4.

8. Kenney C. The best practice: how the new quality movement is transforming medicine. 1st ed. New York: Public Affairs; 2008.

9. JCAHO to Establish Annual Patient Safety Goals. Joint Commission Perspectives; 2002:1–2.

10. The Joint Commission. Improving America's Hospitals: a report on quality and safety: the joint commission; 2007.

Chapter 13
Partners in Progress: Patient Safety in the UK

In 1997, Britons were shocked by a report from the General Medical Council (GMC) of a series of deaths from bungled surgery at the Bristol Royal Infirmary. In response to parents' complaints, the GMC had launched an investigation into the high mortality of cardiac surgery of children at the Infirmary. It found that of 53 children who were operated on, 29 had died and 4 suffered severe brain damage. Three surgeons were found guilty of serious professional misconduct, and two were stricken from the medical register [1].

The public and the profession were shocked that this could happen in the National Health Service (NHS). Richard Smith, editor of the BMJ, wrote, "All changed, changed utterly. British medicine will be transformed by the Bristol case." [2]

Transforming the NHS was already on the mind of Tony Blair and the Labour Party when they took over the government that same year. Britons were unhappy with the quality of care in the NHS, especially long wait times. A recent OECD report had shown that the UK was underperforming its competitors. Blair made improving quality of care and increased funding of the NHS a keystone of his campaign. The Bristol case added fuel to his fire.

© The Author(s) 2021
L. L. Leape, *Making Healthcare Safe*,
https://doi.org/10.1007/978-3-030-71123-8_13

A National Commitment

One of Blair's first acts was to appoint Liam Donaldson chief medical officer (CMO) in 1998. Donaldson was a surgeon who had retrained in public health. He had been CEO of the country's northern regional authority, where he received occasional notifications from hospitals of "accidents" in which patients had been harmed or died from a complication of medical care. As he read them, he recognized that the purpose of the reports was not learning from the incident but to cover the hospitals' leaders backs if the case became public.

These hospital reports were eye-opening for Donaldson, who was previously only dimly aware of the problem. Like your author, another surgeon converted to public health a few years earlier, he began to read about accidents in other industries. He discovered the work of James Reason and human factors experts and became excited about applying lessons from industry to medicine. He asked local managers to report all incidents and set up a database to learn more. He began to develop a list of safety measures that needed to be implemented.

When Blair was elected, Donaldson shared this information and his ideas with him. Shocked, Blair and his new health ministers also

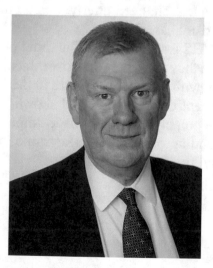

Liam Donaldson. (All rights reserved)

recognized that this was just what he needed politically. He appointed Donaldson as CMO and gave him his full support.

Although the government commitment was new, interest in patient safety in the UK went back at least to 1985 when Charles Vincent began work on avoidable mishaps in medicine, which he published in 1986. Vincent later wrote an editorial in BMJ in 1989 about systems changes [3], followed by a book that he edited with Maeve Ennis and Bob Audley, *Medical Accidents*, in 1993, in which he introduced the concept of applying human factors principles and systems analysis to healthcare [4].

Vincent referenced the findings of the Harvard Medical Practice Study and called for more research into the causes of medical accidents and the development of a comprehensive safety program. Two years later, in 1995, he further expanded these ideas in *Clinical Risk Management* [5]. Risk managers began to think about patient safety, but, as in the USA, the medical profession in general had little interest in these developments. They were fixated on the problem of malpractice litigation and worried that investigation of errors would expose them to more risk. Not much happened.

The Patient Safety Movement

Donaldson would change that. In early 2000, within months of the publication of the IOM report in the USA, he launched the patient safety movement in the UK by releasing his own report, *An Organisation with a Memory* [6].

The report was the product of a panel with a wide-ranging set of disciplines and expertise, including people from other industries. It coupled a comprehensive analysis of the quality and safety problems in the NHS with strong recommendations about what needed to be done. Based on another study done by Charles Vincent [7], it estimated that 11% of hospitalized Britons suffered an adverse event each year, at a cost of one billion pounds for additional hospital stays alone.

An Organisation with a Memory echoed the IOM report in condemning the typical approach when things go wrong of blaming the individual and made the case for a systems approach. The report cited the organizational culture and the lack of an effective reporting system as major barriers. It also acknowledged that some of the existing systems in the UK did work well, especially the confidential inquiries and reporting systems for medical devices.

An Organisation with a Memory called for a fundamental rethinking of the way the NHS approached the challenge of learning from adverse events (AEs). It called for four specific changes: a unified mechanism for reporting and analysis of AE, a more open culture where people can safely report and discuss errors, mechanisms for putting recommended changes in place, and wider appreciation of the systems approach.

About this time, at the urging of Donaldson and BMJ editor Richard Smith, the British Medical Association and the NHS hosted the first UK national symposium on medical error. It was timed to coincide with the publication of a special BMJ issue on patient safety that Smith had conceived of a year earlier and Don Berwick and I edited (Chap. 17). The conference drew a wide audience from Britain and European countries. For many, this was their introduction to the problem of medical errors. Beth Lilja, later the driving force behind the Danish patient safety movement, told me that it was a defining moment for her.

Donaldson came to the CMO job with a passion and an agenda. He recognized that what he had in mind for patient safety would not succeed if it were absorbed into the NHS bureaucracy. The effort needed a full-time commitment and independence. He persuaded the Department of Health to establish an independent Special Health Authority, the National Patient Safety Agency (NPSA). Its mission was to improve patient safety by "encouraging voluntary reporting of medical errors, conducting analysis and initiating preventative measures." [8]

It is worth noting to American readers that the British response to the error threat reflected the ability of the NHS to make changes rapidly and to implement them nationwide. It stands in stark contrast to the USA, where Congress has long been resistant to all forms of regulation and grudging in its support of safety.

The National Patient Safety Agency (NPSA)

The NPSA was designed to identify problems and recommended solutions, not to implement them. There were two major divisions: reporting and solutions. Two experienced administrators, Sue Osborn and Sue Williams, the "two Sues," were given joint responsibility for leading the new agency.

The first priority was to establish the National Reporting and Learning System (NRLS). Like many others, Donaldson believed that a national reporting system was essential to making progress in patient safety. Reporting and analysis could not only lead to increased awareness but also produce actionable recommendations. Getting the NRLS going was a massive information technology challenge that dominated everything else at NPSA.

The NPSA declared its objective was "to promote an open and fair culture in hospitals and across the health service, encouraging doctors and other staff to report incidents and 'near misses'." It was made clear that the purpose of reporting was to enable healthcare providers to learn lessons from each other in order to improve safety—not to identify individuals to punish [9].

The system was set up to receive and analyze reports from all sources (including, later, the public) and to recommend changes. Reporting of adverse events was already well-established in the UK. Hospitals were required to report adverse events to their regional authorities. The NPSA required the reports to also be sent to a central authority, the NRLS, so that the whole NHS could learn from them. The system soon received hundreds of thousands reports, later over a million, annually.

Its success proved to be its undoing. The huge volume and the logistics of categorizing reports impaired its ability to do meaningful analysis as Donaldson had hoped. What the system could do, however, was identify problems requiring action. This information was passed on to the solutions division that then issued alerts with recommendations for implementation of safe practices. NPSA later established a national register to which hospitals were required to report what they did in response to the alerts and why.

Alerts covered the full range of safety issues. *Warning* alerts were issued in response to a new or under-recognized patient safety issue with the potential to cause death or severe harm and asked healthcare providers to coordinate an action plan to deal with them. *Directive* alerts concerned issues for which there were proven effective safe practices. Healthcare organizations were required to implement them. Examples included removal of concentrated potassium chloride (KCl) from nursing units, safe practices for vaccines, blood transfusion competencies, safer patient identification, and the surgical checklist.

The solutions division encouraged the creation of a "no-blame culture" through various publications and extensive educational programs, including training in root cause analysis and disclosure. In 2004 it published *Seven Steps to Patient Safety* that NHS organizations should take to improve patient safety [10]. It emphasized policy measures aimed at removing the blame culture and encouraging the reporting of incidents and near misses without fear of reprimand. The NPSA also advanced safety by training patient safety workers in rapid process change, the just culture, and root cause analysis.

Additional Safety Efforts

In 2001, while the NPSA was actively improving safety, Blair established another arm of the government to address quality of care: the Modernisation Agency. It was challenged to make recommendations to improve quality of care.

The Modernisation Agency appointed "czars" for key issues, such as waiting times, cardiovascular disease, orthopedics, and cancer. Regional strategic health authorities were established as the working arms to manage performance and implement health policy. Don Berwick was enlisted as the only non-UK member of the Modernisation Board to bring in further quality improvement expertise. Using lessons from IHI's experience, clinician-led collaboratives were organized by specialty networks to address specific issues. With funding from the Health Foundation, the Safer Patient Initiative included 20 trusts; it was a large-scale collaborative that worked on five areas: ICU, perioperative care, general hospital care, medication safety, and leadership [11]. Berwick was later knighted by the Queen for his contributions.

A separate UK agency, the National Institute for Health and Clinical Excellence (NICE), also plays an important role in patient safety by assessing the benefits and risks of treatments. It was established in 1999 as an independent organization to produce guidance on public health, health technologies, and clinical practice, which it does by rigorous analysis of evidence. In addition to practice guidelines, it evaluates the safety and efficacy of procedures through its Centre for Health Technology Evaluation.

NICE and NPSA cooperated in risk assessment of new technology, monitoring safety incidents associated with procedures and providing solutions if adverse outcomes are reported. In addition, NICE and NPSA shared reporting in "confidential enquiries" including surgical mortality, maternal and infant deaths, childhood deaths to age 16, deaths in persons with mental illness, and perioperative and unexpected medical deaths.

Despite strong national leadership and extensive efforts to improve patient safety, local leaders were less engaged, and many of the changes were resisted by the medical profession. They roundly bashed the creation of the NRLS, for example, and later objected to the steady barrage of alerts and suggestions "telling us what to do." Safe practices could be mandated, but enforcement was sometimes undermined by resistance and evasion. The public was more supportive but reluctant to abandon the blame mode. When errors were made public, there were still calls for punishment of the individuals responsible.

Support for the NPSA gradually eroded, and in 2005 the two Sues departed and were replaced by Martin Fletcher (a World Health Organization safety leader). He reduced the scope of the agency to focus primarily on the reporting system. NPSA was given responsibility for safety aspects of hospital design and cleanliness and food, as well as safe research practices through the National Research Ethics Service. It took on performance of individual doctors and dentists through the National Clinical Assessment Service (NCAS).

Patient Safety in Scotland

Ironically, in 2008, while the NPSA was under attack, patient safety in Scotland took a giant step forward. Under Derek Feeley's leadership, NHS Scotland launched the *Scottish Patient Safety Programme (SPSP)*, a 5-year national initiative to reduce patient harm. This was the first attempt to implement a patient safety program across a whole healthcare system. Its stated aim was to reduce mortality by 15 percent and adverse events by 30 percent across Scotland's acute hospitals by the end of 2012 [12].

In partnership with IHI, Jason Leitch led SPSP to focus on reducing adverse events in acute care hospitals. It was amazingly successful in reducing the number of cases of bloodstream infections associated with central lines, ventilator-acquired pneumonia, and the length of time patients were staying in intensive care [13, 14]. It also managed one of the most successful implementations of the surgical checklist.

SPSP was one of IHI's most successful initiatives [15]. Don Berwick's later praise was justifiably effusive: "The Scottish Patient Safety Programme, marks Scotland as a leader, second to no nation on earth, in its commitment to reducing harm to patients, dramatically and continually." [12]

Reorganization

Back in England, in 2010, as Liam Donaldson was stepping down after 12 years as CMO, major changes were underway. The Labour Government led by Tony Blair's successor, Gordon Brown, lost a general election, and the Conservative Party took over control. As part of its vaunted commitment to smaller government, it directed each ministry to reduce the number of agencies.

The NPSA was completely abolished for reasons entirely unrelated to its performance or value. Its key functions were transferred to a new division called NHS Improvement; later it became integrated into the central body running the entire health system, NHS England [16]. Safety was relegated to a new agency, the Healthcare Safety

Investigative Branch under NHS Improvement. It conducts independent investigations of patient safety concerns through two programs,
national and maternity. It investigates up to 30 incidents a year and
makes recommendations to improve healthcare systems and processes.

The NRLS was temporarily managed by a London teaching hospital before itself being absorbed into NHS Improvement. The solutions
division of the old NPSA was given to NICE.

The chaos of an NHS reorganization that its CEO said was so big
that "It could be seen from space" made patient safety an "also ran" in
NHS priorities. Under Donaldson's leadership, the UK was one of the
few countries to make a meaningful national commitment to safety
and back it up with structural changes and funding. His strong commitment gave safety visibility and stature. This was lost with the abo-
lition of the NPSA and the redesign of the CMO post to no longer
have responsibility for quality and patient safety in the NHS.

But all was not lost. The arrival of a new health secretary, Jeremy
Hunt, in 2012 brought a new passion and concern for patient safety at
the political level. Hunt reached out to high-profile victims of harm,
righting serious injustices, and stimulated new policies in patient
safety in the NHS. He also promoted action at the global level by initiating a series of global ministerial summits. Patient safety is still on
the agenda even though pursued with less vigor than in the past.

Conclusion

Managing patient safety, like all of healthcare in the UK, was a political process. While this made rapid implementation of changes possible, the downside was that it needed to be owned by the leadership
and frontline staff in the NHS. Thus, patient safety had rapid ups and
downs according to the motives and values of the political party in
power and the healthcare workforce's perceptions of it. It could not
live up to one of Deming's fundamental tenets for success: "constancy
of purpose for improvement." When governments changed, it was
buffeted and tangled up by the dead hand of bureaucratic change. In
spite of all this, the progress in patient safety in Britain was impressive and, importantly, continues.

References

1. Vincent C, Benn J, Hanna GB. High reliability in health care. BMJ. 2010;340:225–6.
2. Smith R. All changed, changed utterly. BMJ. 1998;316:1917–8.
3. Vincent C. Research into medical accidents: a case of negligence? BMJ. 1989;299:1150–3.
4. Vincent C, Ennis M, Audley RJ. Medical accidents. 1st ed. Oxford. New York: Oxford University Press; 1993.
5. Vincent C. Clinical risk management. London: BMJ Books; 2001.
6. U.K. Department of Health. An organisation with a memory: report of an expert group on learning from adverse events in the NHS. London; 2000.
7. Vincent C, Neale G, Woloshynowych M. Adverse events in British hospitals: preliminary retrospective record review. Br Med J. 2001;322:517–9.
8. Secretary of State for Health. The national patient safety agency (establishment and constitution) order 2001 no. 1743: National Health Service; 2001.
9. U.K. Department of Health. Building a safer NHS for patients: implementing an organisation with a memory. London: Department of Health; 2001.
10. National Patient Safety Foundation. Seven steps to patient safety: a guide for NHS staff. London: The National Patient Safety Agency; 2003.
11. The Health Foundation. Learning report: safer patients initiative. London; 2011.
12. Scottish Patient Safety Programme. The improvement hub. Accessed 12 Apr 2020, at https://ihub.scot/improvement-programmes/scottish-patient-safety-programme-spsp/.
13. Hospital patient safety improving. BBC News, 9 September 2009. Accessed 12 Apr 2020, at http://news.bbc.co.uk/2/hi/uk_news/scotland/tayside_and_central/8245738.stm.
14. Crosshouse Hospital reports 18% drop in mortality rates. BBC News. 28 February 2011.
15. Haraden C, Leitch J. Scotland's successful national approach to improving patient safety in acute care. Health Aff. 2011;30:755–63.
16. Transfer of Patient Safety function to the NHS Commissioning Board Authority. NHS; 2012. Accessed 12 Apr 2020, at https://www.england.nhs.uk/2012/05/npsa-transfer/.

Chapter 14
Going Global: The World Health Organization

Where was the World Health Organization on patient safety? Patient safety was taking off in the USA and the UK, and there were stirrings in Canada, Australia, Denmark, Spain, and a few other European countries, but what about the rest of the world? What about developing countries? With fewer resources, their needs for attention to medical harm might well be even greater.

Enter Liam Donaldson. After establishing the National Patient Safety Agency in the UK, Liam turned his attention and considerable skills to the rest of the world, to the WHO.

He was well-positioned for the task. As Chief Medical Officer of the NHS, he represented the UK to the WHO and was on the executive body. He persuaded them to put patient safety on the agenda for the 2002 World Health Assembly. He made his proposal compelling by pledging annual support of $25 million from the UK.

By good fortune, the Presidency of the European Union around that time was on rotation to the UK. Liam also persuaded the UK government to make patient safety a priority for its Presidency. This meant that the European Commission established and funded a program of work that stretched forward into the future.

It worked. The World Health Assembly passed resolution WHA55.18, which urged countries to pay attention to patient safety and directed the Director-General of the WHO to carry out a series of actions to promote patient safety: development of global norms and

© The Author(s) 2021
L. L. Leape, *Making Healthcare Safe*,
https://doi.org/10.1007/978-3-030-71123-8_14

standards, promotion of evidenced-based policies, and encouragement of research in patient safety [1]. The resolution made the drive for safer health care a worldwide endeavor.

In November 2003, at Liam's urging, the WHO collaborated with the UK to convene a meeting of senior policy makers and international experts from all WHO regions to discuss future international collaboration on patient safety. At the meeting Donaldson proposed the establishment of the World Alliance for Patient Safety.

The World Alliance for Patient Safety

A year later, the World Alliance for Patient Safety was formally inaugurated on October 27, 2004, by the Director-General of the WHO, Dr. Lee Jong-Wook, in Washington, DC, at an event hosted by the Pan American Health Organization. The event was remarkable in that it was the first time that heads of agencies, health policy makers, representatives of patients' groups from multiple nations, and the WHO came together to address the problem of unsafe health care. Donaldson and Carolyn Clancy, Director of the US Agency for Health Research and Quality, gave keynote addresses.

The World Alliance was Liam Donaldson's baby. He envisioned it, he funded it, and he led it for the first 5 years.

The Alliance goals were ambitious: to develop standards for patient safety and assist UN Member States in improving the safety of health care by "raising awareness and political commitment to improve safety and facilitate the development of patient safety policy and practice in all WHO Member States" [2]. The program focused on six areas of action:

1. Global patient safety challenge
2. Patient and consumer involvement
3. Developing a patient safety taxonomy
4. Research in patient safety
5. Solutions that improve safety
6. Reporting and learning to improve patient safety

Before the year was out, the Alliance moved ahead on two initiatives that I was privileged to be involved in: reporting and learning and the global patient safety challenge. These initiatives illustrate the scope and power of the WHO to influence change.

Guidelines for Adverse Event Reporting and Learning Systems

In the USA, the most common reaction to the IOM report was to call for more reporting of errors and adverse events. The same was true internationally. By the time the Alliance was formed 4 years later, 38 countries had indicated to the WHO their interest in developing reporting systems. Indeed, there seemed to be a fixation on reporting as the solution to the patient safety problem. But no country had a system they were satisfied with.

Accordingly, it was reasonable that reporting was one of the six areas of action called for in the Alliance prospectus: "The Alliance will develop best-practice guidelines that can be used to facilitate the development of new reporting systems to improve patient safety and to improve existing reporting systems." The statement that followed of core principles to underlie the guideline development quoted almost verbatim from the paper on reporting systems that I wrote in 2002 for the New England Journal of Medicine [3] as part of our series of patient safety topics. (See Chap. 17.)

So I was not totally surprised when Pauline Phillip called from the WHO and asked me to write the reporting guideline. I was not eager to take on another project at that time and had some reservations about working with the WHO because of its reputation for being excessively bureaucratic, but I was very excited about what Liam was doing with the World Alliance and anxious to help it succeed.

It was also another opportunity to bring some balance and reality to the thinking about reporting. So many people thought reporting was the solution to medical errors: "Just make them report their mistakes and they will be more careful," the thinking went. Not only was it not true—there was no evidence that reporting made people more careful—it also was not the solution to the safety problem. The problem was bad systems, not careless people.

Beyond the conceptual fallacy, the logistics of establishing and managing a reporting system were formidable. The costs were daunting for rich countries and far beyond consideration for developing or middle-income countries. We could provide a reality check.

I agreed to write the guideline on the condition that I share the project with a co-author, who would be paid. I had someone in mind: Susan Abookire, a former student of mine and physician who was currently working in safety at Brigham and Women's Hospital. Indeed, when I approached her, Susan was interested and willingly took on the huge task of digging out the historical information on what already was being done worldwide. We wrote the monograph and shepherded it through the labyrinth of WHO approval. We succeeded despite the resistance of an internal reviewer who considered herself much better qualified to write it and at one point suggested it all be redone!

The document was comprehensive. It described and compared the many types of systems in use worldwide. We spelled out in detail the key components of a reporting system and described the requirements for making it work. Controversial issues such as accountability, public disclosure, and confidentiality were addressed [4].

We reiterated the earlier admonition that the fundamental role of a reporting system is to enhance safety by learning from failures. Reporting must be safe—individuals who report must not be punished or suffer other consequences. Reporting is of little value unless it leads to a constructive response. At a minimum, this requires data analysis to identify hazards. But for significant impact, to justify the effort and expense, the system must include root cause analysis of incidents to uncover the contributing factors and lead to recommendations for systems changes.

We described alternatives to reporting for gaining useful information to improve patient safety, such as WalkRounds, focus groups, focused review on specific problems, failure modes and effects analysis, and analysis of malpractice claims data. Existing data sources, such as that generated by the voluntary National Nosocomial Infections Surveillance System and the US National Surgical Quality Improvement Program, can be used to identify hazards. We described the characteristics of successful systems and provided a checklist for developing a reporting system

The monograph was published the following year, as "draft" guidelines [4]. I never got an explanation of why they weren't given the full WHO endorsement, which suggests it was political. The realistic tone of the document—you need experts, it is expensive, and it isn't worth doing if you are unable to respond to the reports with analysis and system changes—undoubtedly was not what many wanted to hear, both within the WHO and among Member States!

The requirements we laid out for establishing a reporting system were indeed formidable; it was unlikely that many governments would be willing to provide the funds to do it right. At this time in the USA, we had no national system, none of the state mandatory systems were effective, and all of them were underfunded.

A few years later, Pennsylvania implemented a comprehensive reporting and analysis system, wisely funded by a tax on hospitals. It has yielded valuable information and stimulated change. Other states have improved their systems with variable results. Britain, on the other hand, had already made a substantial investment in a national reporting system when they established the National Patient Safety Agency.

The majority of members of the WHO are low- and middle-income countries. If they took the Guidelines seriously, they would quickly recognize that there were better ways to deploy their limited resources. That, of course, was the lesson that was implied: there are more effective ways to improve patient safety for far less. Perhaps not exactly what the WHO had in mind when it conceived the project. Nonetheless, the "draft" guidelines are still the WHO publication on reporting 15 years later.

Patient and Consumer Involvement—Patients for Patient Safety (P4PS)

Liam Donaldson's passion for patient safety was rooted in his deep concern for the victims—the injured patients. He was moved by his personal experience as a physician, as well as the writings of Charles Vincent, one of the first to call attention to the psychological impact of unanticipated harm on the patient [5]. On the various occasions when I had the opportunity to hear Donaldson speak, I was impressed that he started every talk on patient safety with a story of a patient. That was the point, that was why we were here.

The Alliance's second major early initiative, **Patients for Patient Safety**, was his mechanism for involving patients in the solution. Launched in 2004, it was based on the recognition that the patient and family have unique information because they are the only ones present through the entire continuum of care, which may have involved care from multiple providers at different institutions. Those who have experienced harm have special insights concerning systems failures. It would seem obvious that they should play a central role in efforts to improve the quality and safety of health care around the world. Patients for Patient Safety (P4PS) would tap that resource.

Founding leaders included Margaret Murphy from Ireland, who also advised the UK National Institute for Healthcare Research, Stephanie Newall from Australia, and Sue Sheridan and Helen Haskell from the USA. All of them had lost children or a spouse as the result of medical errors, and all were, and still are, active and effective leaders in changing policy in their local and national environments. They were motivated to give meaning to their tragedies by sharing their experiences and advocating for change.

The WHO convened the first Patients for Patient Safety workshop in London in 2005. Participants developed the "London Declaration" that enunciated the common vision and commitment for positive engagement of patients in their care. It called for honesty, openness, and transparency, making reduction of health-care errors a basic human right, and for promoting programs for patient safety and patient empowerment by dialogue with all partners (Appendix 14.1).

At this meeting, P4PS created a global network of patients, consumers, caregivers, and consumer organizations to support patient involvement in patient safety programs, both within countries and in the global programs of the World Alliance for Patient Safety [6].

The Patients for Patient Safety network has continued to grow. By 2012 it had 250 members in 52 countries. They are champions for patient engagement and empowerment on hospital boards, medical school councils, governmental policy groups, and professional conferences around the world. The patient's voice is being heard.

Support of Patient Safety Research

At the outset the Alliance wanted to create a proper evidence base for patient safety, an entirely new field of health services research. David Bates of Harvard University was charged with setting out research priorities in the WHO's three bands of countries: high-, middle-, and low-income [7].

The Alliance's first major research initiative was an ambitious project to estimate the extent of medical harm in developing countries. The WHO recognized that to convince people in the developing world that medical errors were a serious problem, they would need to show them the extent of the problem in their own countries. Data from advanced western countries would not do it.

Many of us thought this would be an exercise in futility. The most serious limitation in the MPS—the factor that raised the most questions about its validity—was that much of the data came from poor medical records, those with few progress notes. In the USA, this was especially a problem in small rural hospitals. The records in hospitals in developing countries would surely be worse.

And the logistics! Imagine getting cooperation from such a diverse group. Well, the WHO was undaunted, and Ross Wilson of Australia agreed to take it on and attempt to recreate the MPS in these unpromising environments.

The objectives of the study were to assess the frequency and nature of adverse events in patients in developing or transitional economies and to determine whether the established method for review of records would work in resource poor health-care systems in which medical records might be less comprehensive.

Ten Ministries of Health initially volunteered, but two later withdrew in the face of objections from hospital leaders who feared damage to their reputations. The eight countries that participated were Egypt, Jordan, Kenya, Morocco, Tunisia, Sudan, South Africa, and Yemen. The WHO appropriated $30,000 for each country to conduct the study, a retrospective review of randomly selected medical records from hospital admissions during 2005 in a convenience sample of 26 hospitals. These Middle Eastern and African countries had a combined population of nearly 265 million, about a third of whom lived below the poverty line. The average health expenditure was $133 per person.

The research team used the Medical Practice Study approach in which records are screened using 18 explicit criteria, followed by review of those records that screened positive by a senior physician who would determine if there were an adverse event and evaluate its preventability and resulting disability.

Of the 15,548 records reviewed, 8.2% showed at least 1 adverse event (range 2.5—18.4% by country), of which 83% were judged to be preventable and 30% were associated with death of the patient. About 34% of these adverse events were from therapeutic errors in relatively non-complex clinical situation [8].

Disturbing as these results were, they were undoubtedly underestimates because of poor record keeping in the hospitals. Nursing notes, pathology reports, and procedure notes were not available in some countries. Many hospitals started a new record each time a patient presented, so earlier clinical information was not available, limiting the rate of positives in the primary review.

Further, because the results came from a "convenience sample," i.e., hospitals that volunteered to participate, not ones that were randomly chosen, the data cannot be used to estimate national rates for the studied countries. In addition, research teams noted that some of the hospitals that volunteered were those that were generally regarded as providing some of the best care in that country. Thus, the overall national injury rates were undoubtedly higher.

Like their American predecessors years before in the Medical Practice Study, reviewers had difficulty recognizing systems problems such as lack of availability of information or equipment, bad protocols, poor hand hygiene, etc. Most events were attributed to inadequate training and supervision of clinical staff or to the failure to follow policies or protocols.

Nonetheless, some important conclusions could be drawn. The authors concluded that the problem of unnecessary harm "will not be solved only by providing more staff and equipment, even if that were immediately possible. Basic clinical processes of diagnosis and treat-ment need broad attention, aided by the provision of clinical policies and protocols standardized on best practice and supervised in their implementation." [8]

Despite its limitations, the study accomplished its objective of arousing awareness of the extent of medical harm. It undoubtedly made them more receptive to doing something about it. For that, the Alliance had a plan: a global patient safety challenge.

The Global Patient Safety Challenge

Liam Donaldson's purpose in setting up the World Alliance was to advance patient safety globally, to get all countries involved. The Global Patient Safety Challenge was the action area to make that hap-pen. The idea was to identify a significant universal safety problem and then catalyze worldwide commitment by policy makers, health-care workers, and patients to implement a safe practice that would address that problem and significantly reduce harm.

It was, to say the least, ambitious! There were only two criteria for selecting the practice, but they were formidable: it had to be a practice that would have a measurable impact on safety, and it must be possi-ble to implement the practice worldwide—in all environments, from rural clinics in developing countries to sophisticated modern aca-demic medical centers in Western cities.

The first Global Patient Safety Challenge fits the bill. It focused on preventing health-care-associated infections. It was led by Didier Pettit, an epidemiologist from the University of Geneva. The cam-paign was launched at WHO Headquarters in Geneva Switzerland in October 2005 and titled "Clean Care is Safer Care." Ministers of health from all WHO Member States were called on "to make a for-mal statement pledging to tackle health care-associated infection within their country." [9] To "catalyse and sustain strong and visible leadership and stewardship by government, health authorities and professionals, and minimize complacency" [10].

They were asked to do that by improving hand hygiene (washing or disinfecting your hands before touching a patient). Pettit had brought together over 200 leading specialists in infection prevention and patient safety. They decided that improving hand hygiene could be a powerful and feasible intervention. They developed the safe practice, *Guidelines on Hand Hygiene in Health Care* [11], and a plan for worldwide adoption.

Expert task forces addressed critical implementation topics, such as strategies to promote greater patient involvement and global implementation of the disinfectant. They developed indications for glove use and reuse and addressed the religious, cultural, and behavioral aspects of hand hygiene [12].

Then the specialists took the crucial step that would make hand disinfection possible in low-resource environments: they found an inexpensive way to make a disinfectant for dipping hands which could be readily produced anywhere.

In 2007 and 2008, the Challenge team pilot tested the new hand hygiene guidelines at 6 pilot sites involving 43 hospitals in Costa Rica, Italy, Mali, Pakistan, and Saudi Arabia [13]. Compliance increased overall from 51.0% before the intervention to 67.2% after.

Significant improvement of hand-hygiene compliance was seen in all sites, across all professional categories, and for all indications for hand hygiene. It was greater in low-income and middle-income countries, which had lower compliance rates before the study. Improvement was sustained: 2 years after the intervention, all sites reported

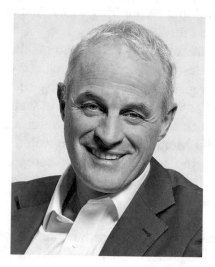

Didier Pettit. (All rights reserved)

continuing or further improvement, including in some cases national scale-up.

Subsequently, over 50 countries ran successful hand hygiene national campaigns, and almost 20,000 health facilities in 177 countries eventually joined the campaign. The need for supporting infection prevention and control improvement was clear. *Clean Care is Safer Care* generated so much momentum and so great a sense of solidarity across the world that it led the WHO to institute a new, formalized infection prevention and control global unit. That unit is still active 10 years after the launch, renewing engagement of thousands of health workers around hand hygiene every year on May 5.

The Alliance Challenge also motivated health organizations in the West. The nationwide movement to improve hand hygiene in American hospitals has been the most successful patient safety initiative. Compliance rates now approach 100% in many hospitals.

The first Global Patient Safety Challenge represented a proven change model that mobilized the world around infection prevention through: (a) awareness-raising about the burden of the problem to engage stakeholders, (b) an approach to engage nations through demonstrable commitment, and (c) the availability of evidence-based guidance and implementation tools to drive improvement.

The second Global Patient Safety Challenge also had a big impact. It tackled surgical safety and resulted in the development of the surgical checklist. That is a more complicated story and is told in the next chapter.

Later Years

Despite the considerable success of these programs, by 2008 the World Alliance was merged into the WHO's mainstream management structure. While this strengthened its authority in relation to Member States and their health systems, the free-thinking and freewheeling style of the World Alliance was lost. This slowed its pace and meant that ideas and actions were subjected to scrutiny within the WHO's governance structure that sometimes had a stultifying effect. In addition, not unlike within the NHS in Britain, there were periods of reorganization within the WHO that created uncertainty in patient safety leadership.

Fortunately, Donaldson remained in his external advisory role as WHO Patient Safety Envoy and helped to build a powerful second phase to the global patient safety program. This included starting a third WHO Global Patient Safety Challenge, currently underway, *Medication Without Harm*, to address the widespread systems problems in medication processes everywhere [14].

Medication Without Harm asks all WHO Member States and professional bodies to commit to reducing severe avoidable medication-related harm by 50% globally within 5 years by taking action to manage medication safety in three areas: high-risk situations, polypharmacy, and transitions of care [15]. Hopefully, it will have an effect similar to its highly successful predecessors.

In 2019, the World Health Assembly adopted a fresh resolution on patient safety: WHA 72.6, *Global Action on Patient Safety*. This secured the future of patient safety as a global health priority for the next 10 years, ensuring that it would not succumb to further organizational change or the whim of new leadership [16].

Conclusion

The World Alliance for Patient Safety had a huge impact on reducing medical harm worldwide. It represented the WHO at its best: a catalyst for change that also provides practical expertise and financial support for those in need. The Global Patient Safety Challenges have saved millions of lives, not just in developing countries but also in Western countries with sophisticated health-care systems. They have stimulated other efforts such as practices to reduce maternal mortality in childbirth.

The Alliance and WHO's continuing programs in patient safety have also "changed the conversation" worldwide. Victims of health-care harm and their families now have a voice and are being heard. Preventing harm by changing systems is not just a theory, it saves lives. Even in situations with very limited resources, it is possible to make changes that make a difference. The patient safety experience provides insight into what the United Nations can do when nations pull together. An important lesson in these troubled times.

Appendix 14.1: The London Declaration

We, Patients for Patient Safety, envision a different world in which health-care errors are not harming people. We are partners in the effort to prevent all avoidable harm in health care. Risk and uncertainty are constant companions. So we come together in dialogue, participating in care with providers. We unite our strength as advocates for care without harm in the developing as well as the developed world.

We are committed to spread the word from person to person, town to town, country to country. There is a right to safe health care, and we will not let the current culture of error and denial continue. We call for honesty, openness, and transparency. We will make the reduction of health-care errors a basic human right that preserves life around the world.

We, Patients for Patient Safety, will be the voice for all people, but especially those who are now unheard. Together as partners, we will collaborate in:

- Devising and promoting programs for patient safety and patient empowerment
- Developing and driving a constructive dialogue with all partners concerned with patient safety
- Establishing systems for reporting and dealing with health-care harm on a worldwide basis
- Defining best practices in dealing with health-care harm of all kinds and promoting those practices throughout the world

In honor of those who have died, those left disabled, our loved ones today, and the world's children yet to be born, we will strive for excellence, so that all those involved in health care are as safe as possible as soon as possible. This is our pledge of partnership.

References

1. World Health Assembly. WHA55.18 quality of care: patient safety. Geneva: World Health Organization; 2002.
2. WHO welcomes key United Kingdom support for global patient safety Spress release]. London/Geneva: World Health Organization; 2005.

3. Leape LL. Reporting of adverse events. N Engl J Med. 2002;347(20):1633–8.
4. Leape LL, Abookire SWHO. Draft guidelines for adverse event reporting and learning systems: from information to action. Geneva: World Health Organization; 2005.
5. Vincent C, Pincus T, Scurr J. Patients' experience of surgical accidents. Qual Health Care. 1993;2:77–82.
6. Patients for Patient Safety: What's New? World Health Organization. https://www.who.int/patientsafety/patients_for_patient/en/. Accessed 19 Apr 2020.
7. Bates DW, Larizgoitia I, Prasopa-Plaizier N, Jha AK. Global priorities for patient safety research. BMJ. 2009;338:b1775.
8. Wilson R, Michel P, Olsen S, et al. Patient safety in developing countries: retrospective estimation of scale and nature of harm to patients in hospital. BMJ. 2012;344:e832.
9. Support from WHO Member States and autonomous areas: pledges to combat health care-associated infections. World Health Organization. https://www.who.int/gpsc/statements/en/. Accessed 19 Apr 2020.
10. World Health Alliance for Patient Safety. Global patient safety challenge: 2005–2006. Geneva: World Health Organization; 2005.
11. WHO Guidelines on Hand Hygiene in Health Care: First Global Patient Safety Challenge, Clean Care is Safer Care. Geneva: World Health Organization;2009.
12. Pittet D, Allegranzi B, Sax H, et al. Evidence-based model for hand transmission during patient care and the role of improved practices. Lancet Infect Dis. 2006;6(10):641–52.
13. Allegranzi B, Storr J, Dziekan G, Leotsakos A, Donaldson L, Pittet D. The first global patient safety challenge "clean care is safer care": from launch to current progress and achievements. J Hosp Infect. 2007;65(Suppl 2):115–23.
14. Donaldson LJ, Kelley ET, Dhingra-Kumar N, Kieny M-P, Sheikh A. Medication without harm: WHO's third global patient safety challenge. Lancet. 2017;389(10080):1680–1.
15. The Third WHO Global Patient Safety Challenge: Medication Without Harm. World Health Organization. https://www.who.int/patientsafety/medication-safety/en/. Accessed 21 Apr 2020.
16. World Health Assembly. WHA72.6 global action on patient safety. Geneva: World Health Organization; 2019.

Chapter 15
Just Do It: The Surgical Checklist

For the second Global Patient Safety Challenge, the WHO chose making surgery safer. My involvement was minor. One day, a year or so after the hand hygiene program started, I received a call from Pauline Kelly, my friend from the Reporting Guidelines project. The World Alliance leaders had decided to do a Patient Safety Challenge on a surgical topic. This made good sense, since surgical mishaps were well recognized as a major cause of mortality worldwide. Nearly half of all AEs discovered in the Medical Practice Study were related to a surgical operation. She asked me if I thought Atul Gawande would be willing to lead it.

My immediate reaction was that it was unlikely. By then, by virtue of his insightful New Yorker articles and his first highly successful books *Complications* and *Better*, Atul was already a celebrity and very much in demand. In addition, he was establishing a center for patient safety research and still practicing surgery. He was a very busy man. But, no harm in asking him, I said. If he would do it, it would be a very successful project.

The topic, safe surgery, was certainly an appropriate global public health problem. Nearly 300 million surgical operations are performed annually around the world. In industrialized countries the rate of major complications has been estimated at 3–16% of surgical procedures, with a death rate of 0.4–0.8% [1, 2].

Studies in developing countries suggest a much higher death rate of 5–10%. This translates to an estimate that 7 million surgical patients

© The Author(s) 2021
L. L. Leape, *Making Healthcare Safe*,
https://doi.org/10.1007/978-3-030-71123-8_15

suffer significant complications each year and 1 million die. Approximately half of these appear to be avoidable [1]. Surgical mortality is 10–100 times higher than maternal mortality from childbirth.

A week or so after my phone call from the WHO, Atul walked into my office. "WHO wants me to do a Global Patient Safety Challenge on a surgical problem. What do you think?" (This is encouraging, I thought: he is willing to consider it!) Well, I said, recalling the reporting guidelines experience, the WHO is very bureaucratic, so working with them can be frustrating at times. On the other hand, they are serious about safety, and if you succeeded in developing an effective intervention it could improve the care of millions of patients around the globe. If you can put up with the grief, you could make an important contribution. He said he would think it over.

To WHO's and my delight, and the world's benefit, Atul decided to take it on. In January 2007, the Safe Surgery Saves Lives initiative began. Atul assembled a team that compiled a background document of safety practices with known benefits to surgical patients. The document established targets for improvement and the specific practices necessary to achieve these targets [3].

An international group of nearly 100 experts was then convened to review the background document and suggest additional topics to be considered. This group included surgeons, anesthesiologists, nurses,

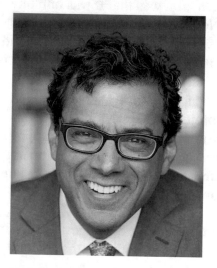

Atul Gawande.

patients, experts in infectious disease, engineers, and organizational leaders who represented the range of practice environments around the world, from primitive developing countries, such as Ghana and Mongolia, to Western democracies, such as New Zealand and the USA.

They identified four areas of potential improvement in surgical safety: surgical site infection prevention, safe anesthesia, safe surgical teams, and measurement of surgical services. They decided to implement a surgical checklist.

The idea of using a checklist to reduce harm was not new. Commercial aviation had used them for years, and Peter Pronovost had recently brought the term to national attention with his pathbreaking work eliminating central line infections [4]. Nor was the concept of a surgical checklist unprecedented. It had been tried with some success at Columbus Children's Hospital, the University of Toronto, Johns Hopkins, and by Kaiser hospitals in southern California [5] and in Australia [6].

The checklist built on another idea that was catching on in the USA to avoid wrong-site and wrong-patient errors: a "time out" at beginning of an operation. In 2004, the Joint Commission launched its Universal Protocol for Preventing Wrong Site, Wrong Procedure, Wrong Person Surgery. It comprised three sets of steps: preoperative verifications, marking the operative site, and a "time out" immediately before the operation.

As the Safe Surgery Saves Lives checklist was developed, each potential step was carefully considered by the international group, and each draft checklist was subjected to a trial by a clinical team. Issues with logistics, timing, and team interactions were worked out, and confusing language was clarified. It was then trialled in a variety of other settings.

Expert working groups were also created to review the available scientific evidence and write a supporting document, *Guidelines for Safe Surgery*, which the WHO issued in 2009 [7]. It focused on critical steps that should be universally followed, such as making sure it is the right patient, having blood available if needed, and briefing the team. And, consistent with the WHO mandate, these were practices that could be implemented in any operating room regardless of the sophistication of the environment.

It's not that simple, of course. The "checklist" they devised is a series of steps to be taken at three critical junctures in care: before anesthesia is administered, immediately before incision, and before the patient is taken out of the operating room. Success at implementing these steps depends on full participation of every member of the team, especially the surgeon.

Before induction of anesthesia, members of the team orally confirm the surgical site and procedure and that the patient has verified his or her identity and has given consent. The team confirms that the surgical site is marked, the pulse oximeter is on, and that all members of the team are aware of the patient's allergies. If there is a risk of blood loss of 500 ml or more, appropriate access and fluids are available.

Before skin incision, the entire team (nurses, surgeons, anesthesia professionals, and all others participating in the care of the patient) orally confirms that all team members have been introduced by name and role and reconfirms the patient's identity, surgical site, and procedure. The surgeon reviews critical and unexpected steps, operative duration, and anticipated blood loss. The anesthesia staff reviews concerns specific to the patient and confirms that prophylactic antibiotics have been administered if indicated. The nursing staff reviews confirmation of sterility, equipment availability, and other concerns. The team confirms that all essential imaging results for the correct patient are displayed in the operating room.

Finally, in the third stage, before the patient leaves the operating room, the nurse reviews aloud with the team the name of the procedure; that the needle, sponge, and instrument counts are complete; that any specimen is correctly labeled; and whether there are any issues with equipment to be addressed. The surgeon, nurse, and anesthetist review aloud the key concerns for the recovery and care of the patient.

The use of the checklist was tested in eight hospitals in eight cities (Toronto, Canada; New Delhi, India; Amman, Jordan; Auckland, New Zealand; Manila, Philippines; Ifakara, Tanzania; London, England; and Seattle, WA) chosen to represent a range of economic circumstances and diverse populations. Data was collected from 3733 patients before and 3955 patients after the implementation of the checklist [8].

The results showed that the rate of any complication at all sites dropped by 36%, from 11.0% at baseline to 7.0% after introduction of the checklist; the total in-hospital mortality dropped 47%, from 1.5% to 0.8%. The overall rates of surgical-site infection and unplanned reoperation also declined significantly. Interestingly, ensuring the correct identity of the patient and site through preoperative site marking and oral confirmation was new to most of the study hospitals.

The results made headlines. To the average person it just made sense. Of course, you would want to be sure you were operating on the right person and doing the right operation. Of course, you would introduce yourself to all the members of the team. If use of the checklist can reduce surgical mortality by 47%, then why wouldn't all hospitals start using it immediately?

The WHO agreed. On January 14, 2009, the checklist was made public, and the WHO launched the *Second Global Patient Safety Challenge: Safe Surgery Saves Lives* with the aim of persuading hospitals everywhere to adopt the checklist. Its use was mandated or strongly encouraged by several governments, including those of the UK and the Netherlands [9]. By the end of 2009, the surgical checklist was being used in 10% of American hospitals and over 2000 hospitals worldwide [5]. In 2017, the WHO reported that the checklist was being used by a majority of surgical service providers around the world [10].

Reports appeared documenting the results of implementing the checklist. There were some impressive successes [11–15]. The Veterans Health Administration provided extensive training and staged implementation and demonstrated an 18% decrease in mortality after 1 year [12]. In the Netherlands, six high-performing hospitals showed reductions of 39% in complications and 48% in mortality [11]. In the UK, results were mixed, but generally positive [16]. A 2013 meta-analysis of seven controlled studies of checklist implementation showed a 41% reduction in complications and a 23% decrease in mortality [17].

But some studies showed little or no effect. Strangely, the point of some reports seemed to be to prove that it was a bad idea [18]. Compliance was a problem everywhere, especially by surgeons. Use of the checklist was not turning out to have the impact that the initial study indicated was possible.

The reasons were not obscure. Implementing the surgical checklist is not nearly as simple as it seems on the surface. The issue is not the technical challenge of getting people to tick off boxes on a list, but the social challenge of changing human behavior [9]. And the checklist represented a major change in how everyone in the operating room functioned. The successful implementation by Peter Pronovost of a checklist to prevent CLABSI was far simpler. It dealt with a single established procedure and far fewer participants, but even doing that was difficult [19].

As quality improvement specialists know, the crucial element in implementing a new safe practice is teamwork. All stakeholders have to be involved in the process change for it to work. Unfortunately, this was still a relatively foreign concept among physicians, especially surgeons, whose definition of a good team was often having assistants who knew what to do and did what they were told to do.

Getting people to be good team players has been the biggest challenge for improving patient safety overall. The surgical checklist put that idea front and center. Successful hospitals implemented it in the way it was intended: as a set of reminders carried out by a team that worked together to prevent errors. They had the will to succeed and leadership at the top and at the team level.

In a 2015 retrospective analysis, Haynes et al. noted several other elements that were crucial to success [20]. First, the checklist must be modified by the local team to meet its needs. Although the authors stressed this in the initial report, it was typically ignored by teams that failed. They didn't make it *their* checklist. They didn't take ownership of the checklist. As a result, they felt that it was something they *had* to do, not something they *wanted* to do.

Second, because the changes called for are extensive, implementation of a checklist should be started on a small scale to work out remaining kinks in the process. This pilot process also uncovers "champions," the respected local surgeons who are key to success of the full rollout.

Third, training sessions are required for all participants to enable them to understand and become comfortable with the new ways. Successful programs typically devoted months to training prior to beginning the implementation. Fourth, the implementation team regularly observed the use of the checklist in practice and provided and received feedback from the clinicians [20].

Most hospitals need help to implement the checklist. They lack the resources and expertise to lead the effort and build teams. As shown by the experience with the Massachusetts Coalition implementation of reconciling medications and communicating critical test results (see Chap. 8) and Peter Pronovost's work implementing a checklist to eliminate central line infections, statewide or system-wide collaboratives are effective ways to provide local teams with direction, coaching, and the opportunity to learn from each other [9].

The barriers to implementation of the checklist—the causes of failure—are largely social. The most common has been resistance by surgeons who were loath to give up their hallowed role as "captain of the ship." Most thought they already had a good team and were not keen about involving others. Some felt that use of memory aids is an admission of weakness or lack of skill or knowledge, others that standardization is a limit to their clinical judgment [21]. Some gave dismissive answers to queries and complained that the process delayed the operation (although the checklist can be completed in 2 minutes); some just refused to participate [22].

Self-introductions were awkward for surgeons, and for other members of the surgical team, as was speaking up. In a system with a long tradition of steep interpersonal hierarchy, it was contrary to their concepts of their roles and what they had been taught. So, when surgeons pushed back, few resisted. Some had a fear of legal responsibility if a complication occurred after they had signed a form. But the biggest change required was in the surgeon's behavior.

A year or two after the checklist was in use, I asked Atul how it was going. He was pleased with the national uptake, he said, although he was concerned that in too many operating rooms surgeons still weren't on board. Too often it was left to the nurse to check the boxes, just one more thing they were required to do.

"Do you know what part of the checklist surgeons find hardest to do?" he said. "Asking all the member of the team to introduce themselves." This step is crucial to the fundamental point of the checklist: converting the many participants in the operating room into a team that worked well together, supported one another, and in which each individual felt personal responsibility for the patient and making sure everything went right.

I was not surprised. In my 27-year surgical career, I had never done that. Nor had any other surgeon I knew. I thought I had a great team: my scrub nurse and circulating nurse had been with me for years, and we worked well together and enjoyed each other. Our several pediatric anesthetists were good friends of mine, and we worked well together with few conflicts. But I never paid any attention to those other people in the operating room who were assisting the nurses or anesthetists, running for blood, getting more instruments, etc.

The idea of involving them in the operation, much less expecting others to take responsibility for my doing the right operation on the right patient, never occurred to me, nor to any of my colleagues. If the idea had come up, we would have rejected it. We were, after all, the "captain of the ship," and it was everyone else's job to do our bidding.

For example, over my years as a pediatric surgeon I performed hundreds of inguinal hernia repairs in children. I was sure that one day I would operate on the wrong side. I really worried about that. It never occurred to me to share that worry with others of the team or ask them to help me make sure it didn't happen. It never did happen, but that was just good luck.

The surgical checklist changed all of that. If the team took it seriously, if they could indeed function as a team, then everything that takes place in the operating room is everyone's responsibility. Clearly, having many eyes on the question of right patient, right operation, right site makes a difference. It takes a team to make care safe. The checklist is a tool that can make that happen.

Conclusion

The surgical checklist story is in many ways the story of patient safety. It is built on a practice borrowed from other industries, notably aviation, where its effectiveness in preventing errors is well-established. It derives its power from its theoretical basis—the human factor principle of avoiding reliance on memory—and from its practical effect: reinforcing teamwork that is essential for safe practice. Thanks to the work of Gawande and others, it has been successfully adapted for use in health care. When used properly, as in the VA, the Netherlands, and Scotland, the surgical checklist is a powerful tool for reducing harm and mortality.

But using the surgical checklist properly has been an immense challenge. Requiring that it be used has not generally been a successful strategy. The system is too easily gamed. If the surgeon is not on board, it is easy to go through the motions and have the nurse ensure that all the boxes are ticked. The larger point of the checklist—to encourage a conversation about important practices and empower all members of the team to take responsibility—is lost.

Teamwork is the heart of successful voluntary adoption of the surgical checklist. Developing meaningful teams is also arguably the most fundamental culture change needed overall to make health care safe. As noted in earlier chapters, major efforts in team training and reinforcement of teamwork in collaboratives have yielded impressive improvements, including the implementation of the surgical checklist, but we still have a long way to go. For now, the surgical checklist, like all of patient safety, is still a work in progress.

References

1. Weiser TG, Regenbogen SE, Thompson KD, et al. An estimation of the global volume of surgery: a modelling strategy based on available data. Lancet. 2008;372:139–44.
2. Kable AK, Gibberd RW, Spigelman AD. Adverse events in surgical patients in Australia. Int J Qual Health Care. 2002;14:269–76.
3. Weiser TG, Haynes AB, Lashoher A, et al. Perspectives in quality: designing the WHO surgical safety checklist. Int J Qual Health Care. 2010;22:365–70.
4. Berenholtz S, Pronovost PJ, Lipsett PA, et al. Eliminating catheter-related bloodstream infections in the intensive care unit. Crit Care Med. 2004;32:2014–20.
5. Gawande A. The checklist manifesto: how to get things right. 1st ed. New York: Metropolitan Books; 2010.
6. Wolff AM, Taylor SA, McCabe JF. Using checklists and reminders in clinical pathways to improve hospital inpatient care. Med J Aust. 2004;181:428–31.
7. World Health Organization. WHO guidelines for safe surgery: safe surgery saves lives. Geneva: World Health Organization; 2009.
8. Haynes AB, Weiser TG, Berry WR, et al. A surgical safety checklist to reduce morbidity and morality in a global population. NEJM. 2009;360:491–9.
9. Leape LL. The checklist conundrum. N Engl J Med. 2014;370:1063–4.
10. Safety P. WHO surgical safety checklist. Inte Arch. 2014. Accessed 30 Apr 2020, at https://web.archive.org/web/20141008162408/https://www.who.int/patientsafety/safesurgery/checklist/en/.
11. von Klei WAHR, van Aarnhem EEHL, et al. Effects of the introduction of the WHO "surgical safety checklist" on in-hospital mortality. Ann Surg. 2012;255:44–9.

12. Neily J, Mills PD, Young-Xu Y, et al. Association between implementation of a medical team training program and surgical mortality. JAMA. 2010;304:1693–700.
13. de Vries E, Hollmann M, Smorenburg SM, Gouma D, Boermeester MA. Development and validation of the SURgical PAtient Safety System (SURPASS) checklist. Qual Saf Health Care. 2009;18:121–6.
14. Weiser GT, Haynes BA, Dziekan RG, Berry RW, Lipsitz AS, Gawande AA. Effect of a 19-item surgical safety checklist during urgent operations in a global patient population. Ann Surg. 2010;251:976–80.
15. Scotland NHS. Healthcare quality strategy for NHSScotland. The Scottish Government: Edinburgh; 2010.
16. Pickering SPRE, Griffin D, et al. Compliance and use of the World Health Organization checklist in UK operating theatres. Brit J Surg. 2013;100:1664–70.
17. Bergs J, Hellings J, Cleemput I, et al. Systematic review and meta-analysis of the effect of the World Health Organization surgical safety checklist on postoperative complications. Chichester: Wiley; 2014. p. 150–8.
18. Urbach D GA, Saskin R, et al. Introduction of surgical safety checklists in Ontario. NEJM; 2014.
19. Dixon-Woods M, Bosk CL, Aveling EL, et al. Explaining Michigan: developing an ex post theory of a quality improvement program. Milbank Qtrly. 2011;89:167–205.
20. Haynes BA, Berry RW, Gawande AA. What do we know about the safe surgery checklist now? Ann Surg. 2015;261:829–30.
21. Fourcade A, Blache J-L, Grenier C, Bourgain J-L, Minvielle E. Barriers to staff adoption of a surgical safety checklist. BMJ Qual Saf. 2012;21:191–7.
22. Vats A, Vincent CA, Nagpal K, Davies RW, Darzi A, Moorthy K. Practical challenges of introducing WHO surgical checklist: UK pilot experience. BMJ. 2010;340:b5433.

Chapter 16
Spreading the Word: The Salzburg Seminar

Salzburg! The name conjures up images of the annual world-famous Salzburg Festival and *The Sound of Music*, with its magnificent castle and the glorious singing of Julie Andrews. The birthplace of the divine Mozart.

What is less well known about this charming city is that it is also the home of The Salzburg Global Seminars, the "home to change makers" since 1947. Founded to bring participants together from around the world for weeklong meetings to explore a single subject, the Salzburg Global Seminar is an independent not-for-profit organization. (See Appendix 16.1 for the intriguing history of how the seminars came into being in the years immediately following WWII.)

The seminars are a mix of lectures, discussions, workshops, papers, and presentations held at Schloss Leopoldskron—the "Sound of Music" palace—an idyllic and secluded spot conducive to thought and insight.

In April of 2001, the Salzburg Seminar, *Patient Safety and Medical Error*, Session 386, became a reference point in the history of patient safety through the seminar on medical error.

This chapter is brief, but it illustrates how a single event—a weeklong intensive interaction on a single subject—can raise people's consciousness, alter their beliefs, and, in some cases, change their careers. All that happened at Salzburg in 2001 as the patient safety movement was getting underway.

© The Author(s) 2021
L. L. Leape, *Making Healthcare Safe*,
https://doi.org/10.1007/978-3-030-71123-8_16

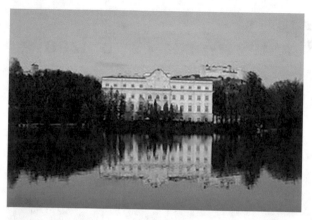

Schloss Leopoldskron. (Reprinted with permission from Salzburg Global Seminar. All rights reserved)

As with many things in quality and safety, having a Salzburg Seminar on medical error was Don Berwick's idea. He had attended an earlier one in 1998 organized by Tom Delbanco, *Through the Patient's Eyes: Collaboration between Patients and Health Care Professionals*, and thought it would be an ideal way to move thinking ahead in patient safety. I thought it was a splendid idea! Fortunately, others did too, and we were able to secure funding and attract a stellar faculty to plan the event.

Our announcement for the session was ambitious:

The Seminar is "intended to provide a forum for an exploration of possible scenarios for making medical facilities safer places for work and for care. To this end, the session will examine the causes, consequences, and methods of improvement of patient safety, with particular emphasis on the American and European experience.

Among the issues to be addressed: the sociologic and technical characteristics of medical care, and the systems that allow them to function as high reliability organizations; the role of effective cooperation, communication, and mutual support among the healthcare providers, the role of the patient in the healthcare process; the influence of individual human factors in healthcare delivery, such as professional training, psychological and physical stress, and principles of designing systems for safety.

The session will seek to bring together a diverse group of individuals involved in various aspects of the medical process, including administrators, healthcare workers, representatives from regulatory agencies, as well as specialists in the field of safety."

The timing proved to be felicitous. The BMJ special edition on medical error the previous year got worldwide attention, bringing the issue to the forefront for the first time for many people. We attracted 62 participants ("Fellows") from 28 countries, including more than a third from non-western countries: Argentina, Armenia, Bulgaria, China, Egypt, India, Israel, Japan, Kenya, Malta, Mexico, Palestine, Philippines, Romania, Russia, South Africa, Sudan, Turkey, and Zimbabwe (Appendix 16.2).

The Fellows varied widely in their knowledge and experience. The environments from which they came and to which they would return spanned the spectrum of awareness and opportunity. But we all had one thing in common: in all countries, the response to an error was to blame the individual. That was a common language we all understood, and that was what we wanted to change.

Our faculty was from "central casting": the recognized thought leaders Jim Reason and Charles Vincent from the UK, safety guru Rene Amalberti from France, Tom Nolan from Associates in Process Improvement, Maureen Bisognano from IHI, Richard Cook from the University of Chicago, Don, and I. We took turns giving talks in the mornings followed by plenary discussions. The major work occurred in four working groups to which participants were assigned. They met in the afternoons for discussions moderated by the faculty.

The four working groups took on separate major challenges to making health care safe: Leadership and Culture Change; Education, Training and Supervision; Personal and Organizational Accountability;

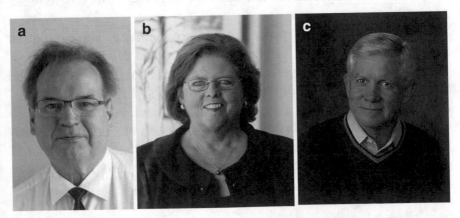

(a) Rene Amalberti, (b) Maureen Bisognano, and (c) Tom Nolan. (All rights reserved)

and Design of Process and Systems. Interspersed in the afternoon sessions were occasional breaks, but we worked most of most days and continued discussions informally in the evenings.

Another important feature of the Seminar was a series of informal presentations by Fellows on subjects for which they had special expertise or experience. Eleven in all, these included regulation, working with consumer advocates, partnering with patients, sleep deprivation and working hours, reporting systems, improving safety in resource-constrained environments, and national funding of safety research.

On the first day, Richard Cook suggested to the faculty that we stimulate the workshop conversations by giving participants a simulation exercise in the form of a "news flash" about a serious situation: a tragic preventable death in their hospital that was published in a local paper's headline above the fold. The Working Groups were instructed to take on the role of C-Suite and Board to discuss their response.

The "news flash" came in the evening. The next day the teams were to make decisions about how they would respond, what their roles were, what they would say, and who would be the best spokesperson within the organization and to the public. Each evening, Richard would tighten the constraint by issuing ongoing press releases of more sensational and damaging speculations and actual findings about the event.

The simulation surfaced a number of issues: just how difficult it was to talk about failure, the state of transparency, accountability, fear of litigation, defensiveness of organizational reputation and assets, the role of the media and the public's right to know, responsibility to the patient's family, and the relationships between family, care team, and hospital.

For some Fellows, this proved to be overwhelming. The simulation succeeded in getting them to begin to understand the complexities of responding to disastrous errors, but how to respond was beyond the capacity of the majority of this diverse group of participants. Most of them were just beginning to think about patient safety and had no experience in dealing with complex issues or failures. For them, it was too intense and emotionally charged. It pushed them into a zone of discomfort and distracted them from what they came to the seminar to accomplish. We stopped the exercise on the third day.

The Working Groups benefited greatly from the diversity of the backgrounds of the participants. Some were experienced and had worked for some time in quality improvement and safety. For others, it was all new. For all, the discussions were deeper—and longer—than any they had previously experienced. The insights and lessons learned were shared with the entire group in the final session of the week when each of the working groups presented their conclusions.

The Seminar had a substantial impact. In large measure it accomplished our objectives of expanding the understanding of patient safety and motivating leaders to advance the cause. It was an incredibly rich and mind-stretching experience in which everyone, faculty and students, learned a great deal and were motivated to work harder—and smarter—to reduce harm.

For many Fellows, it was a generative experience: they left with new lenses through which to view medical error, new ideas for change, and, for many, new commitment to the cause. They began to envision a world in which we stop blaming people for making mistakes and focus on designing sustainable systems to prevent medical error from harming patients.

A number of Fellows, such as Beth Pedersen Lilja of Denmark, Kristoff Viet of Germany, and Julie Morath, Tejal Gandhi, Allan Frankel, and Peter Pronovost of the USA, went on to become leaders who had a significant impact on patient safety. The Salzburg Seminar proved to be a defining experience, referred to years later with much affection.

Appendix 16.1: History of the Salzburg Global Seminars

The *Seminar* was the brainchild of Clemens Heller, a native Austrian attending graduate school at Harvard, who, in aftermath of World War II in 1946, "envisioned a cultural bridge spanning the Atlantic not only by introducing the demoralized Europeans to all sorts of American cultural achievements, but also by stimulating a fruitful exchange between European national cultures and America."

Harvard was unwilling to support the project, but Heller and several friends convinced the Harvard Student Council to be the official sponsor of the Seminar, raised the majority of funds, and obtained permission from the State Department for entrance into Allied Occupied Austria.

By great good fortune, Heller shortly afterward bumped into a friend of his parents, Helene Thimig, the widow of theater producer Max Reinhardt, who owned a summer home in Salzburg named Schloss Leopoldskron. Thimig agreed to rent them the Schloss for the purpose of a summer school.

The Schloss was built in 1736 by Count Leopold von Firmian, Prince-Archbishop of Salzburg. It remained in the possession of the Firmian family until 1837 and then passed through several owners until it was bought in 1918 by Reinhardt, who cofounded the Salzburg Festival. During World War II, the Schloss was confiscated as Jewish property, but after the war it was returned to the Reinhardt Estate.

The first session, officially called "The Harvard Student Council's Salzburg Seminar in American Civilization," lasted 6 weeks in the summer of 1947 and brought together men and women from 18 countries, including countries from behind the Iron Curtain. Faculty included anthropologist, Margaret Mead, economists Walt Rostow and Wassily Leontief, writer and literary critic Alfred Kazin, and others.

The Seminar was formally incorporated on April 20, 1950, by which time it had developed into more than a summer school, and session topics were expanded beyond American Studies. It acquired Schloss Leopoldskron in 1959 [1].

Appendix 16.2: Participants in Salzburg Seminar 386 Patient Safety and Medical Error

Working Group A
LEADERSHIP AND CULTURE CHANGE
(Maureen Bisognano and René Amalberti)

- Ross Baker (Canada)
- James Battles (USA)
- Ahmed Bayoumi (Sudan)
- Jocelyn Cornwell (UK)
- Sally Goebel (USA)
- Erik Jylling (Denmark)
- Harold Kaplan (USA)
- Mariana Lerner (Israel)

- Raymond Mayewski (USA)
- Nagui Mikhail (Egypt)
- Leonard Miron (Romania)
- Julianne Morath (USA)
- Norman Nyazema (Zimbabwe)
- Beth Pedersen (Denmark)
- Peter Pronovost (USA)
- Robert Wells (Australia)
- Alma Yearwood-Dixon (USA)

Working Group B
EDUCATION, TRAINING AND SUPERVISION
(Donald Berwick and Richard Cook)

- DeWitt Baldwin (USA)
- Norberto Barrera (Argentina)
- Guttorm Bratteboe (Norway)
- Allan Frankel (USA)
- Tejal Gandhi (USA)
- Lidia Georgieva (Bulgaria)
- Sandra Huddleston (USA)
- Mauricio Lopez Ramos (Mexico)
- Karine Martirosyan (Armenia)
- Patricia Ogle (South Africa)
- Yasemin Oguz (Turkey)
- Abdalla Shehata (Egypt)
- Richard Smallwood (Australia)
- Lourdes Tejero (Philippines)
- Helfried Waleczek (Germany)

Working Group C
PERSONAL AND ORGANIZATIONAL ACCOUNTABILITY
(Lucian Leape and Charles Vincent)

- Choi Chuen Ha (China)
- Dmitri Elioutine (Russia)
- Michael Fiene (Germany)
- Andrea Gerlin (USA)
- Sven Öhman (Sweden)
- Synnöve Ödegard (Sweden)

- Amos Otedo (Kenya)
- Gajendra Singh (India)
- Anthony So (USA)
- Marianne Sørensen (Denmark)
- David Swankin (USA)
- Kathryn Townsend (USA)
- Joanne Turnbull (USA)

Working Group D
DESIGN OF PROCESS AND SYSTEMS
(Thomas Nolan and James Reason)

- Susan Abookire (USA)
- Nancy Conrad (USA)
- Douglas Eby (USA)
- Kaj Essinger (Sweden)
- Martin Fischmeister (Austria)
- Carol Haraden (USA)
- Yuichi Imanaka (Japan)
- Avi Israeli (Israel)
- Peter Kennedy (Australia)
- Ronald Kirshner (USA)
- Liu Xiaohong (China)
- Mohammed Massoud (Palestinian
- Authority)
- Vin McLoughlin (Australia)
- Josephine Sollano (USA)
- Carina Svensson (Sweden)
- Christian Thomeczek (Germany)
- Josanne Vassallo (Malta)

Reference

1. Eliot T, Lois. The Salzburg seminar: the first forty years. Ipswich: The Ipswich Press; 1987.

Chapter 17
Publish or Perish: British Medical Journal Theme Issue, New England Journal of Medicine Series

"Publish or perish!" The governing principle of academia. Trite though it may be, true it also is. At any research university—and that is where medical schools are and where those who do research in patient safety work—you do not get promoted if you don't publish.

Medical journals publish science, or at least they try to. Was this new patient safety stuff science? There were those who did not think so. It was "soft stuff"—not as bad as psychiatry, perhaps—but "touchy-feely" interpersonal stuff. It didn't seem to fit the mold of medical practice that many doctors embraced of treatment based on scientific evidence. This may have been part of the reason that the results of the Medical Practice Study were ignored when they came out, as were the recommendations in *Error in Medicine* a few years later.

In the "great awakening" of patient safety, in the post-Annenberg and pre-IOM days of patient safety when the NPSF was being formed, the Executive Session was underway, and IHI was establishing its breakthrough collaboratives, leaders of the movement were concerned that young investigators would not be able to get their work in the new science of patient safety published in leading journals where it needed to be for their academic advancement. Lacking that access would stifle innovation.

Leading American journals, NEJM and JAMA, had published the foundational papers, but little since. They and other journals still did not seem to regard this new field of patient safety as "science." NPSF had begun to fund research projects. Would the results be published?

© The Author(s) 2021
L. L. Leape, *Making Healthcare Safe*,
https://doi.org/10.1007/978-3-030-71123-8_17

The breakthrough came, interestingly, from Britain. This was not altogether surprising: the two foremost thought leaders in patient safety, James Reason and Charles Vincent, were from the UK. Reason had been a featured speaker at Annenberg. The NHS Chief Medical Officer, Liam Donaldson, was beginning his work to bring patient safety to the fore. But it was Richard Smith, editor of the British Medical Journal (BMJ), who got it moving.

It was Richard Smith, you will remember, who in 1998 wrote in response to the Bristol Inquiry, "All changed, changed utterly. British medicine will be transformed by the Bristol case" [1]. Richard was a great fan of Don Berwick and had supported the NHS's involving Don in quality improvement. Smith was intrigued by the rising interest in patient safety.

In February 1999, he invited Don and me to edit a special theme issue of BMJ on medical error. We thought it was a terrific idea!

This was big stuff. Annenberg had been exciting, but it did not lead to much movement other than the founding of the NPSF. The public and the medical profession were still largely unaware of the extent of the problem of medical error or of efforts to implement systems changes. AHRQ hadn't yet been born. Don and I were on the IOM Quality Committee, but it had not issued "The Report." Publication of patient safety papers in BMJ would get doctors' attention. We were excited.

Richard gave us full latitude to select the topics and solicit papers. He asked us to commission five articles and five editorials and issue an open solicitation for an additional four original papers and several brief reports. This was going to be a far bigger publishing effort than anything Don or I had ever been involved in.

We wrote a call for papers—an editorial in BMJ—that laid out the problem and asked for submission of papers. We provided a substantial list of potential topics and indicated that we were interested in innovative topics, as well as authors from industry and other fields in addition to health care. The editorial was published on July 17, 1999 [2].

We then wrote to those we had selected to write commissioned papers. As we anticipated, all accepted. The papers were due by November, and our chosen authors produced them in record time. As we reviewed them, it became clear that this single issue of the journal would give an impressively comprehensive look at this new field of patient safety by the people who were making it happen. It would be a reference issue.

The BMJ special issue was published on March 18, 2000 [3], just months after the release of the IOM Report. Publication was timed to coincide with the first UK national symposium on medical error organized by the British Medical Association and the National Health Service, at which Don and I also spoke.

The papers were awesome: Jim Reason (error management) [4], Saul Weingart (epidemiology) [5], Bob Helmreich (lessons from aviation) [6], David Gaba (anesthesia as a model) [7], David Bates (IT and medication errors) [8], and Tom Nolan (systems changes) [9].

In addition to the commissioned papers and editorials by Dennis O'Leary (accreditation) [10], Jim Reinertsen [11] (disclosure), Michael Cohen (voluntary reporting) [12], and Albert Wu (second victim) [13], the final issue included 13 original papers and reports.

This was the first time that a major medical journal brought together in a single-issue works by international authorities on the major concepts in patient safety and results from empirical studies. Smith gave it a real boot by putting a photograph of a crashed airliner on the cover of that issue of the staid old BMJ!

It had an enormous impact. BMJ is the primary medical journal for all of Europe and is read by many around the world. The special issue put safety on the screen for the first time for many people. At least one of my safety friends, Beth Pedersen Lilja from Copenhagen, later told me that it did that for her—and led her and others to come to the Salzburg Seminar the next year.

NEJM Series on Patient Safety

Later that year, in the fall of 2000, I drafted a letter to the editor of the New England Journal of Medicine (NEJM) asking whether they would be willing to consider publishing a series of essays on issues in patient safety. I showed it to my department chairman, Arnie Epstein, who was an Associate Editor at the NEJM. He was supportive, but he thought a more successful approach might be for him to sound out the editor in chief and the other editors and try to persuade them to take it on. The fact that a major rival, the BMJ, had devoted a special issue to patient safety might have sparked some interest.

I really wanted them to do this. Having your paper published in the NEJM is the official stamp of quality in academic medicine. The Journal has the largest circulation of any medical journal in the world and is trusted by physicians and health policy people as the most reliable source of medical information. As a result, it attracts reports of leading-edge medical research and "breakthroughs."

The IOM report brought national attention to patient safety, but it was a book, and most doctors don't have time to read books. They do read journals, though, and in the USA, the NEJM is at the top of the pile. The American readers of the BMJ Special Issue were mostly academics. This would be an opportunity to reach a broad range of doctors and policy makers and increase their awareness and understanding of the major issues in patient safety. If we did it right, patient safety papers published in the NEJM might make them more likely to accept the changes we were proposing and motivate some to join in the work. It would also, of course, spread the word around the world.

About 8 months after that conversation, I finally got the call. They were interested. Arnie and I met with Jeff Drazen, the Editor in Chief, to negotiate the deal—what the series would consist of, who decided, and how to proceed. It was a bit complicated, but we worked it out, and the Deputy Editor, Robert Steinbrook, was assigned to work with me and Arnie to come up with a proposal.

We agreed that the purpose of the series would be to explain key issues in patient safety and to stimulate interest and debate that would influence health policy. We would choose topics that were central to safety and provide fresh analysis, showing how new approaches could provide remedies. The series would include up to 12 papers, published monthly. The proposal was accepted.

The process was much more complicated than it had been with the BMJ, where Don Berwick and I were given carte blanche to pick the subjects and authors and were able to do it quickly. With the NEJM, we had to convince the editors of the worth of each subject and the competence of our chosen author to deliver. The papers would be subject to the usual lengthy review process.

I developed a list of 14 potential topics and wrote a brief on each one, outlining the issues of interest and the questions to be addressed by the paper. These would also be the instructions for the authors.

Arnie, Robert, and I had extensive discussions about whom to invite to write the papers. We read previous papers written by candidates and consulted widely with colleagues about their suitability. If the papers were to be definitive statements of the current state of the art, the authors needed to be unquestioned experts.

We recommended 12 topics to the editors. After some discussion they decided to start with 6 and later consider expanding that number. I was disappointed, but "half a loaf…." We narrowed it to six and gave the editors a brief on each one with the proposed author. They were accepted, and I invited the authors to write the papers. Fortunately, we did ultimately get 12 papers published.

The process took a year, but the series finally began in October 2002 with a bang: five papers in one issue of the Journal. The editors decided to take advantage of the recently aroused interest in a specific safety issue, resident work hours. The Accreditation Council on Graduate Medical Education (ACGME) had announced they would be requiring an 80 hours per week limitation of resident work hours as of July 1, 2003. The rule had sparked a vigorous and sometimes acrimonious debate within the profession. The editors decided to focus on that issue, which, interestingly, had not received much attention in the IOM report.

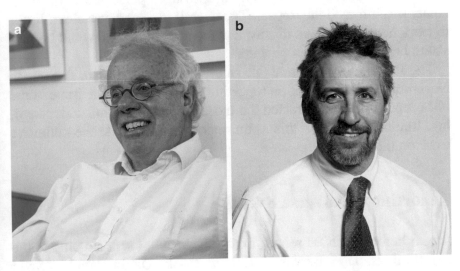

(a) Richard Smith, and (b) Arnie Epstein.

So, in addition to our overview editorial about the series and David Gaba and John Howard's commissioned paper on physician fatigue, the issue contained an editorial on rethinking medical training by Drazen and Epstein, a Sounding Board article on duty hours by Debra Weinstein, and a Health Policy Report on the debate over resident's hours by Steinbrook.

Gaba and Howard's paper, *Fatigue among Physicians and the Safety of Patients*, reviewed the scientific evidence of the effects of fatigue on performance and the efforts to limit MD hours [14]. They analyzed the new ACGME regulations and their consequences. Drazen and Epstein's *Rethinking Medical Training – The Critical Work Ahead* emphasized the enormous importance of the issue and that it was an opportunity to rethink residency training. The measure of success will be whether it is improved [15].

Debra Weinstein's *Duty Hours for Resident Physicians* explored the consequences of hour reduction and the need to reengineer the system of care [16]. Steinbrook's *The Debate Over Resident's Work Hours* provided facts about residency numbers, reviewed the arguments for and against the change, and examined the details of the requirements and problems in implementation [17].

Having multiple papers on the same subject might seem like over-kill, but it was not. The overlapping messages presented in different contexts reinforced the impact. The overall message was clear: limits to work hours were here to stay, and the consequences would be sub-stantial and difficult to cope with.

The Journal then featured one safety paper each month. The one in November was my paper on reporting [18]. This was the issue in the IOM report that had attracted the most interest—and misunderstand-ing. Immodestly, I saw this as an opportunity to write the definitive work on the subject!

Reporting of Adverse Events

A year before the IOM report, in October 1998, I sent a memo to the key thinkers, Don Berwick, Richard Cook, David Woods, David Bates, David Gaba, David Cullen, and Jeff Cooper, asking whether we should work on developing a proposal for a national medical adverse event reporting system. I extolled the virtues of the Aviation Safety Reporting System that we were all familiar with and asked if we should have something like it.

They agreed to consider it. There was an obvious problem with this idea: the Aviation Safety Reporting System gets 30,000 reports a year at a cost of $two million. Extrapolation from our incident studies suggested we could have as many as three million. Do the arithmetic!

In lieu of such a national system, we considered the alternative of hospital level reporting. To succeed would require major efforts by CEOs to create an environment where nurses and others felt safe reporting. Even if it were limited to sentinel events or sampling events one day a month, it would yield more reports than they could handle. A confidential system reporting near misses would face similar barriers. We decided not to pursue it further.

Writing my paper for the NEJM did not go well. Because their whole process around producing the papers was so controlling, I was unsure of whether what I was writing was appropriate, so I sent a draft to Jeff Drazen for his suggestions before finalizing the paper. Was it what he wanted? To my dismay, we miscommunicated, and rather than giving me advice, he sent the draft out for reviews! It was not ready, and by the time I found out it was too late to call it back.

One of the reviewers was the former editor of the Journal, Arnold (Bud) Relman. We were old friends, but that didn't inhibit his professionalism. He chopped away at it. He was particularly offended that I made a reference to something he had said or written without giving citation credit. I had planned to do that, of course, but this was a draft. I called him, explained that the paper was a draft, and apologized. His review, of course, was very helpful. I rewrote the paper, and it survived the final round of reviews.

The paper, *Reporting of Adverse Events*, analyzed the objectives, potential, practices, success, and limitations of current reporting systems, both voluntary and mandatory [18]. It analyzed the characteristics of successful reporting systems. I noted that a *national* voluntary reporting program that provides meaningful analysis of events and feedback of useful information (such as the aviation reporting system) would be quite expensive and, therefore, unlikely to be developed. Existing state mandatory reporting systems had limited value for the same reason. On the other hand, numerous voluntary specialty-based and system-wide reporting systems were developing and seemed to be quite successful.

At the time of the report, 20 states had mandatory reporting systems that varied widely in requirements. The publication of the list of "Never Events" by the NQF the previous year led some states to standardize mandatory reporting around clearly defined and non-debatable events. It also stimulated others to create reporting systems. By 2010, 27 states and the District of Columbia had mandatory reporting systems.

In December, the NEJM published a survey they had commissioned from Bob Blendon: *Views Of Practicing Physicians And The Public On Medical Errors* [19]. In January 2003, the series resumed on a monthly basis with Atul Gawande's *Risk Factors for Retained Instruments and Sponges after Surgery* [20], John Burke's *Infection Control – A Problem for Patient Safety* [21], Charles Vincent's *Understanding and Responding to Adverse Events* [22], and David Bates and Gawande's *Improving Safety with Information Technology* [23]. The commissioned paper on malpractice did not survive the review process; it was replaced by a paper by Tejal Gandhi, *Adverse Drug Events in Ambulatory Care* [24].

The Journal decided this was enough for now. I was disappointed because I thought several other subjects deserved airing: Organizational Change, Nursing, Institutional and Professional Oversight, Regulation, and the VA as a case study. However, the papers published in the series were excellent: informative, provocative, and authoritative. I think they made a difference.

Patient Safety and Quality Journals

The embrace of patient safety by the premier medical journals did indeed seem to have the desired effect of providing academic respectability for the new field of patient safety. Other mainstream journals and specialty journals began to publish more safety-related articles. Junior faculty could now get their papers published.

It is important to note, however, that within the quality and safety community, there were several major outlets that had been publishing research papers for some time. Three deserve comment: the Joint Commission Journal on Quality and Safety, BMJ's Quality in Health Care, and the Journal of Patient Safety.

Joint Commission Journal on Quality Improvement and Safety

The Joint Commission was an early leader in the quality improvement movement. In 1974 it created one of the first journals dedicated to quality improvement, the Quality Review Bulletin (QRB). The name was changed to the Joint Commission Journal on Quality Improvement in 1993, and then, as the patient safety movement got under way, to the Joint Commission Journal on Quality Improvement and Safety in 2003. Published monthly, the Journal has been the major venue for publication of actual protocols and safety practices, such as the two from the Massachusetts Coalition on Reconciling Medications and Communication of Critical Test Results [25, 26].

BMJ's Quality and Safety in Health Care

In 1992, 8 years before the BMJ special issue, its editor, Richard Smith, decided to give greater emphasis to the burgeoning field of quality improvement and created a subsidiary journal, Quality in Health Care. It soon became a major journal for publication of quality of care research, rivaling or surpassing the Joint Commission's journal.

The journal added patient safety to its remit in 2011 when it changed its name to Quality and Safety in Health Care and hired Kaveh Shojania as editor. Currently, it publishes more articles than any other quality or safety journal and is a major voice for patient safety research.

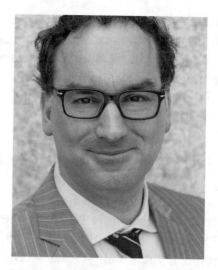

Kaveh   Shojania.   (All   rights reserved)

The Journal of Patient Safety

The latest entry to the field, the Journal of Patient Safety, was created as the official journal of the National Patient Safety Foundation in 2005 under the leadership of Nancy Dickey, former Chairman of the Board of the AMA. As a new journal, it had trouble attracting papers from researchers because of low readership, but it was gaining impact until the Denham scandal (Chap. 5). He had published a number of his own papers, later review of which showed numerous conflicts of interest.

In 2014, David Bates took over as editor. Under his leadership, the Journal has prospered. Although it is a quarterly journal, it now publishes a large number of papers in each issue and has proven to be a valuable patient safety resource.

Conclusion

Academic journals are the lifeblood of research. "If it isn't published, it didn't happen" may be a bit of an exaggeration, but not much. New ideas have to be communicated to get traction; word of mouth and presentations at meetings are not enough to do the job. Most importantly, the peer-review process filters out most (not all) bad research; good studies prompt others to replicate them and often inspire new ideas. All of these journals—the prestigious and the patient safety-oriented—have, in fact, established patient safety as a discipline that is here to stay.

References

1. Smith R. All changed, changed utterly. BMJ. 1998;316(7149):1917–8.
2. Berwick DM, Leape LL. Reducing errors in medicine [editorial]. BMJ. 1999;319(7203):136–7.
3. Leape LL, Berwick DM. Reducing error, improving safety [special issue]. BMJ. 2000;320(7237):725–814.
4. Reason J. Human error: models and management. BMJ. 2000;320(7237):768–70.
5. Weingart S, Wilson R, Gibberd R, Harrison B. Epidemiology of medical error. BMJ. 2000;320(7237):774–7.
6. Helmreich RL. On error management: lessons from aviation. BMJ. 2000;320(7237):781–5.
7. Gaba D. Anaesthesiology as a model for patient safety in health care. BMJ. 2000;320(7237):785–91.
8. Bates DW. Using information technology to reduce rates of medication errors in hospitals. BMJ. 2000;320(7237):788–91.
9. Nolan TW. System changes to improve patient safety. BMJ. 2000;320(7237):771–3.
10. O'Leary D. Accreditation's role in reducing medical errors. BMJ. 2000;320(7237):727–8.
11. Reinertsen J. Let's talk about error. BMJ. 2000;320(7237):730.
12. Cohen MR. Why error reporting systems should be voluntary. BMJ. 2000;320(7237):728–9.
13. Wu A. Medical error: the second victim. BMJ. 2000;320(7237):726–7.
14. Gaba DM, Howard SK. Fatigue among clinicians and the safety of patients. N Engl J Med. 2002;347(16):1249–55.
15. Drazen JM, Epstein AM. Rethinking medical training--the critical work ahead. N Engl J Med. 2002;347(16):1271–2.
16. Weinstein DF. Duty hours for resident physicians--tough choices for teaching hospitals. N Engl J Med. 2002;347(16):1275–8.
17. Steinbrook R. The debate over residents' work hours. N Engl J Med. 2002;347(16):1296–302.
18. Leape LL. Reporting of adverse events. N Engl J Med. 2002;347(20):1633–8.

19. Blendon RJ, DesRoches CM, Brodie M, et al. Views of practicing physicians and the public on medical errors. N Engl J Med. 2002;347(24):1933–40.
20. Gawande AA, Studdert DM, Orav EJ, Brennan TA, Zinner MJ. Risk factors for retained instruments and sponges after surgery. N Engl J Med. 2003;348(3):229–35.
21. Burke JP. Patient safety: infection control - a problem for patient safety. N Engl J Med. 2003;348(7):651–6.
22. Vincent C. Understanding and responding to adverse events. N Engl J Med. 2003;348(11):1051–6.
23. Bates DW, Gawande AA. Improving safety with information technology. N Engl J Med. 2003;348(25):2526–34.
24. Gandhi T, Weingart SN, Borus J, et al. Adverse drug events in ambulatory care. N Engl J Med. 2003;348:1556–64.
25. Rogers G, Alper E, Brunelle D, et al. Reconciling medications at admission: safe practice recommendations and implementation strategies. Jt Comm J Qual Patient Saf. 2006;32:37–50.
26. Hanna D, Griswold P, Leape L, Bates D. Communicating critical test results: safe practice recommendations 2005. Jt Comm J Qual Patient Saf. 2005;31:68–80.

Part III
Getting to Work: Key Issues and How They were Dealt with

Chapter 18
Sleepy Doctors: Work Hours and the Accreditation Council for Graduate Medical Education

On March 5, 1984, Bennington College freshman Libby Zion died at New York Hospital. She had been admitted the night before with vague symptoms and strange jerking motions. After consulting with her family physician, the residents on call gave her intravenous solutions for possible dehydration and prescribed meperidine to control her jerking motions. They then left to take care of other patients. Luise Weinstein, the first-year resident, was responsible for 40 other patients. No sleep for her.

Libby Zion did not improve; she became more agitated. Weinstein ordered restraints, which Zion fought against. Finally, she went to sleep. But her temperature rose, and by 6:30 AM it reached 107 °F. Weinstein took measures to cool her down, but she quickly deteriorated, had a cardiac arrest, and could not be resuscitated.

Her father, Sidney Zion, a lawyer and a writer for the New York Times, was furious. He was convinced her death was due to inadequate care by poorly supervised, overworked residents. In a *New York Times* op-ed piece, he wrote: "You don't need kindergarten to know that a resident working a 36-hour shift is in no condition to make any kind of judgment call—forget about life-and-death." He decried the lack of supervision of the residents and accused the doctors of murder. He launched an unremitting public campaign for justice [1].

A full investigation later concluded that the probable cause of death was a reaction between the prescribed meperidine and an antidepressant she was taking, phenelzine. This interaction was not well-known,

© The Author(s) 2021
L. L. Leape, *Making Healthcare Safe*,
https://doi.org/10.1007/978-3-030-71123-8_18

and, in fact, at a hearing 2 years later several chairmen of departments of medicine at prominent medical schools stated they had never heard of the interaction prior to this case.

Sidney Zion pursued the legal challenge, however, and in 1986 a grand jury charged the residents with negligence. However, after multiple reviews and conflicting findings by state regulatory bodies over several years, an appeals court in 1991 cleared them of all charges [2]. Zion then filed a civil suit which in 1995 concluded with a judgment that the primary care physician and the residents pay Zion $375,000 [2].

Residency Training

The system for training doctors goes back to the 1890s, when William Stewart Halsted, the professor of surgery at the Johns Hopkins Hospital, formalized the training of surgeons. Halsted believed that total immersion in the care of patients was the best way to learn about disease and treatment and to develop a sense of commitment to the patient.

After completing medical school, surgical trainees at Hopkins were required to literally live at the hospital—the origin of the term "resident"—and were discouraged from marrying. Supervised by senior physicians called "Attending Physicians," they were responsible for all aspects of care, including menial tasks such as drawing blood for tests, changing dressings, and transporting patients for tests. It was a long process: up to 10 years for some.

Other specialties adopted the residency concept, gradually modifying it to require 30 hours in-hospital on alternate days, the custom at the time of the Libby Zion case. Surgical training typically required 5 years, medical specialties, three. Residents (also called "house officers") were not paid for their services—after all, they were getting a free education—but they got free uniforms and room and board while in the hospital.

Although they were budding professionals, hospitals often treated them like military academy plebes. An apocryphal story that I heard while a surgical resident at the Massachusetts General Hospital many years later was that a former hospital director was so incensed with residents standing around with their hands in their pockets that he had the pockets of their uniforms sewn shut!

The number of residencies increased as the number of specialties expanded dramatically in the mid-twentieth century. In addition to supervised clinical experience and bedside teaching, programs provided teaching conferences. Few residents were paid anything until the 1960s, when they began to receive a meager "stipend" to meet personal expenses—nothing for living expenses outside the hospital, such as food and rent. Hospitals found it convenient to ignore the reality that now most residents were married, and some had children.

Forty years later, in 2001, the mean salary for residents was $40,000 a year, an average of $9.61 an hour for the typical 80-hour week [3]. Residents' expertise, skills, and dedication enable faculty at teaching hospitals to take care of very sick and complicated patients without hiring help or needing to be present all the time. The "purpose" of residency training may be education, but its practical effect—and attraction for the hospital and its doctors—is the 24/7 service doctors in training provide at below minimum wages.

The sleep deprivation and high workloads of busy acute clinical care practice pose a threat to patient safety for any physician, but especially for residents during training. It has been demonstrated, and we all know from personal experience, that judgment and performance suffer when we are up all night or are excessively fatigued from overwork. There is no reason to believe that physicians have some special immunity to these effects. Other critical industries such as commercial aviation and nuclear power recognize the effects of sleep deprivation and strictly limit work hours. Why should medicine be different? The Zion case forced the public and the profession to confront these issues.

Early History—What Happened After Zion

Following the grand jury indictment in 1986, Health Commissioner David Axelrod (the same person who later funded the Harvard Medical Practice Study) established a blue-ribbon committee headed by Bertrand Bell, the "Bell Commission," to investigate the training and supervision of doctors. It recommended limiting resident work hours and improving supervision [4].

In 1989 New York State adopted the Commission's recommendations and legislated that residents could not work more than 80 hours a week or more than 24 consecutive hours. It also required that they have round-the-clock supervision by attending physicians. Two hundred million dollars was appropriated to hire additional ancillary help and board-certified physicians to assist New York hospitals in compliance [5, 6].

It is worth noting that although it is broadly accepted, the 80-hour limit was not at the time evidence-based. Later studies showed, however, that working more than 80 hours was linked to increased depression, suicide, and needlestick injuries of residents.

On the national level, the professional organization responsible for oversight of most residency and fellowship training programs, the Accreditation Council for Graduate Medical Education (ACGME), took notice. The ACGME is a private, not-for-profit organization that sets standards for US graduate medical training (residency and fellowship) programs and accredits training programs based on compliance with these standards. A resident must successfully complete training in an accredited institution to be eligible for certification in their specialty and licensure to practice.

Within ACGME, resident duty hour standards are set across all specialties by the Board of Directors in concert with the chairs of the 30 specialty review committees in the *common program requirements*. Additional specific and more detailed standards are proposed by the individual Residency Review Committees for each specialty. In addition, there are many subspecialties (such as gastroenterology, nephrology, and cardiology in Internal Medicine) that propose their own standards. In 2018, there were approximately 830 ACGME-accredited institutions sponsoring approximately 11,200 residency and fellowship programs in 180 specialties and subspecialties [7].

In 1988, ACGME spoke up with whispered voice to suggest limiting call to every third night and to permit—not require—its individual specialty Residency Review Committees to incorporate requirements related to work hours in their standards. It did not mandate, as part of the shared requirements, that all specialties adopt a common standard. Not surprisingly, its general request had limited effect. Over the next 2 years, only six specialties—none of them surgical—instituted a limit of 80 hours per week.

New York State did little better. With over 100 teaching hospitals, its hospitals train 15% of the resident physicians in the USA, but it did not initially vigorously enforce its 1989 regulations. This led New York City Public Advocate, Mark Green, in 1994 and 1997 to investigate compliance and report widespread violations. A Department of Health survey in 1998 of 12 hospitals in New York City found that 37% of residents worked more than allowed and 77% of surgical residents worked more than 95 hours per week [8]. The state fined four hospitals $20,000 each and increased the maximum fine to $50,000. Two years later, the state funded and issued a contract for monitoring hospitals and fining them for noncompliance [9].

The pressure for reform continued to build. In April 2001, the NYC residents' union, the Committee of Interns and Residents of the SEIU (CIR), the Public Citizen Health Research Group, the American Medical Student Association, and Dr. Bertrand Bell, petitioned the Occupational Safety and Health Administration to establish and enforce a federal work hour standard for residents [10]. It didn't happen.

In November 2001, a bill was introduced in the House of Representatives to limit work hours of residents to 80 hours a week and to provide for federal enforcement [11]. Meanwhile, the Association of American Medical Colleges (AAMC) issued a policy statement recommending limits on work hours. The ACGME became more active in enforcement; in 2002 it withdrew accreditation of the general surgery program at Yale-New Haven Medical Center because of excessive work hours [12]. Finally, seeking to forestall the pending federal regulation, the ACGME decided it was time to act.

2003 ACGME Regulations

In 2002 the ACGME announced new regulations of resident hours and workloads, to take effect July 1, 2003 [13]. Although most people had seen it coming, it still aroused great consternation. The ACGME had already gradually stiffened requirements, limiting overnight on-call duty to every third night and requiring residents to have 1 day off every 7 days worked. A number of non-surgical specialties had imposed an 80-hour work week limit.

The surgeons, however, had rejected the hour limits. The Residency Review Committee for Surgery gave hospital surgical program directors responsibility for "appropriate" duty hours. They stressed that continuity of care must take precedence without regard to time of day, call schedules, or number of hours already worked. Work weeks of 100–120 hours were still common [14, 15].

The new regulations made the 80-hour week mandatory for all specialties and added a 24-hour limit for on-call duty. Hospitals were required to monitor work hours and reduce residents' responsibility for patient care support services of no educational value, such as drawing blood for tests, starting intravenous lines, and transporting patients [16]. The ACGME would monitor compliance.

These stronger standards, however, fell short of the AMA and AAMC recommendations for shorter on-call hours, or those in the legislation proposed by Congress. Nonetheless, both the AMA and the AAMC endorsed the changes. The new rules were met with skepticism from CIR, Public Citizen, and the New York Times [17]. They also aroused strong feels within the profession—pro and con—the latter especially among the surgeons.

The Duty Hours Debate

The arguments for hour and workload limitations are basically two: that it will reduce injuries and that it will improve residents' mental health and well-being. The evidence of the potential harm to patients from sleep deprivation is abundant. Many studies over the years of its effects on various populations have shown the risk of sleep deprivation [18, 19], including a memorable study that demonstrated that impairment of performance after 24 hours of sustained wakefulness is equivalent to having a blood alcohol concentration of 0.10% [20].

Specific studies of medical residents' performance also confirm its ill effects [21]. One controlled study of first year residents showed that those with 24-hour sleep deprivation made 36% more serious errors than those who worked 16 hour days, and they made over 5 times as many serious diagnostic errors [22]. Other studies showed residents made twice as many mistakes detecting cardiac arrhythmias when sleep deprived and twice as many technical errors in simulated laparoscopic surgery [23].

A survey of residents showed that 41% reported fatigue as a cause of serious mistakes; of those, 31% were fatal [22]. A meta-analysis of studies by the ACGME found that after 24–30 hours of sleep depriva-tion, clinical performance of residents dropped from the 50th to the 7th percentile of performance when rested [24].

Sleep deprivation is also hazardous to the residents themselves. During night call, they are twice as likely to suffer a needlestick injury [25]. Driving home after an "all-nighter," the chance they will sustain a motor vehicle crash that injures the resident or others is increased by 168% [26], and the risk that the accident will be fatal is also increased.

The second argument in favor of shorter hours is that resident well-being is enhanced. Learning is improved by the fact that residents are sufficiently awake and alert to benefit both from clinical experience and from formal educational activities. It was a common experience for residents to fall asleep during conferences or sometimes even while standing on rounds. (Your author remembers having this experience.)

Mood is also improved. Fatigue increases depression, anxiety, con-fusion, and anger that lead to detachment and lack of compassion for patients [21]. With adequate rest, attitudes and overall mental health improve. Finally, more humane hours permit the resident to maintain a balance between personal and professional lives, which would give them a better attitude toward their work and their patients.

The arguments against the proposed limits came largely from the general surgeons and surgical specialists, who raised issues of learn-ing and responsibility. They were concerned that disruption of conti-nuity of care by shorter work hours and more frequent shifts would deprive the trainee of the opportunity to see a clinical episode evolve and participate in all aspects of care [27]. Residents would miss important learning opportunities. They would not participate in enough operations to develop the needed skills and judgment.

They held out the specter of a surgical resident being forced to drop out of an operation because his time was up. They decried "shift med-icine." They worried that young surgeons wouldn't develop a sense of responsibility for their patients. Following the patient through the night and when fatigued was, they maintained, essential to the incul-cation of accountability and professionalism [27]. Others agreed: these are critical issues; their fears were justified.

Surgical residents also agreed. They live for the operating room. As we used to joke when I was a surgical resident, "The only problem with being on every other night is that you miss half of the good cases." It is difficult for the public or non-surgical physicians to fully appreciate the nature of surgical residency or its allure for residents. Participating in a surgical operation is an exhilarating experience. You see inside the human body, handle its organs, and restore its integrity by removing disease or repairing an injury. There is nothing like it in the world.

Surgical residents want to be able to do it themselves, and they can see they need to practice—a lot. They become almost obsessive about "doing more cases." Like all doctors, they want to do a good job, to become competent. They are willing to pay the price in high workloads and long hours, although they worry about its effect on their ability to give good care. A surgical resident once shared her feelings with me, "The thing wrong with having too many patients is that it keeps me from giving them the best care possible."

Years later, surgeons still have strong feelings about their residency years. They look back with nostalgia at the long hours, midnight operations, and heroic efforts to save the life of a badly injured trauma victim. They learned by doing, and it was exciting. In retrospect, some may resent the time it took away from their families, but they have no question it was worth it. These experiences reinforce their mindset about training. As we see daily on the political scene, once established, mindsets are hard to change. Evidence, facts, and even compelling contradictory data don't do it.

Other concerns were that the residents would not have time for reading and reflecting on what they were learning from their clinical experience and that shorter shifts would require more frequent hand-offs of care to another doctor, which would cause *more* errors [27]. These were all important issues that needed to be addressed.

Interestingly, in the debate that followed, no one brought up the fact that most countries in the European Union follow its recommendations of a maximum of 48 hours per week and 13 hours maximum shifts. Are European surgeons poorly trained? Do they have poorer outcomes? There is no evidence they do.

But implementing the new rules would require substantial adjustments by hospitals. The purpose of residency training may be education, but residents also provide many services for the hospital that are of no educational value that can be performed by those with far less training. Eliminating these non-educational services was now essential—and long overdue. Filling the gap by hiring more residents was not an option since CMS would not likely fund it. The choices were to increase the workloads of the attendings or to hire more doctors and physician's assistants. A 1994 study estimated that the national cost of these changes would be $1.4–1.8 billion [28].

Some, however, saw that redesigning the system of care to shift resident responsibilities to others would provide an opportunity to better align clinical responsibilities with other educational needs and to rethink the nature of the workplace. The burgeoning patient safety movement was making clear that health-care organizations badly needed to reform their work practices and change their attitudes toward work. It was time to recognize exhaustion not as a sign of dedication but as a risk to patient safety [21].

Regarding responsibility and dedication, Jeff Drazen, editor of the NEJM pointed out, "The role models that trainees see and the integrity of the environment in which they work appear to be far more important for instilling the professional ethos than the duration of the on-call schedules." [27]

What Happened: 2003–2008

Sadly, few surgical training programs and hospitals saw it that way. Most did not see the requirements as an opportunity to improve graduate medical education, but as a threat to the status quo. They refused to change. However, the ACGME required programs to report compliance based on regular reports by the residents of the hours they worked.

The residents were in a bind two ways. If they reported longer hours than permitted, they would incur the ire of their supervisors, jeopardizing both their clinical experience and recommendations for positions after training. And if the program was found in violation, it could lose its accreditation, making the resident ineligible to become board-certified. Program directors made it clear that they expected the reports to show compliance. So residents falsified their reports.

The extent of this deception came to light in 2006, when the Harvard Work Hours Study Group published the results of a confidential study of reporting by first year residents in 700 programs. It showed gross discrepancies: 83.6% reported work hours that were in violation of the ACGME standards. Working shifts greater than 30 consecutive hours was reported by 67.4%, working more than 80 hours a week was reported by 43%, and 43.7% reported not having 1 day in 7 off duty [29].

The ACGME, however, relying on the "official" reports from the program directors reported near-universal compliance with the ACGME standards during the same reporting period, maintaining that only 5.0% of programs were not compliant and that only 3.3% of residents reported violations of the 80-hour rule [29].

Apparently, the leaders of some Residency Review Committees were concerned about responsibility, continuity, and dedication, but it was okay for program directors to force residents to lie. The new rules weren't being observed, and everyone knew it.

The IOM Panel

Other forces were at work. As noted, a series of research studies had emerged that documented the effects of sleep deprivation on errors and harm to patients [26] and harm to residents [25, 26]. Other studies showed that shorter work hours reduced serious medical errors [22, 30, 31] and improved residents' health and education [32]. The CIR continued to press for enforcement. Congress again took notice. In 2007, the House Committee on Energy and Commerce, responding to the evidence linking medical errors to sleep deprivation and overwork and noncompliance with hour limits, requested the IOM to conduct a study and make recommendations.

The IOM convened a distinguished panel of patient safety and quality experts, policy makers, consumer representatives, physicians, nurses, and program directors, who deliberated and had hearings over an 18-month period. In December 2008 it issued its report, *Resident duty hours: Enhancing sleep, supervision and safety* [33]. The IOM called for new measures that would (1) focus not just on the number of hours worked, but on alleviating fatigue and loss of sleep, (2) increase supervision by senior physicians, (3) improve processes for transferring responsibilities from physicians going off duty to those coming on, and (4) stiffen enforcement by initiating federal oversight of the ACGME regulations [33].

It also called on programs not to reduce hours without putting sufficient funding and resources in place to allow for the reduction of hours without overburdening those residents left behind in the hospital. It estimated the total additional cost at $1.7 billion per year.

The IOM Committee took special aim at violations of current duty hour rules, noting that non-adherence to duty hours "is substantial and underreported, and that more intensified monitoring is necessary immediately." It noted "residents fail to accurately report their duty hours for multiple reasons, including fear of repercussions from their supervisors or, at the extreme, fear of causing a training program to lose its accreditation."

It called on the ACGME to address this issue by making unannounced audits of duty hour compliance and implementing protection for whistleblowers. It called on CMS to conduct periodic reviews of ACGME's duty hour monitoring and on the Joint Commission to include adherence data in its surveys and accreditation process.

The IOM's specific recommendations were built on the existing regulations and were consistent with the lessons learned from sleep research and recent studies of residents' work. It called for a maximum of 80 hours duty a week, no more than 16 hours without sleep, maximum on-call duty one night in 3, one full day off each week and 48 hours off once a month, 12 hours off after a night shift, and 48 hours off after 3 or 4 consecutive nights.

The IOM had spoken. The report was hailed not just for the duty hours standards but also for its emphasis on supervision of residents and external oversight of the ACGME. In addition to the IOM panel recommendations, there was mounting public pressure to do something. People were concerned about being harmed by a sleep-deprived doctor. How would the ACGME respond?

ACGME Duty Hour Task Force

We would soon see. When the ACGME implemented its first set of regulations in 2003, it promised a 5-year review. That time had come, and, with the IOM report and the continuing threat of Federal regulation, the ACGME needed to act. In 2008, it commissioned a 16-member Duty Hours Task Force composed of its members, trustees, medical educators, and a consumer, to review relevant research, hear testimony, and draft new standards.

There was concern that limited hours had created a "shift mentality" that conflicted with the physician's moral and professional responsibility to the patient, that programs' focus on duty hours diverted their attention from making needed changes in the learning environment, and that residents were conflicted about leaving patients to comply with the rules [34].

The Task Force discussed the need for enhanced supervision and faculty oversight, improving handovers, and the need to increase attention to patient safety. Research showed that the 2003 regulations had not led to increased hours of sleep. It also showed that reduced hours had no effect on mortality.

Regarding hours, would they heed the IOM recommendations? The leadership was ready to move. The Council of Review Committee Chairs was not so sure. The early signs were not encouraging. At the ACGME June 2009 Congress devoted to duty hours, many representatives of specialty societies spoke out against implementing the IOM recommendations.

Harvard Conference on Duty Hours

Meanwhile, many safety leaders thought the IOM recommendations deserved a broader review, with input not just from leaders of graduate medical education but also from those most affected: patients and residents, nurses, hospitals, and training directors, as well as policy makers and others. The changes proposed by the IOM would affect hundreds of thousands of physicians and residents, over 1000 hospitals, and have a global budget in the billions [35]. Implementing them would be a huge challenge.

The organized voice of residents, the CIR/SEIU, representing 13,000 residents in New York, was particularly concerned about what the ACGME would do. To put pressure on hospitals to implement the IOM recommendations regardless of what the ACGME required, they thought a persuasive strategy would be to provide advice from experts and evidence from those who had successfully implemented hours and workload changes.

At CIR's behest and funding, the leaders of sleep science and resident hours research, Chuck Czeisler and Chris Landrigan, and I convened a 2-day work hours conference at Harvard Medical School in June 2010, *"Enhancing sleep, supervision and safety: What will it take to implement the Institute of Medicine recommendations?"*

Attendees included quality improvement experts, medical educators, hospital administrators, consumers, regulators, sleep scientists, patient advocates, policy makers, a resident, a medical student, and two members of the IOM committee that produced the report. We also had representatives from AHRQ, JCAHO, CMS, and AHA, as well as training directors who had successfully implemented changes in their training programs to meet the 2003 requirements.

A recent survey had shown the disconnect between public perception and reality. The vast majority of the public had no idea that doctors worked 24 hours or more without sleep. When informed of this, only 1% supported it. Eighty percent supported a limit of 16 hours. Importantly, 81% believed that the patient should be informed if the doctor treating them had been working for more than 24 hours: 80% would want a different doctor. Ninety one percent favored strict rules to assure direct on-site supervision by attendings [36].

Roundtable discussions were held on eight topics: workload and supervision, work hours, moonlighting, physician safety, handovers and quality improvement, monitoring and oversight of the ACGME, financial support for implementation, and future research. The head of ACGME, Tom Nasca, himself a supporter of more humane working conditions, addressed the group.

The most memorable feature of the conference was the presentation of three case studies by training directors of programs in internal medicine, obstetrics, and surgery who had successfully developed new programs that functioned well within the hour limits. They showed that the objectives of training could be met and that residents attended more conferences and had higher morale. Both residents and faculty at these institutions were pleased with the results.

In its report, *Implementing the 2009 Institute of Medicine Recommendations on Resident Physician Work Hours, Supervision, and Safety*, the conference made 27 recommendations of necessary and practical steps that are needed to make the new limits work [35]. It concluded that innovators had demonstrated that hours and workloads can be reduced without compromising clinical experience or inhibiting the learning of responsibility, but regulation and financial incentives were needed to facilitate spread.

The ACGME Response

Just a week after the conference, on June 23, 2010, the ACGME Duty Hours Task Force issued its recommendations. It rejected most of the IOM duty hour recommendations except for a maximum duty period of 16 hours for first-year residents (only) and on-site supervision of first-year residents by faculty [34].

The 80-hour work week was retained, as well as limiting on-call duty to every third day (except for "night floats," who were limited to six consecutive nights), and 24 hours off duty every 7 days. However, there was a loophole: programs could apply to be more "flexible" in integrating service with teaching, which could include increasing work hours to 88 hours a week.

The recommendations of the Task Force were accepted by the Council of Review Committee Chairs, and in September 2010 the ACGME Board of Directors approved new rules that would go into effect July 1, 2011.

The patient safety community was disappointed. The reaction focused on duty hours. Most didn't believe the ACGME was making a commitment to ensure adequate supervision and a better learning environment.

In fact, the major thrust of the ACGME report was not about duty hours; it was about the learning environment. The Task Force was explicit: "The goal of the ACGME's new approach to duty hours is to foster a humanistic environment for graduate medical education that supports learning and the provision of excellent and safe patient care. The graduate medical education community has a moral responsibility to prepare residents to practice medicine outside the learning environment, where they will be unsupervised, must think independently, and must function when fatigued" [34].

"Paramount is an environment characterized by supervision customized to residents' level of competence, faculty modeling of fitness for duty, and the provision of high-quality care in a team setting and an institutional culture of safety." The new standards reflected this commitment.

The seriousness of the commitment of the ACGME to changing the learning environment was made clear by the significant expansion of its role. It would establish a new program of annual site visits of sponsoring institutions that would be separate from accreditation and would not focus just on duty hour compliance but also on supervision and the provision of a safe and effective environment for care and learning.

This was a big change, and it should have a major impact on residency training and patient safety. It is what Sidney Zion called for 25 years earlier.

The recommendation of the Duty Hours Task Force for evaluating the learning environment did not arise de novo. Ten years earlier there had been discussions at ACGME about how to improve the design of residency and fellowship programs through the use of a developmental framework and move the accreditation system to a focus on outcomes using a continuous quality improvement philosophy [37].

In 2009, ACGME CEO Tom Nasca convened a group of healthcare quality and patient safety experts, chaired by Carolyn Clancy, director of AHRQ, and Timothy Flynn, the chair of the ACGME Board of Directors, to make recommendations on how residency programs could be motivated to do a better job in training residents in patient safety.

One of the problems was that Graduate Medical Education programs were often managed at the department level, while quality and safety efforts were carried out at the hospital level from which the residents were not commonly included. How could they be integrated?

The group recommended that ACGME conduct an additional type of on-site visit, separate from and unrelated to accreditation visits. These visits would evaluate the learning environment, the residents' progress in achieving competencies, how they were integrated into the quality and safety activities of the hospital, and how programs were dealing with concerns about disparities and transitions in care.

CLER

To implement this ambitious program, Nasca brought Kevin Weiss, a member of the quality and safety workgroup and an immediate past CEO and president of the American Board of Medical Specialties into ACGME to develop the program. ACGME labeled it Clinical Learning Environment Review (CLER).

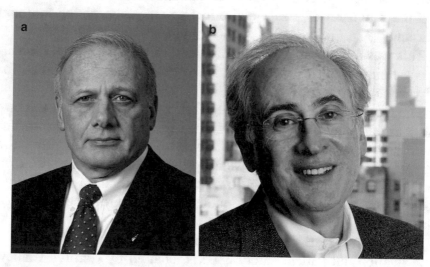

(a) Tom Nasca and (b) Kevin Weiss

The core of the CLER Program is a commitment to formative assessment and feedback regarding a residency training program's engagement in six focus areas: patient safety; health-care quality; care transitions; supervision; fatigue management, mitigation, and duty hours; and professionalism. The CLER Program required biannual formative assessment by each accredited sponsor of graduate medical education. It was designed to provide direct feedback to teaching hospitals and health-care organizations and to inform the ACGME accreditation process on issues in the six focus areas [38].

Training programs were now labeled Clinical Learning Environments (CLEs). Through periodic site visits that involve the program directors, residents, and the CEOs, the program aims to stimulate conversations and motivate CLEs to build upon their strengths and internally address opportunities for improvement.

Visits focus on six areas of concern: (1) the engagement and demonstration of meaningful participation of residents in the patient safety programs of the institution; (2) the engagement and demonstration of meaningful participation of residents in the institutional quality of care activities and participation in programs related to reduction of disparities in clinical care conducted by the institution; (3) the establishment and oversight of institutional supervision policies; (4) the effectiveness of institutional oversight of transitions of care; (5) the effectiveness of duty hours and fatigue mitigation policies; and (6) activities addressing the professionalism of the educational environment [39].

Milestones

In addition to the CLER program, ACGME established the milestone program. ACGME standards require residency and fellowship program directors to periodically assess each individual resident and fellow. These assessments use a variety of tools, including direct observations; global evaluation; audits and review of clinical performance data; multisource feedback from peers, nurses, patients, and family, simulation; self-assessment; and in-service training examinations [40].

ACGME requires semi-annual assessment of each resident and fellow on their progress in achieving *milestones* in the six domains of clinical competency that had been described as relevant for all medical practice by the ACGME and the ABMS in 1999. (See Chap. 20 for a discussion of the six competencies.)

Residency programs had for some time been required to configure curricula and evaluation processes in the framework of the six competencies under the Outcome Project, launched in 2001. Achieving the competencies was, in fact, the *purpose* of the programs. Under the ACGME, the training programs would ensure achievement of the six competencies. Certification programs, under the ABMS, would ensure that physicians maintained them.

Implementing outcome-based, i.e., competency-based, education into residency training was a big challenge for programs. Program directors and faculty had struggled since the launch of the Outcome Project to understand what competencies meant and what they looked like in practice [39]. They had different ideas of how to do it and different sets of skills for making the changes. There was wide variation between specialties and between programs within a specialty.

The concept of developmental milestones grew out of this need to move the outcomes project forward and deal with these variations. Milestones use narratives to describe the educational and professional trajectories of residents from the beginning of their education through the achievement of competency and the ability to enter into the unsupervised practice of medicine [40]. They define the stages in achieving competency for each of the six domains (Boxes 18.1 and 18.2).

Box 18.1 Milestone template

Milestone description: template

Level 1	Level 2	Level 3	Level 4	Level 5
What are the expectations for a beginning resident?	What are the milestones for a resident who has advanced over entry, but is performing at a lower level than expected at mid-residency?	What are the key developmental milestones mid-residency?	What does a graduating resident look like?	Stretch goals – exceeds expectations
		What should they be able to do well in the realm of the specialty at this point?	What additional knowledge, skills, and attitudes have they obtained?	
			Are they ready for certification?	

Ref. [40]

Box 18.2 Milestones for systems-based practice 1: patient safety and quality improvement

SBP1: Patient safety and quality improvement				
Level 1	Level 2	Level 3	Level 4	Level 5
Demonstrates knowledge of common patient safety events	Identifies system factors that lead to patient safety events	Participates in analysis of patient safety events (simulated or actual)	(simulated or actual)	Actively engages teams and processes to modify systems to prevent patient safety events
Demonstrates knowledge of how to report patient safety events	Reports patient safety events through institutional reporting systems (actual or simulated)	Participates in disclosure of patient safety events to patients and families (simulated or actual)	Discloses patient safety events to patients and families (simulated or actual)	Role models or mentors others in the disclosure of patient safety events
Demonstrates knowledge of basic quality improvement methodologies and metrics	Describes local quality improvement initiatives (e.g., community vaccination rate, infection rate, smoking cessation)	Participates in local quality improvement initiatives	Demonstrates the skills required to identify, develop, implement, and analyze a quality improvement project	Creates, implements, and assesses quality improvement initiatives at the institutional or community level

Ref. [40]

"Simply stated, the Milestones describe performance levels residents and fellows are expected to demonstrate for skills, knowledge, and behaviors in the six clinical competency domains. They lay out a framework of observable behaviors and other attributes associated with a resident's or fellow's development as a physician. The Milestones' primary purpose is to drive improvement in training programs and enhance the resident and fellow educational experience." [39]

Milestones were officially launched in 2013 in seven core specialties (emergency medicine, internal medicine, neurological surgery, orthopedic surgery, pediatrics, diagnostic radiology, and urology) as a component of the new accreditation system. The remaining core disciplines and the majority of subspecialties implemented the milestones a year later.

The CLER program and the Milestones have transformed residency training from an apprentice system—"do what I do"—measured by time served, into an educational system measured by competency achieved through planned experiences that include not only technical competency and knowledge, but experience in quality and safety and systems improvement.

Duty Hours

What happened about duty hours? Opposition to the 80-hour limit died a quiet death as evidence piled up against it. The ACGME funded two randomized trials that compared programs that strictly adhered to the rules to those with the flexible ones. The results showed that violations of 80-hour rules were linked to increased depression, suicide, and harm, such as needlestick injuries [25]. They also showed no differences in outcomes among surgery programs, leading to the conclusion that they should be bound by the same hour limits [41].

The other bit of evidence that the 80-hour limit was not harmful came from New York. The state had been strictly enforcing the 80-hour limit, with substantial fines, for a long time. No one could prove that physicians trained in New York were less competent. Skeptics began to come around. At the 2015 ACGME conference of Review Committees and others interested in graduate medical education, every medical organization agreed on the 80-hour limit. Shortly afterward it was adopted as a standard. The ACGME now cites programs if more than one resident in a program has violated the 80-hour limit.

Is the issue of duty hours settled, then? Hardly. Why is an 80-hour work week acceptable? Why is 13 hours a day, 6 days a week, with 1 weekend off a month considered humane given the damage it does to residents' well-being and family life? Talk about "normalizing deviance"!

Why do we turn a blind eye to the experience of the rest of the Western world—the EU limits that show competent and caring doctors can be trained in 48 hours a week? Forty-eight versus eighty! A world of difference. Could we train good—excellent—doctors in 48 hours a week, or at most 60? Of course we could.

They might even be better doctors. One of the major lessons in patient safety is that you can't expect health-care workers to care about patients' safety when you don't care about worker safety. Why do we think that treating doctors inhumanely will lead them to be kind and caring for their patients? Perhaps patients' complaints about how they are treated by their physician stem from how we treat the doctors during their formative training years.

Conclusion

What do we make of all this? The conflict over duty hours subsided with the "victory" of the 80-hour work week. On the other hand, the aggressive stance of the ACGME regarding the learning environment has been a welcome change and the CLER program has had an impact.

The implications for patient safety are also profound. A major stumbling block in advancing patient safety has been the lack of buy-in by most physicians; they don't "own" it. As Kevin Weiss points out, the profession doesn't "own" anything until it makes it an expectation of training and builds it into the training standards for the profession. That is where we agree on the definition of what the next generation must know and be able to do. Where we agree on who we are. The requirements for accreditation are therefore essential to how the profession is able to establish professional identity for all those who enter the profession (Kevin B. Weiss, MD, personal communication, May 20, 2020).

The groundwork was laid when the ABMS and ACGME agreed on the six domains of competency that included systems-based practice. The turning point was when ACGME expectations for training programs based on the six competencies became *requirements*. After evidence showed that programs were falling woefully short, the first CLER report outlined the needs for learning in quality and safety. These were later cut and pasted as requirements for accreditation.

Thanks to Tom Nasca and the ACGME, residency training has changed more in the past 20 years than in all of the previous 100. It is finally beginning to become more about education than service, about creating good physicians, not exploiting them. We now aspire to educate the whole physician, one who is skilled and expert, works well with others in teams, and communicates well with patients and colleagues.

The duty hours issue still needs work. We still have sleepy doctors. It's time to say good-bye to the 80-hour week and create a more humane environment. But we've made immense progress, and we are almost certainly turning out better doctors.

References

1. Lerner BH. A case that shook medicine: how one man's rage over his daughter's death sped reform of doctor training. The Washington Post. 2006; Lifestyle.
2. Sack K. Appeals court clears doctors who were censured in the Libby Zion case. The New York Times. 1991;B:2.
3. 2001 AAMC survey of housestaff stipends, senefits and funding. Washington, DC: AAMC; 2001.
4. New York State Department of Health's Ad Hoc Advisory Committee on Emergency Services. Supervision and residents' working conditions. New York; 1987.

5. New York Codes, Rules, and Regulations, Title 10 Section 405.4 Medical Staff (10 CRR-NY 405.4). In: New York State Department of Health, ed; 1988.

6. Lees DE. New York state regulations to be implemented. Anesth Patient Saf Found Newsl. 1988;3(3)

7. Accreditation. Accreditation Council for Graduate Medical Education (ACGME). https://www.acgme.org/What-We-Do/Accreditation. Accessed 6 June 2020.

8. Resident assessment: compliance with working hour and supervision requirements. New York: New York State Department of Health; 1998.

9. Health Care Reform Act of 2000, Bill No. A09093/S06187. In: New York State Assembly.

10. Gurjala A, Lurie P, Wolfe S. Petition to the occupational safety and health administration requesting that limits be placed on hours worked by medical residents (HRG Publication #1570). Public Citizen. https://www.citizen.org/article/petition-requesting-medical-residents-work-hour-limits/. Published April 30, 2001. Accessed 6 June 2020.

11. H.R.3236 – Patient and Physician Safety and Protection Act of 2001. In: House of Representatives 107th Congress 1st Session, ed: U.S. Congress.

12. Barnard A. Surgery residents' long hours draw warning for Yale. The Boston Globe. 2002;A1.

13. Philibert I, Friedmann P, Williams WT. Education AWGoRDHACfGM. New requirements for resident duty hours. JAMA. 2002;288(9):1112–4.

14. Daugherty SR, Baldwin JDC, Rowley BD. Learning, satisfaction, and mistreatment during medical internship: a national survey of working conditions. JAMA. 1998;279(15):1194–9.

15. Schwartz RJ, Dubrow TJ, Rosso RF, Williams RA, Butler JA, Wilson SE. Guidelines for surgical residents' working hours: intent vs reality. Arch Surg. 1992;127(7):778–83.

16. Report of the ACGME Work Group on Resident Duty Hours. Chicago: Accreditation Council for Graduate Medical Education; 2002.

17. Sleep-Deprived Doctors. The New York Times. June 14, 2002; Editorials/Letters: A36.

18. Gabehart RJ, Van Dongen HPA. Circadian rhythms in sleepiness, alertness, and performance. In: Kryger MH, Roth T, Dement WC, editors. Principles and practice of sleep medicine. 6th ed. Philadelphia: Elsevier; 2011. p. 388–95.

19. Dinges DF, Pack F, Williams K, et al. Cumulative sleepiness, mood disturbance, and psychomotor vigilance performance decrements during a week of sleep restricted to 4-5 hours per night. Sleep. 1997;20(4):267–77.

20. Dawson D, Reid K. Fatigue, alcohol and performance impairment. Nature. 1997;388(6639):235.

21. Gaba DM, Howard SK. Fatigue among clinicians and the safety of patients. N Engl J Med. 2002;347(16):1249–55.
22. Landrigan C, Rothschild J, Cronin J, et al. Effect of reducing interns' work hours on serious medical errors in intensie care units. N Engl J Med. 2004;351:1838–48.
23. Czeisler CA. Medical and genetic differences in the adverse impact of sleep loss on performance: ethical considerations for the medical profession. Trans Am Clin Climatol Assoc. 2009;120:249–85.
24. Weinger MB, Ancoli-Israel S. Sleep deprivation and clinical performance. JAMA. 2002;287(8):955–7.
25. Ayas NTB, Barger LK, Cade BE, Hashimoto DM, Rosner B, Cronin JW, Speizer FE, Czeisler CA. Extended work duration and the risk of self-reported percutaneous injuries in interns. JAMA. 2006;296(9):1055–62.
26. Barger L, Cade BE, Ayas NT, et al. Extended work shifts and the risk of motor vehicle crashes among interns. N Engl J Med. 2005;352:125–34.
27. Drazen JM, Epstein AM. Rethinking medical training--the critical work ahead. N Engl J Med. 2002;347(16):1271–2.
28. Stoddard JJ, Kindig DA, Libby D. Graduate medical education reform: service provision transition costs. JAMA. 1994;272(1):53–8.
29. Landrigan CPB, Barger LK, Cade BE, Ayas NT, Czeisler CA. Interns' compliance with accreditation council for graduate medical education work-hour limits. JAMA. 2006;296(9):1063–70.
30. Lockley S, Cronin JW, Evans EE, et al. Effect of reducing interns' weekly work hours on sleep and attentional failures. N Engl J Med. 2004;351:1829–37.
31. Levine AC, Adusumilli J, Landrigan CP. Effects of reducing or eliminating resident work shifts over 16 hours: a systematic review. Sleep. 2010;33(8):1043–53.
32. Reed DA, Fletcher KE, Arora VM. Systematic review: association of shift length, protected sleep time, and night float with patient care, residents' health, and education. Ann Intern Med. 2010;153(12):829–42.
33. Ulmer C, Wolman D, Johns M. Resident duty hours. Washington: The National Academies Press; 2009.
34. Nasca TJ, Day SH, Amis ES. The new recommendations on duty hours from the ACGME task force. N Engl J Med. 2010;363(2):e3.
35. Blum AB, Shea S, Czeisler C, Landrigan CP, Leape L. Implementing the 2009 Institute of Medicine recommendations on resident physician work hours, supervision, and safety. Nature Sci Sleep. 2011;3:47–85.
36. Blum AB, Raiszadeh F, Shea S, et al. US public opinion regarding proposed limits on resident physician work hours. BMC Med. 2010;8(33). Published online 2010 Jun 1. https://doi.org/10.1186/1741-7015-8-33.
37. Nasca TJ, Philibert I, Brigham T, Flynn TC. The next GME accreditation system — rationale and benefits. N Engl J Med. 2012;366(11):1051–6.
38. Clinical Learning Environment Review (CLER). Accreditation Council for Graduate Medical Education (ACGME). https://www.acgme.org/

What-We-Do/Initiatives/Clinical-Learning-Environment-Review-CLER. Accessed 6 June 2020.

39. Holmboe ES, Edgar L, Hamstra S. The milestones guidebook: ACGME; 2016.
40. Holmboe ES, Yamazaki K, Edgar L, et al. Reflections on the first 2 years of milestone implementation. J Grad Med Educ. 2015;7(3):506–11.
41. Rosen KA, Loveland AS, Romano SP, et al. Effects of resident duty hour reform on surgical and procedural patient safety indicators among hospitalized veterans health administration and medicare patients. Med Care. 2009;47(7):723–31.

Chapter 19

A Conspiracy of Silence: Disclosure, Apology, and Restitution

When patients are harmed by their treatment, they want three things from their doctor: they want the doctor to tell them what happened, say they are sorry, and tell them what will be done to keep it from happening to someone else. "What happened" is an acknowledgment that something went wrong, followed by an explanation of why it happened, and some guidance on what the future holds. If they have additional medical expenses or a disability, they also want compensation. Sadly, none of this happens most of the time [1].

The psychological harm following injury can be devastating. Feelings of fear, betrayal, anxiety about the future, and anger are common. Yet this aspect of patient safety was scarcely mentioned in the medical literature or in discussions prior to the patient safety movement. An exception was the work of Charles Vincent, who wrote in 1994 about why patients sue doctors. He described the mix of feelings of fear, loss of trust, and not knowing what happened [2]. In fact, for the patient the psychological trauma often exceeds the physical. It is those feelings, not pain or a long convalescence, that they remember years later.

In 2003, Gallagher conducted focus groups of patients to learn about their experiences and opinions about disclosure. They corroborated Vincent's findings. He found that becoming aware of an error in their care made patients "sad, anxious, depressed, or traumatized." Patients feared additional errors, were angry that their recovery had been prolonged, and were frustrated that the error was preventable

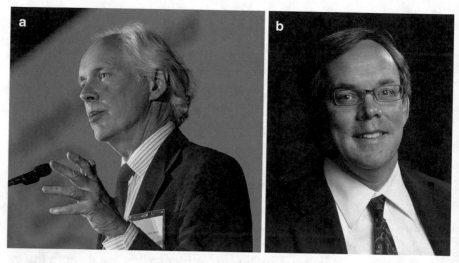

(a) Charles Vincent and (b) Tom Gallagher.

[3]. Patients said they would be less upset if the doctor disclosed the error compassionately and apologized.

While medicine seemed to pay little attention to patients' feelings, there was a continuing thread in the medical literature over the years about the effects that errors had on the physician. Perhaps the most powerful was by David Hilfiker, who in 1984 wrote a poignant piece in the New England Journal of Medicine, "Facing Our Mistakes," that described his personal anguish dealing with his patients and his own feelings after harming a patient by his error [4]. In 1985 and in 1988, Vincent reported on the devastating effect that making an error has on physicians [5]. In 1991, Albert Wu wrote of the problems house officers had in talking about mistakes and coined the term "second victim," [6] and in 1992, Christensen wrote of the profound effects of their errors on physicians [7].

The second victim's emotional state is potentially harmful to the patient as well. It clouds the physician's judgment, increasing the risk of committing a second error. It makes empathetic communication difficult at just the time when it is most important.

But neither of these powerful forces—the devastating effects of unexpected harm on patients and on their physicians—was much in the discussion about communicating with patients after an error, either before or after the IOM report. Instead, the arguments tended to be framed in terms of duty: honest disclosure is the "right thing to do," it is the "ethical" thing to do, "we have a professional obligation to be honest with our patients," etc.

Not that it is the kind thing to do, the healing thing to do, the human thing to do. Nor that effective and empathetic communication is the *necessary* thing to do, that it is the appropriate medical *treatment*— effective and science-based—for this second injury we had caused.

And, although principles were declared and practices for disclosure were recommended by elite medical organizations, including the AMA and the Joint Commission, they lacked force; open and honest communication following medical harm remained the exception, not the rule.

As noted previously, the most powerful—and most remembered— event at the very first patient safety meeting, the 1996 Annenberg Conference, was the presentation of the case of Ben Kolb, a boy who died from a medication mix-up in the operating room. What was memorable to the audience was that the hospital was open and transparent about it from the beginning, admitting error and apologizing. It was memorable because it was so rare. Few medical people in the audience thought such a case would be handled that way in their institution.

The very word used to describe these conversations, *disclosure*, tells much about the problem. It clearly implies ownership and choice. Information about the details of what happened and possible wrongdoing is deemed to belong to the physician, not the patient; it is the physician's choice whether, and how much of, this secret information should be *disclosed* to the patient. The high-flown rhetoric about honesty, honor, and professionalism and the duty to disclose reinforce the concept that the information belongs to the physician.

Not surprisingly, this idea is totally rejected by patient advocate groups, who reasonably ask, "Whose body is it anyway?"

Important as these concerns are, they have traditionally had little bearing on what actually happens. Rationality, empathy, logic, duty, and, sadly, even ethics play a distant second fiddle to the real reasons that doctors are not open and honest with their patients: shame and fear. Shame silences doctors, but fear drives the debate: the fear of being sued for malpractice.

Malpractice

It is not an irrational fear. The conventional wisdom for decades was that you made mistakes because you weren't careful enough. It was your fault, doctor. This thinking was reinforced by the lawyers and the courts, who took the position that an error is *by definition* a failure to meet the standard of care; failure to meet the standard of care in turn is the definition of negligence, of malpractice.

This is not true, of course. Making a mistake is not negligence, it is part of normal human behavior. That is the point of the patient safety movement. But the lawyers didn't believe that. They would have us believe that if you admit to making a mistake, or even if you acknowledge that something went wrong, you are asking to be sued for malpractice.

Defense lawyers—those who worked for hospitals and doctors—saw their responsibility as protecting the doctor or hospital from being sued regardless of whether there was negligence. The way they sought to do that was to get the doctors to "stonewall" from the beginning: tell the patient nothing, don't admit error, and, by all means, never apologize. Liability insurers, anxious to minimize losses, reinforced this message. Many even told physicians that if they admitted error, their insurance would not cover them.

Doctors went along. Admitting error, especially an error that has hurt your patient who trusted you, is painfully difficult. Being told by an authority not to admit anything gave them cover for not doing something they really didn't want to do. If the lawyers recommended it, then perhaps it was all right, even though it did violate their code of professionalism and even though deep down they knew it was wrong.

A word about malpractice suits. When a claim is filed, a protracted period of several years or more follows during which the physician must go back over the case in minute detail in multiple interviews with lawyers and depositions from the opposing side, while constantly dreading the trial itself. Often, the physician does not believe he did anything wrong. In fact, he may not even have made a mistake, or if he did, it was no worse than anyone else's, and he certainly didn't intend harm. But intent has nothing to do with it in tort law. (If the injury were intended, it would be criminal assault.)

Nor does the fact that we now know that almost all errors result from multiple systemic factors. In addition, in the USA, the focus of medical liability has long been on the physician, so that is who insurance policies cover. That is where the money is, so that is who the malpractice lawyer goes after. Medical negligence is about the individual not meeting the standard of care, defined as "what a reasonably prudent specialist should do under the same or similar circumstances."

Although safety experts hold that in most cases it is the hospital that should be held liable since it is responsible for the systems that fail and cause harm, that is a relatively new concept and still not widely accepted. Moreover, most hospitals were, until recently, charitable organizations for which states have traditionally provided immunity or very limited liability.

In a malpractice trial, the plaintiff's lawyer's task is to convince the jury not only that the doctor's action harmed the patient, but that the physician was careless, even reckless. The trial is an exercise in public humiliation, drawn out over a week or more: not only did the doctor do a bad thing, he or she is a bad person. No wonder doctors dread it and do whatever they can to avoid it.

Medicine is the only profession consistently subjected to this type of humiliation. Not just a few, but *most* physicians are sued at least once in their professional career, and some, especially those in the high-risk specialties such as vascular surgery and neurosurgery, are sued multiple times. The average neurosurgeon is said to spend 25% of their time in malpractice litigation.

In addition to fear of being sued for malpractice, doctors had other reasons to perpetuate a "conspiracy of silence." Admitting a mistake, most believed, would undermine their patient's trust of the physician. Colleagues would think less of them. Both their professional and their public reputations would be tarnished, perhaps irrevocably damaged. Referring relationships might be diminished and their income suffer.

But the most powerful deterrent to open communication is shame. The roots are deep within the physician's psyche, the product of the high-achieving personalities that are attracted to medicine. It is enhanced by an educational system that sets perfect performance as the standard and of a cultural environment that reinforces it. Admitting—to yourself or to others—that you have made a serious error is admitting that you have failed to live up to your own standard of perfect performance to prevent harm to your patient.

For the physician, making a serious error is not just a practice failure, it is a character failure. The shame can be overwhelming. With their self-esteem so at risk, it is not surprising that physicians develop defense mechanisms, such as denial that an error occurred or displacement of blame to an underling. Failing that, they desperately want to keep it a secret.

When I first began to comprehend the power of approaching medical errors as systems failures in the early 1990s, it seemed to me that a systems approach would not only reduce harm to patients, it would immensely benefit physicians. If doctors bought into the concept that errors are caused by systems failures, not personal failures, the burden of shame and guilt would be lifted from their shoulders, enabling them to be open and honest with their patients. While this is attractive in theory, in practice it has yet to happen on any significant scale.

Not only have malpractice concerns totally dominated the thinking about disclosure, some have argued that full disclosure would significantly *increase* the number of liability suits and total costs. Their reasoning held that if all patients were informed about an error, a significant number of patients who otherwise would not have known would be added to the pool of patients who might sue [8].

The Contrarians

The first chink in the wall of silence appeared in 1999, about the time *To Err Is Human* came out. Steve Kraman and Ginny Hamm published the experience from the Veterans Administration Hospital in Lexington, Kentucky, which in 1987 had instituted a policy of full disclosure and compensation following harm from a negligent medical error. A review of 88 cases from 1990 to 1996 revealed total hospital annual payments were less than half the rate in previous years [9].

Unfortunately, although the entire VHA adopted a disclosure policy that patients be informed of unintended outcomes, it did not extend Kraman's program to the entire system. VHA continued the practice of not explaining why things went wrong and not apologizing.

In Colorado, COPIC, the state's largest liability insurer, in 2000 developed the "3Rs" (recognize, respond, resolve) program of "no-fault" compensation to forestall litigation. It provides patients up to $30,000 for out-of-pocket health-care expenses and lost work time. They do not offer explanations or apologies and make the offer only in cases where the patient has not filed a claim. It is a structured service recovery operation, in effect an expansion of long-standing insurance practices aimed at loss control. It has been effective in reducing litigation, however. In one reported 5-year period, it handled over 3000 cases and reduced payouts and lawsuits dramatically [10, 11].

The real breakthrough came a few years later when Rick Boothman, Chief Risk Officer of University of Michigan Health System, reported their experience with a program he instituted in 2001 of responding to claims by admitting fault and offering compensation if internal investigation revealed "that the injury resulted from care that fell below expectations." The program was not limited to disclosure but linked to quality and safety efforts and expanded to identify injuries by various means. If an error was found, fault was admitted, and compensation was given for lifelong medical expenses, lost wages, and other costs—all without the patient needing to file a claim.

Analysis of results over a 5-year period following full implementation of the program showed a reduction of suits by 65% and decreases in legal costs and payouts to patients by more than 50% each. Total liability costs per year dropped from $3 million to $1 million [12].

Boothman emphasizes that the more important impact was on the culture. Full disclosure after unplanned clinical outcomes became the leading edge of changing the culture within the organization to increase transparency. Transparency is the key to a learning culture that facilitates internal reporting of adverse events and dealing with disruptive behavior and other performance problems. Full and open case investigations are necessary if we are to learn from our mistakes and advance the systems thinking that safety requires [13]. Boothman observed that in those organizations in which open disclosure failed, leadership did not connect it to their core mission and did not actively support adoption against the skeptics [13].

So, the arguments against full disclosure and apology were wrong: patients weren't more likely to sue, they were *less* likely to sue. And the costs went down not up. Trust depends on honesty, so it is not surprising that patients' trust in their physicians is enhanced, not diminished, by the doctor's forthright admission of failure and taking responsibility for it. Being honest is not only the morally and ethically right thing to do, it is the smart thing to do.

An interesting sidebar: at a lawyers' conference on malpractice that I attended about this time, a prominent Houston plaintiff's lawyer boasted about the number of patients who came to him to sue their doctor and then said, "Ninety percent of them wouldn't be there if the doctor had just told them what happened and said he was sorry!"

Physicians agreed in principle but had trouble doing it. They were cautious about how much to tell patients and believed that apology would be used as evidence of liability. They chose their words carefully, sometimes acknowledging the harm but not disclosing the error, why it happened, or what would be done to prevent recurrences. They were unlikely to discuss minor errors or near misses [3].

But things were beginning to change. At about this time, Gallagher issued a call for action by physicians, hospitals, certifying boards, accrediting bodies, medical societies, and medical educators to develop policies for disclosure, train physicians in communication, and provide support for patients and doctors [14].

Also in 2005, two senators, Hillary Clinton and Barack Obama, introduced the National Medical Error Disclosure and Compensation (MEDiC) Act that emphasized open disclosure, apology, early compensation, and analysis of the event. It was offered as a means of addressing both patient safety and the problems with the liability system. Although it never passed, it put the issue on the national agenda [15].

Doing It Right

Responding appropriately after a serious harmful event is not as simple as it may seem to those who have never had to do it. It is a highly emotionally charged moment for the patient and the physician. The patient is frightened, and if the harm resulted from an error the physician may be overwhelmed with feelings of shame and guilt. It is not a situation conducive to thoughtful supportive communication. The patient needs immediate reassurance from their doctor, primarily that they will be all right, and an explanation of what happened, but the initial talk is not the time to speculate on causes or details of what happened. They need to know *what* happened, not yet *why* it happened.

The physician should be honest and transparent, acknowledge that something has gone wrong, and explain what happened and what is being done to counter its effects. They should express regret—"I'm sorry this happened to you"—but avoid commenting on the cause of the event or apologizing, because investigation may reveal information that contradicts the initial assumptions of culpability. The patient should be told that an investigation will be carried out and the results will be given to them as soon as it is completed.

If investigation reveals that the injury was caused by an error, the physician needs to apologize. As the person responsible for the patient's care, the doctor in charge is the one to apologize, even if the error was made by a resident, a nurse, the pathologist, or someone else. The patient looks to their personal physician to make sure care is safe. The other person should accompany the physician if appropriate.

The CEO or other high-ranking administrator should also be there to apologize for the failure of the hospital's systems to prevent the injury. Although the patient understandably holds the person who made the error responsible, since errors result from systems failures, it is important for the patient to hear that from someone other than the physician, from whom it would seem self-serving.

A meaningful apology must include three elements: remorse, accountability, and amends. The physician must communicate their genuine deep feelings of sorrow, "I feel terrible about what happened." They must also take responsibility, "We let you down, it should not have occurred." The exact words are not critical, but it must come from the heart. Mere words, however "correct," will not do.

Meaningful apology also includes making every possible effort to make up for the injury. This means financial compensation for all expenses related to the injury, present and future. In addition to medical expenses, these include lost wages, extra household costs, and long-term effects of disability. Without restitution, apology is a gesture.

These are difficult conversations, and they will not occur unless there is serious advance planning. Physicians need to be trained in disclosure—which is not easy since it is so painful for them—and they need support in the moment. They need help in apologizing. Fortunately, for most physicians these conversations occur rarely, but that means they need coaching and support when they do.

This is where the hospital comes in. Ideally, the risk management department has shifted its focus from limiting liability to limiting (emotional) harm to both the patient and the doctor and is integrated with the quality and safety programs and nursing and physician administration. If not, a team needs to be developed in the quality and safety group. A training program is essential for teaching physicians how to communicate in this difficult situation, and it should be required for all physicians, who will find it difficult and painful.

Hospitals must also have support systems for both the patient and the doctor, as well as the nurse and support staff. Open, honest disclosure diminishes the patient's fears and anxiety, but it doesn't take it away. The patient needs comforting and understanding. So does the doctor. Even if they succeed at communicating with the patient after a serious event as a result of their training and excellent coaching, the shame and guilt don't go away. A colleague's arm around the shoulder and a reassuring word can go a long way, but more is needed. A system is needed to make sure both patients and doctors get emotional support in these first traumatic days.

Some years ago, a seriously injured patient in Boston, Linda Kenney, began to create that system. From her own experience, Linda recognized that the best support would come from a peer – someone who had been through a similar experience. With Rick VanPelt, the anesthesiologist involved in her episode, she founded Medically Induced Trauma Support Services (MITSS) to help hospitals develop peer support systems both for patients and families and for clinicians and staff. Thousands of people have been trained by this program, which is now a division of the Betsy Lehman Center for Patient Safety [16] .

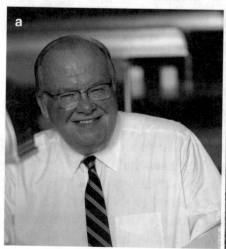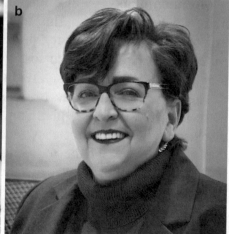

(a) Rick Boothman and (b) Linda Kenney.

Truly effective support requires changing the institution's culture away from punishment to learning—the basic challenge of the safety movement. Away from the hushed comment and pointed fingers, from "Isn't it too bad about Charlie" or "We all make mistakes" to a culture that really does look at an adverse event as a "treasure," an opportunity to learn how the system failed—and fixes it. A culture that recognizes that, with rare exceptions, the physician is not the cause of the error but the victim of it.

When Things Go Wrong—The Disclosure Project

Gallagher's work and Kraman's and Boothman's experiences changed the discussion in the patient safety world but seemed to have little impact on the practice in hospitals. Most of the principle players: hospitals, doctors, defense lawyers, and liability insurers were skeptical. The VA and Michigan were "different." Too risky to take a chance—although, of course, it was "the right thing to do."

Harvard hospitals were no exception. The ones that I was close to were not changing their policies or practices. CRICO, the Harvard hospitals' umbrella liability insurance company that funded our early error research, was proud of its record defending doctors and saw no need to change. Despite my entreaties and those of others, they and the hospitals were loath to take a chance. They gave lip service to full disclosure but did little to facilitate it. I stewed about this for some time. I would teach my students about the importance of honesty, communication, and apology, but I knew it wasn't happening.

How to get it moving? Perhaps if it were possible to get the leadership of all of the Harvard hospitals to agree on a uniform policy of full disclosure, apology, and restitution, it would stimulate their staff to actually do it. And if Harvard hospitals had success, perhaps that might persuade others that it was feasible and safe.

To see if this idea had any traction, I ran it by some of my frontline colleagues and friends: the safety leaders at the five major Harvard teaching hospitals. I asked them whether they were interested in exploring the issues about disclosure and apology. All responded enthusiastically.

The first meeting of what became the Disclosure Working Group was on May 10, 2004. Quality and safety leaders from the five hospitals were joined by two representatives from the Risk Management Foundation (RMF) of CRICO, and one from the Institute for Healthcare Improvement (IHI):

- *Janet Barnes*, nurse and risk manager at Brigham and Women's Hospital (BWH)
- *Maureen Connor*, risk manager at Dana-Farber Cancer Institute (DFCI)
- *Connie Crowley-Ganser*, vice president for quality at Boston Children's Hospital
- *Frank Federico*, pharmacist and quality leader at IHI
- *Bob Hanscom* and *Luke Sato* from CRICO/RMF
- *Cy Hopkins*, a quality and safety leader at Massachusetts General Hospital
- *Hans Kim*, quality specialist at Beth Israel Deaconess Medical Center

Review of their current institutional policies revealed that only three of the five hospitals had a written disclosure policy, and only one had a training program for physicians regarding disclosure. Clearly, we had work to do. Perhaps if we could spell out in detail what was needed and show how to do it, we would get buy-in.

At the second meeting a month later, we were joined by three new members, all physicians, Arnold Freedman, from DFCI, David Roberson from Children's, and Rick Van Pelt from BWH. John Ryan, the key CRICO/RMF lawyer, would join us at the next meeting. At this meeting, we made an important decision: in keeping with the systems concept, the policy should not focus on errors, but on adverse events.

At the July meeting, we made an even more important decision. Rather than limit our efforts to disclosure policy, we would craft a comprehensive document that addressed all aspects of responding to unanticipated events. No such statement existed; there were major assertions about disclosure (ASHRM, Minnesota Children's Hospital, etc.), and papers written about supporting patients and physicians, but no statements, policies, or recommendations that embraced all of the issues. Such a statement could have a major educational impact within our institutions at all levels. Much of the information and the rationale behind it would be new for many physicians.

The organizing principle, setting the "tone" of the statement, would be, "What is the right thing to do?" We defined the "right thing" as the institution taking responsibility to make things right by being open, informative, supportive, and restorative. We would try to break the mold of hospitals and doctors thinking about what is in their best interest to what is in the best interest of the patient.

We also agreed that the document needed to start off with the moral/ conceptual justification for this work. We are talking about much more than just disclosure or dealing with malpractice or the "business case." It is about hospitals meeting their obligation to respect patient's integrity, be sensitive to their needs, and earn their trust. This is the "do the right thing" part. Something like, "We hold these truths to be self-evident, that all patients are entitled to ... " (though not quite so grand—nor stolen!).

A bit late, but fortunately not too late, we suddenly realized that our group was missing the key stakeholder: the patient! To our great good fortune, Mary Dana Gershanoff and Gary Jernegan, co-chairs of the Dana-Farber Pediatric Patient & Family Advisory Council, were pleased to join us. When I told Tom Delbanco, an old friend and nationally respected physician patient advocate at BIDMC, about what we were doing, he expressed strong interest, so we asked him to join us as well. I was delighted, for his contributions were bound to be significant.

By March, we had a consensus document that we were happy with. We framed it in three parts: The Patient and Family Experience, The Caregiver Experience, and Management of the Event, with chapters on relevant issues. Each topic was organized into three sections: what should be done, why (the reasoning and evidence), and the specific recommendations. Following Tom Delbanco's recommendation, we titled it *When Things Go Wrong* [17].

When Things Go Wrong

The Patient and Family Experience

Three issues were addressed: communicating with the patient, support of the patient and family, and follow-up care of the patient and family.

The initial communication should occur promptly, within 24 hours. Patients have a right to be fully and promptly informed of any incident as soon as it is recognized. The physician responsible for the patient's care should acknowledge the event, take responsibility for it, express regret, and explain what happened. When results of the investigation are available, they should be communicated by the responsible physician and involve the CEO or CMO in serious cases. If an error was found, the physician apologizes.

Support of the patient and family addresses their psychological, social, and financial needs. Patients should be asked about their feelings, provided with psychological support, and given attention to their continuing medical care. Immediate financial assistance should be given if needed. Hospitals should consider paying for all future expenses due to permanent disability and continuing medical treatment.

Follow-up care after discharge from the hospital requires the care team to provide continuing psychological and social support by maintaining communication through scheduled follow-up visits and telephone calls.

The Caregiver Experience

Like patients and families, caregivers are significantly impacted, emotionally and functionally, following an adverse event. They need support to recover and to communicate appropriately with the injured patient. Hospitals need to have training programs in communication with patients when things go wrong, and how to deal with their own feelings. They also need "just in time" coaching when events occur and training in supporting colleagues when in need.

Management of the Event

The hospital needs to have an incident policy that sets expectations and provides guidance for the staff to improve patient safety by learning from adverse events and changing systems.

The *elements* of the policy are a commitment to open and honest communication, provision of just-in-time guidance, education of caregivers in empathetic communicating, provision of emotional support, and systems of documentation and reporting.

The *initial response* is first to stabilize the patient and eliminate any remaining threat, to secure implicated drugs and equipment, and to provide a substitute provider if needed. The care team must be promptly briefed to ensure consistent communication with the patient and family. The person to communicate with the patient and family is decided upon. An investigation should be done quickly while memories are fresh. The event is reported to the appropriate hospital authority.

Analysis of the event is essential for several reasons: to prevent, if possible, a recurrence in a future patient, to satisfy the patient's right to know what the causes were and what is being done to remedy them, and to disseminate the learnings to other health-care organizations. Analyses should be multidisciplinary and nonjudgmental. The objective is to uncover the multiple factors that contributed to the event and, where possible, develop systems changes to make it less likely that the event will recur.

Documentation of the event is essential, as is *reporting*. The reporting policy should define the process for responding, identify who is to be notified, how, and by whom. Reporting must be safe for the caregiver and should lead to investigation and corrective action. When required, file reports with regulators.

We were pleased with our product. Nothing like this had been done before. We hoped it would motivate all of the Harvard hospitals, and others, to make major changes in how they handle patient harms. We made it clear up front that this was a call to action. Now to find out if anyone would respond to the call!

Getting Support

I went on a major selling job. RMF arranged a meeting with the Chief Medical Officers of all 14 Harvard-affiliated hospitals. I asked them to read the draft; discuss it with their local physicians, nurses, administrative leaders, and hospital counsel; and circulate it widely among staff. We asked them to tell us if this was an appropriate approach and to tell us how to make it better—within a month. They did—and we received a deluge of comments from many people in many of the hospitals. We were pleased that all were supportive of the effort, and we got a lot of good advice. This was the first step in building stakeholder support.

John Ryan, our legal representative from RMF, arranged for me to meet with the risk management lawyers from the major hospitals to get their input. At the meeting, I was pleased, and frankly a bit surprised, to find they had no problems with what we had written. That was a good sign!

However, they did have a concern that some doctors might apologize right away for something that was found on investigation to not be due to an error. Coming back to the patient later with a different story would be difficult. We changed the document to emphasize that the initial communication should be an expression of regret about the event. Apologizing would take place later if appropriate.

The committee member from each institution and I then met with all of the hospital CEOs and their key leaders, such as the CMO, CNO, and COO to discuss the paper and ask for their endorsement. We found them overall quite receptive. The CEOs of two of them, BWH and Children's Hospital sent me letters of support.

In July, an unfortunate thing happened. Liz Kowalczyk, a health reporter for the Boston Globe contacted me. She got wind of our project—hardly a surprise, since by now probably over 100 people had seen the draft—but she had not seen the draft. I told her that we would welcome an article on the final version, after the hospitals had approved it, but because of the sensitivity of the subject, they would have a negative reaction to anything coming out before all issues had been settled. It would make it harder to get them to sign on. I asked her to hold off for now. Despite that, she went ahead and published a substantial article on July 24.

As predicted, there were some strong reactions—particularly the MGH. Their CEO, Peter Slavin, was furious. I met with him and assured him that we had released no information and would not until everyone was signed on.

By September, we had incorporated many suggestions and had the revised, final version of the report. I then sent it to the CEOs with the request that "your institution endorse the principles and concepts in the document and commit to implementing them in your hospital." Recognizing that this would require approval at various levels, from medical executive committee to the Trustees, we asked for a response by December 1.

By November 15, we had a letter of endorsement signed by all seven of the Partners hospitals' CMOs! By mid-December, we knew we would get letters from all the rest, so we made plans to publish in the spring.

After getting the endorsement from the hospitals, I went to Harvard Medical School to see if we could also get them to endorse it and be the organization to publish it. I thought the combination would be very powerful—a statement coming from the school and all of its teaching hospitals.

They requested I provide letters from all of the hospital CMOs, which was easily done, and present it to the Academic Council. The meeting went well, there were no difficult questions, and I left thinking they were supportive. In the end, however, they decided not to endorse it. Having "jumped through all the hoops," I was very disappointed. It was yet another example of how difficult it is to navigate the political aspects of this sensitive subject.

Fortunately, their refusal did not hold us back nor have any long-term impact. Paula Griswold of the Massachusetts Coalition for the Prevention of Medical Errors Coalition was delighted to publish it. RMF agreed to pay for printing and mailing costs.

When the printed copies arrived, I went for maximum distribution. Copies were sent to the leaders of all of the hospitals, members of the Coalition, CRICO/RMF, IHI, NPSF, BCBS, as well as the head of every national organization with a stake in patient safety (AMA, ANA, AONE, Leapfrog, CAPS, advocacy groups, etc.) and to every person I knew in patient safety anywhere in the world.

It was well received. As we hoped, this comprehensive statement by an authoritative source gave those working in patient safety what they needed to start making disclosure and apology work in their hospitals. We hoped we had kick-started the process. Later feedback and citations in fact did indicate that it was widely disseminated and had significant influence.

National Progress in Communication and Resolution

While we were working to move communication and resolution ahead, the National Quality Forum (NQF) also had a committee working on it, although none of us were aware of it. Eight months after we published our report, the NQF issued a new Safe Practice on disclosure. The key elements were that the patient should be provided the facts about the event: whether there was an error and the results of event analysis, the physician should express regret and give formal apology if the outcome was caused by error or system failure. Institutions were to integrate disclosure, patient-safety, and risk-management activities and establish a support system with coaching and emotional support for patients and staff [18].

The NQF action changed the ballgame. The NQF cannot require any institution to implement its Safe Practices, but it is the respected source that regulators and overseers, such as the Joint Commission [19], AHRQ, and the Center for Medicare and Medicaid Services look to for establishing standards. Activity picked up.

In 2007, Stanford University Medical Network launched a claims management process called Process for Early Assessment, Resolution and Learning (PEARL). Although, like COPIC, it was not a full program that included apology and appropriate compensation for all injured patients, it did reduce suits and costs. They reported that in the first 3.5 years after implementation, claim frequency dropped 36%, with a cost savings of $3.2 million per fiscal year.

At the University of Illinois Medical Center at Chicago (UIMCC), Tim McDonald and David Mayer developed the "Seven Pillars" program derived from work done at Michigan to integrate communication with system improvement [20]. Mayer was Associate Dean for Education who had a deep interest in patient safety. In 2005 he started the Academy for Emerging Leaders in Patient Safety, a week-long program on patient safety at Telluride for medical students. There were 20 students. The program has since been expanded to include residents and is now given in four locations to over 150 a year.

In the Seven Pillars program, quality improvement efforts were directed to define or improve systems for all seven stages of the process: reporting, investigation, communication and disclosure, apology and remediation, system improvement, data tracking and analysis, and education and training.

They later reported that from 2002 to 2013, the intervention at UIMCC nearly doubled the number of incident reports, reduced the number of claims by 42%, reduced legal fees and costs by 51%, and reduced the number of lawsuits by 47% [21, 22].

In 2009, at the direction of President Obama, the US Department of Health and Human Services authorized AHRQ to launch a demonstration project on communication and resolution programs under its $23 million Patient Safety and Medical Liability grant. UIMCC and the University of Washington (UW) were among four health systems piloting chosen. UIMCC's demonstration project demonstrated that it was possible to package training and tools to disseminate the Seven Pillars approach to DRP to community hospitals settings. The UW intervention trained 1300 health-care providers in teaching skills in disclosure and apology [22].

But the full application of Boothman's work did not take off until Alan Woodward, an emergency physician and past president of Massachusetts Medical Society who was passionate about medical liability reform, and Kenneth Sands, chief quality officer of Beth Israel Deaconess Medical Center, developed a plan for getting widespread adoption of programs by involving all stakeholders.

They obtained a 1-year planning grant from AHRQ to create a roadmap for implementing a statewide Communication and Resolution Program (CRP) model. They interviewed dozens of key stakeholders in the medical liability arena and identified 12 significant obstacles to implementation and developed strategies to overcome each. The roadmap provided a guide for action [23].

Woodward then did something quite remarkable to assure success: he brought the lawyers on board. He persuaded the Massachusetts Bar Association and the Massachusetts Academy of Trial attorneys to join the Massachusetts Medical Society to promote CRP programs statewide. Not just to participate but to join in leading the new effort. This was not to be just a doctors' patient safety project.

Their first task was to create a more supportive legal environment. They developed consensus language for legislation that mandated sharing of all pertinent medical records, a 6 month pre-litigation resolution period, strong apology protections, and the obligation of hospitals to disclose any significant adverse outcome [24]. Given the support of the key parties, the legislature accepted their language without change as part of the 2012 comprehensive medical reform act, setting the stage for moving ahead with the new approach.

To implement the roadmap, the group formed the Massachusetts Alliance for Communication and Resolution following Medical Injury (MACRMI) with representation from statewide organizations with a stake in the medical liability process: physicians, hospitals, patient advocates, insurers, and attorneys.

MACRMI's goal was to develop, implement, and pilot a rigorous Communication, Apology, and Resolution Program (which it calls CARe), collect comprehensive data to assess its impact, and assist its dissemination. Modeled after the University of Michigan Health System's program, CARe promotes early resolution in cases of avoidable medical injury. When unanticipated adverse outcomes occur, patients and their families are provided full explanation of what happened, what it means for the patient medically, what will be done to prevent the error from happening again, and, where appropriate, a sincere apology and adequate and an offer of fair and timely compensation.

To achieve this goal, MACRMI developed an implementation guide with comprehensive resources, including best practices, algorithms, policies and procedures, teaching materials, and tracking tools (all available free on their website: www.macrmi.info). It then tested CARe and the toolkit in a pilot program in 6 hospitals over 3 years, collecting settlement data on nearly 1000 cases as well as patient experience and provider satisfaction survey information.

Data from the study showed that claims and costs did not increase, and more patients were compensated. The median compensation for these cases was $75,000, a number too low for a typical plaintiff's attorney to take the case. Of cases that reached the resolution stage, 41% gave rise to a safety measure that was or was likely to be implemented by the hospital. These included new labeling for high-risk medications, color-coded socks for patients at risk for falls, and a multidisciplinary checklist for breech deliveries [25, 26].

As a result of MACRMI's efforts, 12 health-care institutions in Massachusetts are now using CARe, and a number of others are moving toward it. In addition, several entities in other states are in the process of implementing programs [27].

But the impact of MACRMI is much greater than the early adoption numbers signify. What we are witnessing is the beginning of a culture change in the way we think about and respond to those we harm. A change in thinking not just in a group of hospitals and a physicians' group and a carrier, but in the governor's office, in the legislature, in the plaintiff's bar, in the defense bar and even in the courts. Patient safety—their welfare—and honesty are what CRP programs are about, not reducing losses in malpractice suits.

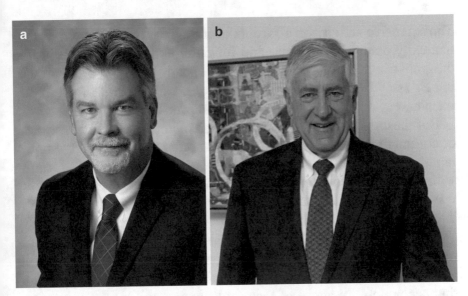

(a) David Mayer and (b) Alan Woodward.

From the experience of those in Massachusetts, Michigan, Washington, and others around the country, AHRQ developed the CANDOR (Communication and Optimal Resolution) initiative to proactively engage health-care providers, patients, and their family in preventable harm communications. It combines early event reporting, analysis, prompt, supportive and compassionate ongoing communication to the patient, fast, fair resolution where warranted, and applying lessons learned to change systems [28, 29].

AHRQ developed a CANDOR toolkit with input from those facilities awarded grants and other experts to help hospitals implement CRPs quickly and promoted its adoption. Several large health-care systems, including CentraCare and MedStar Health, have made commitments to its implementation, and the Medical Professional Liability Association and the Doctors Company have given it strong support [30].

Conclusion

The extensive activity on all fronts over the past two decades has dramatically changed the landscape for communication and resolution programs, increasing awareness of the urgency for change and providing an array of mechanisms to help health-care organizations implement new systems and provide the training and support that are needed.

But the challenges are immense. Implementing an effective system of communication, apology, and resolution is the cutting edge of the larger issue of transparency. Openness and honesty in communicating with patients is difficult in an institution that is not transparent in other ways, such as freedom to discuss errors and a willingness to go public with its mistakes. Creating transparency requires strong leadership.

CRP is also about another crucial aspect of a safety culture that is too often overlooked in the emphasis on reducing blame: accountability. The mindset of doctors and hospital leaders has to change to putting accountability ahead of fears of litigation and loss of reputation. To do this, strong leadership is required. CEOs have to stand up to the lawyers and insurers and insist they play their roles in that mission.

Even with strong leadership and a skilled team, teaching physicians to communicate effectively and empathetically after a serious preventable event is difficult. Unfortunately, lip service to CRP often outstrips true implementation. Needing to fulfill oversight demands, some hospitals initiate program improvements that focus selectively on claims resolution rather than on comprehensive programs of full communication, apology, and restitution that prioritize patient support and opportunities for improving quality and safety. While some patients are helped, many are not, and there is little learning or system change. The culture really doesn't change [31].

For all these reasons, it is not surprising that progress has been slow. From an historical perspective, however, a great deal has happened in a relatively short time. The vice grip of the dishonest and futile legal approach of deny and defend has been broken. Open communication and support are now at least part of the conversation in health-care organizations as the key organizations overseeing their behavior, AHRQ, NQF, TJC, CMS, ABMS, and ACGME, have incorporated it into their standards. The pace has accelerated. A better future is in sight for our patients and their doctors.

References

1. Iedema R, Allen S, Britton K, et al. Patients' and family members' views on how clinicians enact and how they should enact incident disclosure: the "100 patient stories" qualitative study. BMJ. 2011;343:d4423.
2. Vincent C, Young M, Phillips A. Why do people sue doctors? A study of patients and relatives taking legal action. Lancet. 1994;343:1609–14.
3. Gallagher TH, Waterman AD, Ebers AG, Fraser VJ, Levinson W. Patients' and physicians' attitudes regarding the disclosure of medical errors. JAMA. 2003;289:1001–7.
4. Hilfiker D. Facing our mistakes. N Engl J Med. 1984;310:118–22.
5. Vincent C. Research into medical accidents: a case of negligence? Br Med J. 1989;299:1150–3.
6. Wu A, Folkman S, McPhee S, et al. Do house officers learn from their mistakes? JAMA. 1991;265:2089–94.
7. Christensen J, Levinson W, Dunn P. The heart of darkness: the impact of perceived mistakes on physicians. J Gen Intern Med. 1992;7:424–31.
8. Studdert DM, Michelle MM, Gawande AA, Brennan TA, Wang YC. Disclosure of medical injury to patients: an improbable risk management strategy. Health Aff. 2007;26:215–26.
9. Kraman SS, Hamm G. Risk management: extreme honesty may be the best policy. Ann Intern Med. 1999;131:963–7.
10. Gallagher TH, Studdert D, Levinson W. Disclosing harmful medical errors to patients. N Engl J Med. 2007;356:2713–9.
11. Mello MM, Boothman RC, McDonald T, Driver J, Lembitz A, Bouwmeester D, Dunlap B, Gallagher T. Communication-and-resolution programs: the challenges and lessons learned from six early adopters. Health Aff (Millwood). 2014;33(1):20–9.

12. Kachalia A, Kaufman SR, Boothman R, et al. Liability claims and costs before and after implementation of a medical error disclosure program. Ann Intern Med. 2010;153:213–21.

13. Boothman CR, Imhoff JS, Campbell AD. Nurturing a culture of patient safety and achieving lower malpractice risk through disclosure: lessons learned and future directions. Front Health Serv Manag. 2012;28:13–28.

14. Gallagher TH, Levinson W. Disclosing harmful medical errors to patients: a time for professional action. Arch Intern Med. 2005;165:1819–24.

15. Clinton H, Obama B. Making patient safety the centerpiece of medical liability reform. N Engl J Med. 2006;354:2205–8.

16. MITSS: supporting patients and families for more than a decade. Patient Saf Qual Healthc. 2013. Accessed 4 June 2020, at https://www.psqh.com/analysis/mitss-supporting-patients-and-families-for-more-than-a-decade/.

17. When Things Go Wrong: Responding to Adverse Events. A consensus statement of the Harvard Hospitals. Massachusetts Coalition for the Prevention of Medical Errors: Boston; 2006.

18. National Quality Forum. Safe practices for better healthcare: 2006 update. Washington, DC: NQF; 2007.

19. The Joint Commission. Accreditation guide for hospitals. Oakbrook Terrace: The Joint Commission; 2011.

20. McDonald T, Helmchen L, Smith K, et al. Responding to patient safety incidents: the "seven pillars". Quality and Safety in Health Care. 2010;19:e11–e4.

21. Lambert BL, Centomani NM, Smith KM, et al. The "seven pillars" response to patient safety incidents: effects on medical liability processes and outcomes. Health Serv Res. 2016;51:2491–515.

22. Pillen M, Hayes E, Driver N, et al. Longitudinal evaluation of the patient safety and medical liability reform demonstration program: demonstration grants final evaluation report. Rockville: Agency for Healthcare Research and Quality; 2016. Report No.: AHRQ Publication No. 16-0038-2-EF.

23. Bell SK, Smulowitz PB, Woodward AC, et al. Disclosure, apology, and offer programs: stakeholders' views of barriers to and strategies for broad implementation. Milbank Q. 2012;90:682–705.

24. Acts of 2012, Chapter 224: an act improving the quality of health care and reducing costs through increased transparency, efficiency, and innovation. Section 221–223. Boston; The General Court of the Commonwealth of Massachusetts; 2012.

25. Kachalia A, Sands K, Van Niel M, et al. Effects of a communication-and-resolution program on hospitals' malpractice claims and costs. Health Aff. 2018;37:1836–44.

26. Mello MM, Kachalia A, Roche S, et al. Outcomes in two Massachusetts hospital systems give reason for optimism about communication-and-resolution programs. Health Aff. 2017;36:1795–803.

27. McDonald T, Niel M, Gocke H, Tarnow D, Hatlie M, Gallagher T. Implementing communication and resolution programs: lessons learned from the first 200 hospitals. J Patient Saf Risk Manag. 2018;23:73–8.
28. Boothman RC, Blackwell AC, Campbell DA Jr, Commiskey E, Anderson S. A better approach to medical malpractice claims? The University of Michigan experience. J Health Life Sci Law. 2009;2:125–59.
29. Boothman RC. CANDOR: the antidote to deny and defend? Health Serv Res. 2016;51:2487–90.
30. Communication and Optimal Resolution (CANDOR) Toolkit: Patient Safety Tools and Training Materials. Agency for Healthcare Research and Quality. Accessed 8 July 2020, at https://www.ahrq.gov/patient-safety/capacity/candor/modules.html.
31. Gallagher TH, Boothman RC, Schweitzer L, Benjamin EM. Making communication and resolution programmes mission critical in healthcare organisations. BMJ Qual Saf. 2020;29(11):875–8.

Chapter 20
Who Can I Trust? Ensuring Physician Competence

Gwyneth Vives, a scientist at Los Alamos National Laboratory in New Mexico, suffered a complication and bled to death 3 hours after giving birth to a healthy boy in 2001. It was 4 days before Christmas. Vives suffered a vaginal tear and other lacerations during the delivery that caused profuse bleeding. Her obstetrician, Pamela Johnson, was sued for failure to order a blood transfusion for Vives as well as abandonment since she had turned over repair of the vaginal tear to a midwife. Two other patients also sued Johnson. Jean Challacombe alleged that Johnson tore her bowel and uterus while doing a dilation and curettage the same day Vives died. Tanya Lewis accused Johnson of doing an unnecessary hysterectomy.

Johnson had been forced to leave a previous job at Duke University Medical Center in North Carolina because of a "high surgical complication rate" and the "worst QA (quality assurance) file of anyone at Duke." At least three patients had filed claims against Johnson for malpractice. Later, Johnson lied to get her New Mexico license, saying she had never lost hospital privileges, according to an order of the New Mexico Medical Board [1].

"It's not bad people, it's bad systems," we said. But it has been a hard sell. When something bad happens, the natural reaction is to blame, to point the finger at the person who made the mistake, the bad doctor. We now know that this is both wrong and ineffective. Most harm, most errors—probably 95% or more—do, in fact, result from bad systems that lead good people to do bad things. That concept has

© The Author(s) 2021
L. L. Leape, *Making Healthcare Safe*,
https://doi.org/10.1007/978-3-030-71123-8_20

been the main driver of patient safety: to get people to think of errors and harm as the result of faulty systems, not faulty people.

But there are some "faulty" people—doctors whose incompetence or negligence harms and kills patients. "That's not a systems problem," people would say. Ah, but it is. Our doctors are educated and trained by a system, certified by a system, monitored by a system, and disciplined by a system. What are those systems? And do they identify doctors when they begin to fail, assess them, and do something about it— *before* they hurt someone? A prevention system, or at least an early warning system. A reasonable question. Indeed, a vital question.

The System We Have

The system we have for producing a competent physician is composed of several interdependent systems. We have a rigorous *educational* system for medicine. Everyone knows that medical education is very difficult, intense, detailed, and challenging. Medical school is hard to get into, the bar is high, and graduates are well-equipped with scientific knowledge when they emerge. This is followed by 3–5 years of residency training and additional years of subspecialty fellowship training, essentially an in-hospital graded experience organized by specialty and culminating in examination and certification of competence by the specialty board ("Board certification").

The system for ensuring the *continuing* competence of the practicing physician also has several parts. The main responsibility falls to the individual specialty boards, who, in conjunction with their association, the American Board of Medical Specialties (ABMS), attempt to ensure continuing competence for the 85% of physicians who are certified by repeated assessments of their diplomates (the word for those certified) through maintenance of certification programs.

State licensing boards exercise responsibility for continuing competence of physicians through periodic relicensing. All but two rely largely on physicians certifying that they have completed a required number of continuing education courses and truthfully answering relicensing application questions about such things as malpractice claims, other civil lawsuits, criminal charges, illness and substance use, and even whether they have paid their taxes.

At the hospital or practice plan level, the system for ensuring continuing competence is *credentialing*, a process that determines whether a physician has admitting privileges to the hospital (or practice in a group) for their patients. Privileges are conferred annually or biannually by a committee of physician peers based on the recommendation of the department chair.

What's the Problem?

The problem is that these systems are not coordinated, and they don't work very well. Despite the many layers of responsibility and the array of mechanisms for ensuring safe and competent care, too many physicians fall short, and too many patients are harmed. Let's look at the facts.

Direct measures of physician performance are hard to come by. There is no nationally standardized system for routine measurement of outcomes of physicians' treatments. An indirect measure of incompetence is malpractice claims, but only claims that result in a payment to the patient are recorded, about a fifth of claims [2]. In 2019, 8378 payments were made for claims against physicians, down significantly from 16,116 in 2001 [3]. (Perhaps as the result of improved disclosure policies?—see Chap. 19.)

Another indirect measure is disciplinary actions by state medical boards. In 2017, 4081 physicians were disciplined by state medical board, including 1147 reprimanded (i.e., censured), 1343 restricted, and 264 who had their licenses revoked [4].

Malpractice claims and disciplinary actions by state boards capture only the proverbial tip of the iceberg. Most negligence is not reported, and few patients sue (see Chap. 1). For each of these cases, there are dozens that are not reported and many more instances of substandard care that results in patient harm.

More information is available about behavioral problems. Studies of disruptive behavior are disturbing. These include angry outbursts, verbal threats, shouting, swearing, degrading and demeaning comments, and threats of physical force, as well as shaming and sexual harassment [5].

Surveys of nurses show that more than 90% report experiencing such abuse [6], many of them repeatedly. Abuse of medical students is also common. Annual surveys of graduating medical students by the Association of American Medical Colleges (AAMC) show that 12–20% report abuse [7], although other data suggest it is much more common [8, 9]. In one survey of students from twenty-four different medical schools, 64% reported at least one incident of mistreatment by faculty, 76% by residents [10].

Residents in training are also victims. Half of 1791 residents in 1 survey reported being subjected to bullying, belittling, and humiliation [11]. A meta-analysis of 52 studies of residents showed that the prevalence of intimidation, harassment and discrimination was 64% [12].

Patients are also targets of abuse. Surveys show that 13–27% of patients report problems with doctor communication [13]. Patient interviews show the percentage is closer to 50% [14].

Why Doctors Fail

Why? Why do physicians who have successfully completed medical school and a rigorous residency training fail to maintain their competence or develop patterns of disruptive and unsafe behavior that compromise their ability to give high-quality, competent care? There are many reasons. Some succumb to the urge to establish a large practice to fulfill monetary needs or underlying feelings of inadequacy and then find its demands more than they can cope with. Others become overconfident and become unable to acknowledge shortcomings. Some are lazy and just don't keep up.

But for most, the causes are more mundane. Like everyone else, physicians have mental and physical health issues. Major depressive disorders occur in 16% of the public. The extent among physicians is unknown, but higher suicide rates—40% higher than the public for male physicians and 100% higher for female physicians—suggest depression is also probably more common [15].

The extent of physical illness among physicians is also unknown, but a reasonable estimate is that at least 10% of doctors must restrict their practices for several months or more at some time in their 40-year careers because of disabling illness [15]. Nor are physicians exempt from cognitive decline as they age, although we have no data.

Approximately 10–12% of physicians will develop a substance abuse problem at some time in their careers. About half of these are alcohol dependence, the rest, opioids and other drugs [16].

Stress is another factor. Physicians are subjected to unique stresses that can lead to dysfunctional behavior. Overwork, sleep deprivation, decreasing reimbursement, and pressure to see more patients are common. In recent years, the fraction of physicians exhibiting burnout has skyrocketed [17]. Young physicians worry about achieving a work/family balance and paying off their educational debts, which in 2018 averaged $196,520 at graduation. Stress leads to isolation and maladaptive coping strategies, such as alcohol or drug abuse.

Putting this all together, the conclusion is stunning. As John Fromson and I wrote in *Problem Doctors: Is There a Systems-Level Solution?*: "When all conditions are considered, **at least one third of all physicians will experience, at some time in their career, a period during which they have a condition that impairs their ability to practice medicine safely**" [15].

The question is: What do we do about it?

Who Is Responsible for Ensuring Physician Competence and Safety?

Who is responsible for making sure that physicians are competent and safe? The answer is disarmingly simple: physicians. Society has given physicians an implicit contract: it grants them incredible powers to cross otherwise sacrosanct boundaries—to learn our most intimate thoughts and invade our bodies and our psyches—in return for the pledge that the profession will use its knowledge and skills for the good of society. It grants the profession substantial autonomy to determine its own educational standards and the right of self-regulation.

The essence of medicine's contract with society is *professionalism*, the commitment of the physician to place the interests of the patient above their own, to maintain their skills, and to ensure that their colleagues do so as well [18].

One way physicians have met this obligation is through specialty societies, the AMA, and state medical societies, which from their origins have considered improving the quality of practice of their members their first priority—their purpose, really. The American College of Surgeons (ACS), for example, was the first to set standards for hospitals, leading ultimately to the formation of the Joint Commission.

Specialty society annual meetings are largely devoted to learning, both from formal instruction and from research presentations. Larger societies, such as the American College of Physicians, American Association of Family Practitioners, and American Society of Anesthesiologists, have extensive extramural continuing education programs and online resources. State medical societies also sponsor educational programs. These programs assist physicians in accruing specific hours of medical education that are required for relicensure by their state boards of medicine.

Physicians have also met their obligation by developing professional organizations that set standards and exercise oversight. The primary responsibility for ensuring physician competence in the USA rests with two national organizations: the American Board of Medical Specialties (ABMS), whose specialty boards examine and certify practicing physicians, and the Accreditation Council for Graduate Medical Education (ACGME), which sets standards and oversees physician residency education.

American Board of Medical Specialties

Specialty board certification is the essential badge of quality for physicians. For decades, becoming certified required only that the physician pass a rigorous written and oral examination at the conclusion of residency. You were certified for life. That began to change in 1969 when the newly formed Board of Family Medicine required that diplomates be reexamined every 10 years to maintain certified status. The process of recertification gradually spread to other specialties.

By the late 1990s, just as the patient safety movement was beginning to gain momentum, the leadership of the ABMS realized they needed to do much more to ensure their diplomates were competent and to assure the public that was so.

In a rather remarkable joint effort, ABMS and ACGME came together in 1999 to explicitly define physician competence. They described six domains of clinical competency that physicians would be expected to achieve and maintain [19] (Box 20.1). The six competencies were adopted by the individual specialty boards as the basis for assessments of physicians. The ACGME adopted them as the framework for progressive training in a specialty.

Box 20.1 Six Domains of Competency
- *Practice-based learning and improvement*: show an ability to investigate and evaluate patient care practices, appraise and assimilate scientific evidence, and improve the practice of medicine.
- *Patient care and procedural skills*: provide care that is compassionate, appropriate, and effective treatment for health problems and to promote health.
- *Systems-based practice*: demonstrate awareness of and responsibility to the larger context and systems of health care. Be able to call on system resources to provide optimal care (e.g., coordinating care across sites or serving as the primary case manager when care involves multiple specialties, professions. or sites).
- *Medical knowledge*: demonstrate knowledge about established and evolving biomedical, clinical, and cognate sciences and their application in patient care.
- *Interpersonal and communication skills*: demonstrate skills that result in effective information exchange and teaming with patients, their families, and professional associates (e.g., fostering a therapeutic relationship that is ethically sound, using effective listening skills with nonverbal and verbal communication, working as both a team member and at times as a leader).
- *Professionalism*: demonstrate a commitment to carrying out professional responsibilities, adherence to ethical principles, and sensitivity to diverse patient populations.

Adapted from Ref. [19]

In addition, the periodic recertification examinations would be replaced by continuing maintenance of certification (MOC), which required the physician to demonstrate a commitment to lifelong learning, self-evaluation, and improving their practice and to prove it through periodic assessments.

Each specialty board devised its own MOC program, tailoring the six competencies to its individual needs and defining how to meet the requirements. The certifying board would then "continually" determine whether or not the physician is in compliance with its MOC requirements. Finally, there was an answer to the patient's concern, "I know he was competent when he was certified, but is he competent now?"

Boards differed greatly in how they assessed compliance. For most, physicians were required to periodically document that they had maintained the core six competencies. A four-part assessment was designed to test their medical knowledge, clinical competence, communication skills, and quality of care. Approaches have included patient registries, audits, peer review, and comparison to national benchmarks. Another is to give credit for participating in hospital quality improvement projects.

Physicians pushed back. Naturally skeptical, they had to be convinced that the process was relevant to their practices and would improve quality of care at a time when they felt overworked and underpaid. However, by 2012 about half of all certified specialists had complied [20].

Older physicians who had been exempted from the 10-year relicensing requirement when it began also sat this one out. As of 2012, of the 66,689 diplomates of the American Board of Internal Medicine who held only the old time-unlimited certificates, only 1% chose to become recertified through MOC [20].

The concept of the six competencies was truly brilliant. Its explicit definitions made it possible to measure competence for the first time. The ACGME incorporated them in standards for residency training. Medical schools adopted them to structure curricula, and the Joint Commission made them requirements for hospital evaluation of their physicians. CMS gave physicians a bonus on their Medicare reimbursement if they participated in its Physician Quality Reporting System and MOC.

Accreditation Council for Graduate Medical Education

The other professional organization responsible for ensuring competence of physicians is the Accreditation Council for Graduate Medical Education (ACGME) . Not unlike the Joint Commission, the ACGME accreditation process had for years focused on structural aspects of training programs, such as qualifications of the program director and number of teaching cases, plus a few outcomes, especially the percentage of graduates who passed certifying examinations.

Following the development of the six competencies, ACGME in 2001 launched the Outcome Project, which requires residency training programs to configure curricula and evaluation processes in the framework of the six competencies.

In 2011, in conjunction with changes in duty hour limits, a major emphasis was begun to improve supervision and providing a safe and effective environment for care and learning: the Clinical Learning Environment Review (CLER) Program.

Through frequent site visits independent of the accreditation process, CLER focuses on the resident experience and progress in six areas: patient safety; health-care quality and reduction in health-care disparities; care transitions; supervision; fatigue management, mitigation, and duty hours; and professionalism [21]. "Milestones" were developed that describe the skills, knowledge, and behaviors in the six areas that residents are expected to reach at each level as they progress through their training.

These ACGME programs are described in greater detail in Chap. 18.

The Joint Commission

The Joint Commission plays an important role in enabling and ensuring physician competence through its oversight role with hospitals. Not only does it require hospitals to have systems and programs that foster quality and safety, which of necessity involve physicians, hospitals are also required to have programs to oversee and enhance physician performance. See Chap. 12 for more details.

State Licensing Boards

An interesting aspect of self-regulation is state regulation. While that sounds like an oxymoron, it is not. State medical licensing boards have legal authority to hold physicians accountable for competent practice, but for many years they were composed entirely of physicians, who were deemed the only ones qualified to judge other doctors. In recent years lay members have been added in some states, but physicians still dominate.

State boards exercise their authority primarily through licensing. Initial licensing for American medical school graduates requires passing three examinations taken in medical school and the first year of residency. Subsequently, physicians are required to complete a certain number of hours of continuing education annually and pay a fee to renew their licenses. State boards can also require physicians to undergo evaluations to ascertain knowledge and skill and require educational remediation and/or rehabilitation of physicians who have physical, mental, or substance use disorders.

Oversight is typically passive. Rather than actively monitoring or auditing performance of doctors in practice, boards tend to function in a reactive mode, responding to malpractice suits, patient complaints, and the occasional problem physician referred by a health-care organization.

State boards can place physicians on probation, censure, ask them to sign a letter of agreement to change behavior, restrict practice, or remove their license to practice. But they are reluctant to do so. Physicians on boards are very sympathetic to their colleagues, in part because they are aware of their own vulnerability. Of the nearly 600,000 physicians in practice in 2017, only 4081 (0.7%) were disciplined by their state boards [4].

Boards are particularly reluctant to take away licenses because doing so is an existential threat to the physician, rendering them unable to practice. As a result, it rarely happens. Licenses were suspended or revoked for 904 physicians (0.15%) in 2017 [4].

Boards also have a long history of being very forgiving of those with psychoactive substance use disorders. (William Halsted, legendary surgeon at Johns Hopkins Hospital and founder of the residency system, was a known cocaine addict.) Physicians with a substance use problem that interferes with their ability to practice medicine are usually required to enter into a 3–5-year monitoring agreement that includes mandatory random urine testing, workplace monitoring by peers and supervisors, attendance at meetings like A.A. or N.A., and seeing a therapist or alcohol/drug counselor. If they fail to follow through, they may have their license to practice suspended until a significant period of being clean and sober is once again documented.

While these practices accord with current thinking that addiction is a disease and not a moral failing, the difference from other fields, of course, is that impaired physicians put patients at risk. Forgiveness can be carried to extremes. For example, a Virginia psychiatrist was in drug rehabilitation 9 times and relapsed at least 12 times during a 10-year period before the medical board took away her license [22]. In a five-year period, only 1400 physicians across the country were disciplined for substance abuse and reported to the National Practitioner Data Bank [23].

The National Practitioner Data Bank was established by Congress in 1986 to stop doctors from escaping troubled histories by having a central location where any sanctions or malpractice verdicts could be recorded. Names are not made public, but they are available to state licensing boards, hospitals, and other health-care entities, including federal agencies, who are required to consult NPDB prior to hiring.

Nevertheless, hospitals and boards have dragged their feet on complying, reluctant to tarnish a physician's reputation or restrict their ability to practice. Various tactics are employed to circumvent the requirement to report physicians, most commonly the hospital rather than the physician paying the settlement in a malpractice case.

Nearly 54 percent of all hospitals have never reported a disciplinary action to the data bank. For example, in the Vives case mentioned above, no one told the data bank that Pamela Johnson had been forced to leave her job at Duke. Enforcement is no better: no fine or penalty has ever been levied according to the federal Department of Health and Human Services, which oversees the system.

Federation of State Medical Boards

The national voice for state boards is the Federation of State Medical Boards (FSMB). All 71 state medical and osteopathic boards are members. The FSMB is the spokesperson for issues related to regulation and discipline. It proposes policy changes and facilitates collaborative efforts of state boards and other entities. With the National Board of Medical Examiners (NBME), it sponsors the US Medical Licensing Examination that is required of all medical school graduates for medical licensure.

FSMB recommends standards, but it has no enforcement power. In 2004, it promoted a radically new policy—"State medical boards have a responsibility to the public to ensure the ongoing competence of physicians seeking re-licensure"—i.e., meaningful maintenance of licensure like the maintenance of certification programs that were being developed [24].

In 2010, FSMB expanded this to declare that as a condition of license renewal, physicians provide evidence of participation in a program of professional development and lifelong learning based on the six ABMS competencies [25].

It then took the step that quality and safety experts had long called for to align licensing and certification: participation in the MOC process of their specialty board would satisfy the standards for relicensure [26].

FSMB also plays a key role in the assessment and rehabilitation of problem doctors. While many state medical societies have monitoring programs for doctors with alcohol and substance use disorders, fewer address knowledge and skill deficits, personality disorders, technical and cognitive deficiencies, or disruptive behavior.

A joint program of FSMB and NBME, the *Post-Licensure Assessment System* (PLAS), administers a standardized examination of clinical knowledge to physicians referred by state medical boards or by themselves. If results are unsatisfactory, the physician may undergo an additional assessment and then choose (or be required) to participate in a remediation program [27].

Alternatively, physicians may be evaluated by the Physician Assessment and Clinical Education (PACE) Program, founded in 1966 at UC San Diego School of Medicine long before FSMB took on this responsibility. The program assesses physicians referred by state boards as a condition of maintaining their licenses. It conducts a rigorous evaluation of a physician's ability to safely practice medicine. They undergo an oral clinical examination, clinical observation, and physical and mental health screening. PACE offers remedial courses in anger management, communication, professional boundaries, prescribing, and medical record keeping [28].

A number of other programs have been developed in recent years for doctors and other professionals with problems. For all, the goal is to enable dyscompetent professionals to undergo remediation and training so that they can remain in practice.

Unfortunately, there are many barriers to physicians' participation in these programs. Foremost are financial. In our fee-for-service health-care system, the physician is in a triple bind. Not only do they lose income while undergoing rehabilitation, they often have to pay a substantial fee for it, and if they are absent for more than a few weeks, their practice deteriorates as patients find other doctors. In a more rational system, their employer would maintain their salary and pay the costs of rehabilitation.

Another problem is that if residency retraining is needed, it is difficult to find programs that are willing and able to add the physician to their roster of residents, even for a short time. Similarly, their colleagues and hospital may be reluctant to take on responsibility or potential liability for supervising their practice. Doctors are uncomfortable supervising their peers.

Experience shows that performance problems can be solved or significantly ameliorated for the vast majority of physicians. Few need to be, nor should be, removed from practice. We know what to do.

Making it happen is another matter. Rehabilitation and remediation are still very much a work in progress.

New York Cardiac Advisory Committee

Perhaps the most effective—and unique—instrument of state regulation is the New York Cardiac Advisory Committee. In the 1950s, long before there was national interest in improving quality or safety, the Health Department of New York convened a group of respected cardiac surgeons and cardiologists to oversee the newly developing field of cardiac surgery. The committee was an outgrowth of the state certificate of need program that regulated which hospitals could establish new programs. It had the power to limit the number of hospitals performing cardiac surgery. Its responsibility was to establish and maintain high-quality programs geographically distributed to meet the needs of the state's population.

In 1989, responding to the concern that its comparisons of mortality among hospitals were not valid because they were not adjusted for risk, and recognizing the need for a data-based approach, the CAC established the Cardiac Surgical Reporting System (CSRS) to develop risk-adjusted measures and collect data on outcomes of coronary artery bypass graft (CABG) surgery. For the first time, the adjusted outcomes of all cardiac surgeons and all hospitals performing cardiac surgery were measured and reported publicly.

The initial findings showed wide variations in 30-day operative mortality with low-volume surgeons and low-volume hospitals faring the worst. High-outlier hospitals were put on probation. The responses were prompt. The survival of their programs at risk, most of them undertook a variety of actions to improve their programs: establishing full-time chiefs, replacing chiefs and poor-performing surgeons, adding cardiac anesthesiologists and nurse specialists, etc. The results were dramatic. Within 3 years, mortality dropped 41%, giving New York the lowest CABG mortality of any state, a status it has maintained [29].

The reports attracted intense media attention in the early years, causing concern about shaming and government interference. Mortality for hospitals and surgeons were reported in the newspapers.

Was that appropriate? Certainly, the public has a right to know. This notion, now well-accepted and enshrined in Hospital Compare and other public data, was a radical idea at the time and hotly debated. There is little question, however, that the public release of the information was a key motivator for change.

As the CAC began to measure risk-adjusted outcomes of CABG surgery in 1989, they approached our team at RAND to do an appropriateness study of CABG, angioplasty, and coronary angiography. Our earlier work had shown high rates of inappropriate use of these procedures. The CAC and the state health department wanted to know if their efforts resulted in lower rates in New York. With their collaboration we were able to get funding for the study, which we carried out over the next 2 years.

The results confirmed the higher quality of cardiac surgical care in New York. The inappropriate rate for CABG was 2.4%, far lower than the 14% found in a previous study in several other states. Mortality was also low, 2.0%, far lower than the national average of 5.5%. The inappropriate use rate for angioplasty was also low: 4%. These added to the evidence that close oversight and the feedback of risk-adjusted data are powerful motivators for quality [30–32].

The CAC program has continued to be successful. It is a superb example of the power of intelligent, well-managed regulation to ensure quality and safety of health care. Unlike other states, in New York the health commissioner has the authority to require reporting, to carry out audits to verify data quality, and to establish the oversight committee and the power to shut programs down.

Involving the state's leading cardiac surgeons and cardiologists in the advisory committee gave credibility to its decisions and acceptability to the cardiac surgical community. The focus on objective evidence provided a powerful incentive for poor performers to improve [29]. The program is a model of effective regulation.

The Civil Justice System—Malpractice Litigation

Finally, when all else fails, the legal system steps in. Doctors can be sued and forced to pay substantial compensation if their performance can be proven to be negligent. The legal definition of negligence is quite simple: failure to meet the standard of care. Proving that is another matter. In the end, relatively few patients are compensated. The Harvard Medical Practice Study found that fewer than 10% of patients harmed by negligent care ever sued [33]. National studies show that fewer than half of malpractice suits result in a payment to the patient [2, 34].

But negligent care is only responsible for a small fraction of serious medical injury. The vast majority of injured patients have no recourse to the legal system. Malpractice litigation also fails to achieve its other purported objective: deterring bad behavior in the future. There is no evidence this happens. Physicians see cases as one off, bad luck, and unjustified. They often don't believe they have done anything wrong. The process of being sued is devastating for physicians, however, as is discussed in more detail in Chap. 19.

A serious defect of the current system is that malpractice settlements are usually sealed, prohibiting any party from making the information accessible. Not only does this cloak of secrecy prevent the medical team from learning from the event and fixing the faulty systems, it keeps vital information away from state boards and future patients.

Overall, malpractice litigation is an ineffective tool for ensuring or improving physician competence. Interestingly, fewer patients are suing. Malpractice payments dropped from 16,116 in 2001 to 8378 in 2019 [3]. It is tempting to attribute this to a reduction in patient injuries or to improved disclosure practices, but there is little evidence for either.

A far better legal approach would be *enterprise liability*, in which the institution, not the physician, is responsible for compensating patients for the costs of harm. Hospitals and health-care organizations would be sued instead. It makes sense. If, as we maintain, harm results from failed systems (including systems for ensuring physician competence), then it is the party responsible for the systems—the organization—that should be held accountable for their failures. Indeed, if we were really serious about this, we would require hospitals to compensate patients for *all* costs of the harm we have caused, even when no error is identified: no-fault compensation—as was recommended by the Harvard Medical Practice Study 30 years ago.

Hospital Responsibility for Physician Performance

As in politics, all quality is local. Medical specialty boards set standards, examine, and certify; states license and discipline; but meaningful oversight of physician performance, what happens in everyday practice, takes place where care is delivered. For 80% of physicians, that is the hospital. For others it can be their large multispecialty group. But for practitioners in solo or small group practice, such as primary care, psychiatry, and dermatology, oversight is often quite lax.

Hospital oversight is through *credentialing* committees, groups of physicians appointed by the medical staff who annually or biannually decide on admitting privileges and what procedures a doctor may perform. It is awesome power, second only to state licensing. If they are unable to admit patients to a hospital, most physicians cannot practice. They are professionally dead. Every hospital has a credentialing committee. Medical specialty boards are the carrot, credentialing committees are the stick.

The process that most credentialing committees use for carrying out this responsibility is quite simple: they rely on the recommendation from the specialty department chair. Typically, this is a pro forma process unless the department chair recommends against it. Then it can get very messy.

So, where "the rubber hits the road," where the action takes place to ensure physician competence, is the department. The department chair is ultimately responsible for assessing the competence of every member of the department. How do they do it?

Until very recently, assessment has been informal, especially in smaller private hospitals where the chair has little authority. The chair relied on personal knowledge about the physician and feedback from peers. Absent serious complaints from patients or staff about the physician's conduct, approval was routine.

Few department chairs actually reviewed patient outcomes or conducted peer assessment of performance. Annual physical examinations are still not required. Random drug testing is rare and hotly resisted by many physicians as an affront to their professionalism. Cognitive testing is almost nonexistent.

The good news is that methods for monitoring clinical performance have improved greatly in recent years. To be objective, evaluation must be based on data: compliance with standard practices and outcomes, how well patients do. While measuring outcomes is easiest with surgical patients, many "medical" outcomes are now also collected routinely. Individual results can then be compared with national and local norms to identify outliers who need attention.

The Joint Commission now requires that physicians currently on staff have an annual Ongoing Professional Practice Evaluation (OPPE). This is a summary of ongoing data collected for the purpose of assessing a practitioner's clinical competence and professional behavior. Newly hired physicians and those already on staff found to have competency issues on their OPPE are required to have a Focused Professional Practice Evaluation in which the medical staff evaluates the privilege-specific competence of the practitioner [35].

Psychosocial aspects of physician competence—communication skills, interpersonal relations, and ability to collaborate—have long been considered unquantifiable. They have traditionally been assessed informally through conversations with peers and coworkers. Personality or interest tests and the like have been tried and found not to be reliable. But one method of evaluation does produce data that is reliable and has proven to be quite useful: multisource feedback, popularly called "360" evaluations.

Multisource Feedback

Multisource feedback (MSF) is a formalized method of obtaining feedback about an individual's performance from those with whom they interact. Since the late 1990s, it has been used to assess physicians by Lockyer in the Physician Achievement Review (PAR) program in Alberta, Canada [36], but is now being increasingly used in US hospitals. The PACE program in California has used it for some time to evaluate physicians referred for problem behavior.

The process begins by having the physician and their peers, nurses, residents, and patients complete a questionnaire of 10–40 items that assess clinical behaviors, such as communication, collaboration, professionalism, interpersonal, and management skills. Typically, 7–15 individuals in each of these groups complete the questionnaire, rating the physician on a five-point scale. The results are tabulated by group, and mean scores are compared to the physician's self-assessment for each item. The department chairman then reviews the data with the physician to identify areas for improvement. Studies have shown that MSF has high reliability, validity, and feasibility [37].

The impact of the 360 review can be very powerful. In a pilot study some years ago in one department in a Boston hospital, we found that, as in Lake Wobegon, all physicians rated themselves above average for almost all questions. Peers tended to agree, but resident and nurse ratings were sometimes quite a bit lower, especially regarding interpersonal relations. Feedback of this information to the physician was always a surprise and sometimes emotionally very disturbing. Several were reduced to tears. It was a powerful motivation for change.

MSF is increasingly being used in the USA. ABMS now recommends that specialty boards use MSF to assess professionalism and knowledge, and ACGME requires training programs to use multiple evaluators to provide objective performance evaluation of residents. The Pulse 360 Program creates and sells 360 feedback tools and training programs for health care. It is used in over 200 hospitals [38].

Support of Physicians with Problems

With the demands of MOC, methods for evaluation and support are improving. Specialty boards, especially the ABIM, have become more engaged with hospitals in providing continuing education, translating standards into practice, and collecting outcome data to measure performance. Blue Cross Blue Shield Association, CIGNA HealthCare, Humana, and Wellpoint have incorporated them in their quality recognition programs.

But serious behavioral problems are often managed poorly. Department chairs may lack the training and skills to deal with them. Many fear confrontation and avoid it if possible. Peers are reluctant to be involved, valuing their own independence and respecting that of others.

A major barrier is that disciplinary action will often be vigorously resisted by the offending physician, who may even sue the department or the hospital. This leads to bad publicity in the newspapers and requires a number of doctors to spend many hours in depositions or hearings—a messy business, indeed. No wonder doctors shy away from judging their peers.

How Should it Work? The Ideal System

There must be a better way to ensure physician competence and improve quality of care. There is. It is for the hospital (or practice) to perform a meaningful evaluation of every physician every year using a routine, formal, proactive system of monitoring with validated measures, followed by action to remedy shortcomings when they are discovered. Some years ago, John Fromson and I proposed that the system must have three characteristics [15]:

- First, it must be *objective*, i.e., assessment must be based on data: patient outcomes data and compliance with performance standards, not on subjective judgments of personality or motivation.
- Second, it must be *fair*. All physicians in the organization must be evaluated by the same system, not just suspect individuals.
- Third, it must be *responsive*. When problems are identified, they must be treated promptly. There is no point in evaluation if nothing comes of it. Most physicians with problems will only need feedback. They can and will self-correct. Others may need counseling. Some may require referral to an outside program for assessment. Retraining may be needed.

An effective system is proactive. It is based on the notion that subpar performance can be objectively defined, routine monitoring can detect problems early, and the responses to deficiencies will be prompt and constructive.

The point is not to identify "bad apples" and throw them out, but to detect deficiencies early and correct them before patients are harmed, to enable good doctors with minor problems to become better, and to help those with more serious problems to overcome them if possible.

In the ideal system, the department adopts explicit standards, requires compliance, monitors performance, and responds to deficiencies. The department chair reviews performance data with each physician annually, and together they work out a plan for improvement as needed. In some cases, this may require external testing and remediation.

A similar oversight process should be required of larger medical groups and employed physicians. The remaining small number of physicians in solo or small practice might then be required by licensing authorities to take advantage of some mechanism like PACE or CPEP in order to maintain licensure.

Fortunately, as we have seen, the ABMS and specialty boards have worked hard in recent years to develop national standards of competence and behavior and to integrate them into the process of continuing certification. Closer coordination of this oversight with local review and response would lead to greater accountability and improved performance.

Nonregulatory Approaches to Improving Competence

Independent of the impressive changes to improve accountability by the establishment organizations described above, a number of independent voluntary initiatives have taken place over the years to improve the process of physician assessment and improvement. Several deserve special mention.

National Surgical Quality Improvement Program

In 1986, responding to a series of newspaper articles about poor care in Veterans Health Administration (VHA) hospitals, Congress mandated that VHA report risk-adjusted surgical outcomes annually and compare them to national averages. There was a problem, though: there were no known national averages and no known risk adjustment models!

But the VA was uniquely suited to develop them for its population. The VHA is the largest health-care provider in the USA, serving several million veterans and performing surgery in 128 of its 159 Veterans Administration Medical Centers (VAMCs). At the behest of their surgical leadership, a research group at the Brockton/West Roxbury VA Medical Center in Massachusetts led by Shukri Khuri, Chief of Surgery, and Jennifer Daley, an experienced quality-of-care researcher, carried out the National VA Surgical Risk Study from 1991 to 1993. Using data collected from 117,000 major operations in 44 VAMCs, they developed risk adjustment models for 30-day mortality and morbidity rates for noncardiac surgery [39].

They then turned their attention to measurement of surgical outcomes. Surgery is uniquely suitable for measurement of outcomes since there is a clearly defined expected outcome for every operation. Using this validated model for risk adjustment, outcomes could now be measured with some confidence in their validity.

In 1994 the VHA established the National VA Surgical Quality Improvement Program (NSQIP), a reporting and managerial structure for the continuous monitoring and enhancement of the quality of surgical care, under an executive committee led by Khuri and Daley [40].

Surgical clinical nurse reviewers (SCNRs) were trained in the accurate collection and timely transmission of risk adjustment data, consisting of 45 presurgical variables, 17 surgical variables, and 33 outcomes. Logistic regression analysis was used to calculate a predicted probability of 30-day mortality and complications. Risk-adjusted observed versus expected (O/E) outcome ratios were calculated for all types of procedures at the surgical service of each VAMC and overall.

Feedback of these procedure-specific O/E ratios is provided annually to the chief of surgery, director, and chief of staff of each VAMC, and the CMO of each Veterans Integrated Service Networks (VISN), as well as results for all participating hospitals, by code. Hospital leaders know only the code for their hospital.

The executive committee produces an annual assessment of high and low outliers and communicates levels of concern about high outlier status to hospital and VISN, as well as praise and rewards to low outliers. Persistent high outliers are subject to internal and external reviews.

NSQIP also develops and disseminates self-assessment tools to providers and managers and, at the request of a VAMC, organizes consultative site visits to assess data quality and performance.

NSQIP provides management (directors and CMOs of VISN) with advice and expertise in conducting external reviews and site visits and disseminates best practices reported by low O/E hospitals.

The first assessment of results showed that during the period from 1991 to 1997 30-day mortality decreased from 3.1 to 2.8 and morbidity decreased from 17.4 to 10.3. By 2006, postoperative mortality had dropped by 47% and morbidity rates by 43% [41].

The program was well-accepted by the chiefs of surgery who valued the feedback and learned to find and improve deficiencies. From the beginning, NSQIP has been about quality improvement, not judgment. The emphasis is on systems not providers. No individual provider-specific data is transmitted to the central data base.

Several aspects of NSQIP accounted for its success. Most important was the fact that VHA had in place a universal computerized record system, VISTA, that made clinical and laboratory data available for risk analysis. It also had access to the operating room log in every VAMC, so all procedures were automatically and reliably identified.

Second, for data entry it relied exclusively on trained surgical clinical nurse reviewers (SCNRs) who were experienced in practice, data collection, and quality assurance. This gave high levels of credibility, reliability, and validity to the data. Third, inclusion of surgical leaders from the field in the design of the program and oversight led to support by VAMC senior surgeons, administrators, VISN directors, and CMOs.

The private sector took notice. Why not use NSQIP for non-VA surgical departments? Within months of the first report, in 1999, a pilot program was begun in three academic surgical centers, University of Michigan, Emory University, and the University of Kentucky, to determine if the risk adjustment models would work for the more heterogeneous private sector patient populations. They did. Comparison of findings in 2747 patients at these centers with contemporary results in 41,360 patients in the VHA showed no differences in risk-adjusted mortality between the non-VA and VA cohorts [42].

Following this success, the American College of Surgeons (ACS) in 2001 sponsored a pilot program funded by AHRQ in18 private sector hospitals that showed that NSQIP also led to reduced morbidity and mortality in private sector hospitals. In 2004, ACS began enrolling additional private sector hospitals into ACS NSQIP. Within a year, 41 hospitals had joined. By 2018, participants included 568 hospitals in the USA, 96 in Canada, and 38 overseas. Nine of the top 10 hospitals ranked as America's Best Hospitals by *U.S. News & World Report* in 2018 participated in ACS NSQIP [41].

Meanwhile, NSQIP continues to work on improving. More specialty variables were incorporated; additional outcome measurements, such as functional status, quality of life, and patient satisfaction, were developed and incorporated; and structure and process measures were added [43].

Analysis of Patient Complaints

In the early 1990s, Gerald Hickson, Associate Dean for Clinical Affairs at Vanderbilt University Medical Center, and his colleagues found that analysis of written complaints by patients to the hospital was a useful tool for identifying physicians with interpersonal problems. About 2/3 of complaints were about a hospital or practice service or system issue; 1/3 were about a named physician.

While patients often complain about their doctors, it is unusual for them to make a formal complaint in writing [44]; most physicians receive none or only one or two over their entire professional career. But some have more. Hickson wondered if there was a relationship between the number of complaints and the likelihood of the physician being sued. ("Claims" in risk management parlance.)

Indeed, there was. In a six-year period, he found no claims for 81% of doctors who had only one or no complaints. The majority of those with 2–6 complaints also had no claims. But physicians with 4 or more complaints over this period were 16 times more likely to have 2 or more claims than physicians with no complaints. Those with 25 claims or more had a 95% chance of being sued [45].

Hickson realized that patient reports could serve as the basis of an "early warning system" to more rapidly identify and engage with physicians before harm occurred and suits began to accumulate. They could then be helped to overcome their deficiencies. He developed a tiered intervention program, the Promoting Professionalism Pyramid, that defined a process that started with a conversation with a colleague and escalated if needed to formal evaluation and required behavioral change.

Following the first complaint, a colleague would have a "cup of coffee conversation" in which the complaint is shared with the physician in a nonjudgmental way and they are asked to reflect on the event. Often the physician has not recognized the bad behavior and justifies it because of the situation. The colleague makes no judgment, merely delivering the news. But for many, that is all that is necessary: their behavior changes.

At the second level, when there have been additional reports that suggest a pattern of inappropriate behavior, an *awareness* intervention is called for. A respected colleague presents the data to the individual showing how their complaint history compares to that of their peers and gives them the opportunity to respond. Again, in most cases this is all that is needed to lead the physician to change behavior.

For those that do not respond to the awareness intervention, the response moves to the next level. The department chair steps in and makes it clear that the individual must change their behavior. Chairs are trained to work with the physician to define an improvement plan that may range from coaching and counseling to formal outside evaluation and retraining.

If the physician is unwilling to undergo assessment and take responsibility for improving, or if these measures fail, then disciplinary action is required, which can include revoking admitting privileges or reporting to the state medical board [46]. Fewer than 1% fall into this category.

Hickson also developed a comprehensive program at Vanderbilt to reduce disruptive behavior by teaching interpersonal skills and professionalism at all levels: medical students, residents, and physicians. Physician leaders also receive skills training for conducting interventions [46].

He also developed a Comprehensive Assessment Program for Professionals to provide medical and psychological evaluation and treatment planning. Group classes were developed for disruptive behavior, prescribing problems and crossing sexual boundaries [47].

National Alliance for Physician Competence

This was one of the most unusual and exciting ventures I was ever part of, both for its goal, which was to set standards for good medical practice, and for those who participated, who were leaders of the national groups that could make it happen—in education, regulation, professional societies, and others. It was also one of the most frustrating.

The Alliance was organized by James Thompson, President and CEO of the FSMB, an ENT physician and former Dean at Wake Forest School of Medicine. Moved by the IOM reports, *To Err is Human* and *Crossing the Quality Chasm*, Thompson recognized when he took over FSMB that state medical licensing boards needed better methods for determining physician competence, both for licensing and for disciplinary actions. ACGME and ABMS had defined the six competencies, and the ABMS was moving to maintenance of certification. Shouldn't state boards do likewise?

Thompson encouraged the Federation to issue a statement on the need for maintenance of licensure, but much more was needed to make it a reality. He conferred with experts he knew as a former Dean: Donald Melnick, President and CEO of the National Board of Medical Examiners (NBME); James Hallock, CEO of the Educational Commission for Foreign Medical Graduates (ECFMG); and David Leach, CEO of ACGME. They supported his effort but felt that a comprehensive strategy linking licensure to education and specialty certification was needed. The time had come to begin a dialogue about the future of physician education and self-regulation.

On March 24, 2005, they brought together more than 60 leaders and representatives from organized medicine, academic medicine, hospitals, regulatory agencies, the insurance industry, accrediting organizations, payers, and the public in Fort Worth, Texas, for the first "Summit" on Physician Accountability for Physician Competence (PA4PC) (Table 20.1). The goals were to determine (1) how to define a competent physician, (2) how to measure competency, and (3) how medical organizations would assure the public that physicians are maintaining competence throughout the lifetime of their practice [26].

With help from Innovation Labs, and financial support from the NBME, the meeting explored the context within which physicians

Table 20.1 Institutional members of the National Alliance for Physician Competence

The Association of American Medical Colleges
AARP
Accreditation Council for Continuing Medical Education
Accreditation Council for Graduate Medical Education
American Board of Internal Medicine Foundation
American Board of Medical Specialties
American Medical Association
American Osteopathic Association
American Osteopathic Board of Emergency Medicine
Association of American Medical Colleges
Association for Hospital Medical Education
Blue Cross/Blue Shield Association
Christiana Care
Council of Medical Specialty Societies
Crozer-Keystone Health System
Educational Commission for Foreign Medical Graduates
The Federation of State Medical Boards
Iowa Board of Medical Examiners
Michigan Board of Medicine
National Board of Medical Examiners
National Board of Osteopathic Medical Examiners
Oregon Board of Medical Examiners
The Robert Wood Johnson Foundation
Texas A&M Health Science Center

would be expected to demonstrate accountability in the year 2020. What should the system look like? The group was energized and quickly found common ground on the big issues.

In subsequent meetings, other relevant stakeholders, such as patients and content experts like myself, were added to the group. Over the next 2 years, in a series of semi-annual meetings PA4PC drafted detailed definitions of competence and the content for a document, Good Medical Practice, that described the behaviors and values one should expect of a competent physician. A task force worked on simplifying physicians' access to credentialing information for multiple purposes such as licensing and board certification. The group renamed itself the National Alliance on Physician Competence.

The good practice document was our central focus. It was based on the work of the General Medical Council in the UK but reframed in terms of the six domains of competency defined by ABMS and ACGME. There were great debates about terminology. Should the document say doctors "should" do such and such or "must" do it? Ultimately, both were rejected. This would be a statement of who we *are* and what we do—who we *aspire* to be—not because it is required, but because of our values and commitment to our professionalism. We would use simple declarative sentences: "We respect each patient's dignity and individuality"; "We promptly modify our practice to incorporate evidence-based care"; "We apologize promptly to a patient when an error has occurred."

As it came into focus, we realized that the document should begin with The Patient's Perspective: a comprehensive statement of what patients have a right to expect from doctors regarding medical knowledge and skills, communication and interpersonal skills, shared decision-making, access and availability, and ethical integrity. This is the lens through which we see our role, our duty. The *purpose* of competence is to provide optimal patient care.

We finished the first draft, Version 0.1, of *Good Medical Practice – USA*, on August 15, 2007. It described the behaviors expected of all doctors who are permitted to practice medicine. The Patient's Perspective was followed by Duties of the Doctor consisting of one chapter for each of the six domains of competency. It was incredibly detailed, 200 statements in all, providing guidance on every aspect of practice, especially those that are difficult, such as knowing one's limits, giving bad news, dealing with problem colleagues, etc. Simple declarative statements of what good doctors do.

We called on medical educators and regulators to incorporate these principles in everything they do and challenged all physicians to take personal responsibility for making it happen.

The Alliance grappled with the relationship between maintenance of licensure and maintenance of certification and how to engage the practicing community and the public in the effort. To facilitate the licensing and certification processes, it developed a standardized, comprehensive "Trusted Agent/Portfolio System" that would enable physicians to retrieve all needed credentials from a single source.

The Alliance examined how a "continuum of competence" could be established: a system that would start in medical school and continue through residency programs, licensure, specialty certification, hospital credentialing and privileging, and the accreditation of institutions. How would the use of Good Medical Practice and the Trusted Agent/Portfolio System impact long-term maintenance of competency throughout a physician's career?

The last meeting of the National Alliance for Physician Competence Summit was held on July 7–9, 2008. The goal was to prepare to go public. Small groups synthesized and polished models to shift the paradigm for competence. These were then rolled into a single model of 14 components. Others focused on finalizing the renamed *Guide to Good Medical Practice*. Plans were made to "go live" with it in September, when Alliance participants would distribute the document. A draft Alliance website was created. A revised Alliance Participant Agreement was approved.

Then it all fell apart. From the beginning, the AMA had been a reluctant participant. It traditionally opposed anyone telling doctors how to practice and was against giving state boards more power. It declared opposition to the Guide even before it was

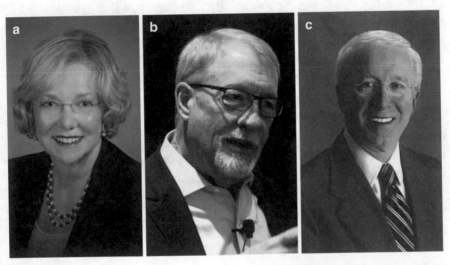

(a) Jennifer Daley, (b) Jerry Hickson, and (c) Jim Thompson. (All rights reserved)

written, maintaining that medicine is full of gray areas that are too difficult to measure. It opposed the concept of maintenance of certification.

At the last two meetings, it sought to undermine the process of the meetings by sending a large number of delegates who raised objections in all the working sessions. Although most of these were rejected by the majority, they disrupted the collaborative process.

Finally, at the last session the AMA withdrew its support. And, much to my surprise, despite the fact that it was the convener, so did the FSMB. It was proving to be too much for the individual state licensing boards. They were reluctant to take on this level of responsibility, and they saw no way to obtain the resources that would be required. The ABMS did not fight for it. It was having enough trouble figuring out how to implement the six competencies. The Alliance was finished. Our "brief shining moment," our Camelot, was over.

The Coalition for Physician Accountability

But Don Melnick, Jim Hallock, and Darrell Kirsch, CEO of the AAMC, were not going to let the concept die. The next year, they formed the Coalition for Physician Accountability to continue the discussion and further the cause. Its membership includes the stakeholders who have direct responsibility for assessment, accreditation, licensure, and certification along the continuum of medical education and practice.

The Coalition provides a forum for dialogue about ways to "promote professional accountability by improving the quality, efficiency, and continuity of the education, training and assessment of physicians" [48]. The Coalition meets twice yearly to analyze critical issues related to the regulation of physician education and practice and to develop consensus on actions to address them.

It functions through its member's endorsement of consensus statements about a diverse group of topics: regulation, innovation in medical school curricula, graduate medical education accreditation, interprofessional education, medical student and physician burnout, use of health information technology, opioid epidemic mitigation, interstate licensure, and a framework for professional competence and lifelong learning. It developed a consensus letter that was sent to Congress regarding maintaining Medicare support of GME, and it sent a letter to the National Coordinator outlining the commitment of Coalition members to promoting the use of health information technology.

Conclusion

Ensuring physician competence is a complex and difficult business. Despite the huge amount of work done by many diverse parties, it is still very much a work in progress. Oversight bodies, the state licensing boards and, especially, the specialty boards, have made substantial improvements in how they function, but the results still fall far short of achieving their objectives.

Why? Why doesn't the system work better? Why don't ABMS and the specialty boards make it work better and require, audit, and enforce adherence to the impressive and innovative processes they developed for maintenance of certification based on the six competencies?

Undoubtedly, there are many reasons, but I suggest that the fundamental reason, the "root cause" if you will, is that it is contrary to human nature for any group to police itself. We have not asked that of the other major industries where safety is critical: aviation and nuclear power. They are closely regulated by specific government agencies.

Do we need a federal agency to regulate quality and safety in health care? I have long believed we do [49]. The federal agencies regulating aviation and nuclear power are good models. The government exercises strict oversight of compliance with its rules, but those rules were developed in collaboration with the industry. Participation leads to buy-in and higher likelihood of compliance. (Recall the New York Cardiac Advisory Committee.) An agency developing regulations for doctors should collaborate with the specialty boards and state boards as well as representatives from professional societies and health-care organizations.

Hospitals should be held accountable for their physicians' performance. They should participate in developing regulations that ensure they are accountable to the public, such as required reporting of adverse events. The Joint Commission should be a partner in this process and play an important role by carrying out the necessary annual or semi-annual audits.

We have made tremendous progress in recent years in defining competence and measuring it. What was formerly implicit and casual can now be defined in an explicit and formal manner. We now know how to enable physicians to realize their full potential and by so doing immensely improve the quality and safety of patient care. The time has come to make it happen.

References

1. Thompson CW. Poor performance records are easily outdistanced. The Washington Post; April 12, 2005.
2. Studdert DM, Mello MM, Gawande AA, et al. Claims, errors, and compensation payments in medical malpractice litigation. N Engl J Med. 2006;354:2024–33.
3. National Practitioner Data Bank (2020): Adverse action and medical malpractice reports (1990 - March 31, 2020). U.S. Department of Health and Human Services, Health Resources and Services Administration, Bureau of Health Workforce, Division of Practitioner Data Bank; 2020.
4. Federation of State Medical Boards. U.S. Medical Regulatory Trends and Actions 2018. Euless, Texas: Federation of State Medical Boards; 2018.
5. Leape L, Shore M, Dienstag J, et al. A culture of respect: I. The nature and causes of disrespectful behavior. Acad Med. 2012;87:845–52.
6. Saxton R, Hines T, Enriquez M. The negative impact of nurse-physician disruptive on patient safety: a review of the literature. J Patient Saf. 2009;5:180–3.
7. Mavis B, Sousa A, Lipscomb W, Rappley MD. Learning about medical student mistreatment from responses to the medical school graduation questionnaire. Acad Med. 2014;89:705–11.
8. Kassebaum D, Culer E. On the culture of student abuse in medical school. Acad Med. 1998;73:1149–58.
9. National Patient Safety Foundation. Unmet needs: teaching physicians to provide safe patient care. Boston: Lucian Leape Institute at the National Patient Safety Foundation; 2010.
10. Cook AF, Arora VM, Rasinski KA, Curlin FA, Yoon JD. The prevalence of medical student mistreatment and its association with burnout. Acad Med. 2014;89:749–54.
11. Chadaga AR, Villines D, Krikorian A. Bullying in the American graduate medical education system: a national cross-sectional survey. PLoS One. 2016;11:e0150246.
12. Bahji A, Altomare J. Prevalence of intimidation, harassment, and discrimination among resident physicians: a systematic review and meta-analysis. Can Med Educ J. 2020;11:e97–e123.

13. Summary of HCAHPS survey results: January 2018 to December 2018 discharges. Centers for Medicare & Medicaid Services, 2019. Accessed 9 July 2020, at https://hcahpsonline.org/globalassets/hcahps/summary-analyses/summary-results/october-2019-public-report-january-2018%2D%2Ddecember-2018-discharges.pdf.

14. Leape LL. Unpublished Work.

15. Leape L, Fromson JA. Problem doctors: is there a system-level solution? Ann Intern Med. 2006;144:107–15.

16. Berge KH, Seppala MD, Schipper AM. Chemical dependency and the physician. Mayo Clin Proc. 2009;84:625–31.

17. Shanafelt TD, Hasan O, Dyrbye LN, et al. Changes in burnout and satisfaction with work-life balance in physicians and the general US working population between 2011 and 2014. Mayo Clin Proc. 2015;90:1600–13.

18. ABIM Foundation, American Board of Internal Medicine, ACP-ASIM Foundation, American College of Physicians-American Society of Internal Medicine, European Federation of Internal Medicine. Medical professionalism in the new millennium: a physician charter. Ann Intern Med. 2002;136:243–6.

19. Board certification: a trusted credential based on core competencies. American Board of Medical Specialties, [Archived February 15, 2020]. Accessed 9 July 2020, at https://web.archive.org/web/20200215154456/https:/www.abms.org/board-certification/a-trusted-credential/based-on-core-competencies.

20. Iglehart JK, Baron RB. Ensuring physicians' competence--is maintenance of certification the answer? N Engl J Med. 2012;367:2543–9.

21. Nasca TJ, Weiss KB, Bagian JP, Brigham TP. The accreditation system after the "next accreditation system". Acad Med. 2014;89:27–9.

22. Thompson CW. Medical boards let physicians practice despite drug abuse. The Washington Post; April 10, 2005.

23. National Practitioner Data Bank. https://www.npdb.hrsa.gov/index.jsp.

24. Federation of State Medical Boards Public Policy Compendium. Federation of State Medical Boards; 2007.

25. Federation of State Medical Boards Public Policy Compendium, policy 250.004 maintenance of licensure: Federation of State Medical Boards; 2011.

26. Thompson JN, Robin LA. State medical boards. J Legal Med. 2012;33:93–114.

27. Directory of physician assessment and remedial education programs. Federation of State Medical Boards. 2020. Accessed 9 July 2020, at https://www.fsmb.org/siteassets/spex/pdfs/remedprog.pdf.

28. Physician Assessment and Clinical Education (PACE). UC San Diego School of Medicine. Accessed 9 July 2020, at http://paceprogram.ucsd.edu/.

29. Chassin MR. Achieving and sustaining improved quality: lessons from New York state and cardiac surgery. Health Aff. 2002;21:40–51.

30. Leape LL, Hilborne LH, Park RE, et al. The appropriateness of use of coronary artery bypass graft surgery in New York state. JAMA. 1993;269:753–60.

31. Hilborne LH, Leape LL, Bernstein SJ, et al. The appropriateness of use of percutaneous transluminal coronary angioplasty in New York state. JAMA. 1993;269:761–5.

32. Bernstein SJ, Hilborne LH, Leape LL, et al. The appropriateness of use of coronary angiography in New York state. JAMA. 1993;269:766–70.

33. Localio AR, Lawthers AG, Brennan TA, et al. Relation between malpractice claims and adverse events due to negligence. N Engl J Med. 1991;325:245–51.

34. Cohen TH. Medical malpractice trials and verdicts in large counties, 2001. Washington, DC: Bureau of Justice Statistics; April 18, 2004.

35. Focused Professional Practice Evaluation (FPPE) - Understanding the requirements. The Joint Commission. Accessed 27 Sept 2020, at https://www.jointcommission.org/standards/standard-faqs/critical-access-hospital/medical-staff-ms/000001485/.

36. Lockyer J. Multisource feedback in the assessment of physician competencies. J Contin Educ Health Prof. 2003;23:4–12.

37. Donnon T, Al Ansari A, Al Alawi S, Violato C. The reliability, validity, and feasibility of multisource feedback physician assessment: a systematic review. Acad Med. 2014;89:511–6.

38. PULSE Program. Physicians Development Program Inc. Accessed 9 July 2020, at https://pulseprogram.com/.

39. Khuri SF, Daley J, Henderson WG. The comparative assessment and improvement of quality of surgical care in the Department of Veterans Affairs. Arch Surg. 2002;137:20–7.

40. Khuri SF, Daley J, Henderson W, et al. The Department of Veterans Affairs' NSQIP: the first national, validated, outcome-based, risk-adjusted, and peer-controlled program for the measurement and enhancement of the quality of surgical care. National VA Surgical Quality Improvement Program. Ann Surg. 1998;228:491–507.

41. ACS NSQIP Hospitals. The American College of Surgeons. Accessed 22 June 2020, at https://www.facs.org/search/nsqip-participants?allresults=.

42. Fink AS, Campbell DA Jr, Mentzer RM Jr, et al. The National Surgical Quality Improvement Program in non-veterans administration hospitals: initial demonstration of feasibility. Ann Surg. 2002;236:344–53.

43. Khuri SF. The NSQIP: a new frontier in surgery. Surgery. 2005;138:837–43.

44. Annandale E, Hunt K. Accounts of disagreements with doctors. Soc Sci Med. 1998;46:119–29.

45. Hickson GB, Federspiel CF, Pichert JW, Miller CS, Gauld-Jaeger J, Bost P. Patient complaints and malpractice risk. JAMA. 2002;287:2951–7.

46. Hickson GB, Pichert JW, Webb LE, Gabbe SG. A complementary approach to promoting professionalism: identifying, measuring, and addressing unprofessional behaviors. Acad Med. 2007;82:1040–8.

47. Vanderbilt Comprehensive Assessment Program. Vanderbilt University Medical Center. Accessed 9 July 2020, at https://www.vanderbilthealth.com/v-cap/.

48. Coalition for Physician Accountability. Accessed 9 July 2020, at http://www.physicianaccountability.org/.
49. Leape LL. Translating medical science into medical practice: do we need a national medical standards board? JAMA. 1995;273:1534–8.
50. Holmboe ES, Edgar L, Hamstra S. The milestones guidebook. Chicago: ACGME; 2016.

Chapter 21
Everyone Counts: Building a Culture of Respect

"The doctor treats me like an idiot." "He doesn't like people who ask questions." "He makes me feel like I'm wasting his time." (from a patient)

"When did you get your MD degree?" "When I want your advice, I'll ask for it." (doctor to a nurse)

"Is that what they teach you in medical school these days?" "Don't you know anything about renal anatomy?" (doctor to a medical student)

What is this all about? How can the noblest of professions, made up of intelligent, hard-working, dedicated people, have within its ranks some who treat others badly in their time of need? Why doesn't "professionalism" for all health-care professionals extend to ensuring that they live up to standards of decency and civility? As we have seen in the previous chapter, the reasons are complex, and disrespectful behavior is but one of many potential failings that doctors may suffer. But its influence is profound.

As the patient safety movement entered its second decade, experience with attempts to change systems led safety leaders to recognize that major progress could not occur without a supportive culture. And it became apparent that the major barrier to creating that culture, the core of the problem, was inappropriate physician behavior. This was, of course, the focus of our work on disclosure and apology: getting physicians to respect the patient's need for, and right to, full information on what went wrong when they were harmed by their care.

The original version of the chapter has been revised. A correction to this chapter can be found at
https://doi.org/10.1007/978-3-030-71123-8_24

© The Author(s) 2021, corrected publication 2021
L. L. Leape, *Making Healthcare Safe*,
https://doi.org/10.1007/978-3-030-71123-8_21

Physician behavior was also the focus of the attempts to reform medical education. The first LLI white paper, *Unmet Needs: Teaching physicians to provide safe patient care*, documented the alarming frequency of demeaning and dehumanizing treatment by faculty that medical students experienced. It came down with a strong recommendation that medical school deans and teaching hospital CEOs adopt a zero-tolerance policy for disrespectful or abusive behavior [1].

What is the patient experience? In my course on quality and patient safety at the Harvard School of Public Health, I collected disturbing data about the patient experience from my graduate students. Each year, at the beginning of the course, to ground their approach to quality improvement in real-world experience, I asked students to interview someone who had a serious medical problem. The students were to ask just two questions: What is it like living with this condition? What has been your experience with medical care? Consistently, over 10 years, nearly half of patients recounted episodes where they were treated in a demeaning or disrespectful way by their doctors, leaving memories that were often still vivid years later.

Even more than patients and students, nurses are on the receiving end of disrespectful treatment by physicians. Almost all nurses can tell stories of disruptive behavior and humiliation. Most of the physicians they work with treat them well, but it occurs frequently enough to poison the atmosphere and cause some to leave nursing.

Although available evidence does indicate that the percentage of doctors who engage in grossly disruptive behavior is small, many more engage in less flagrant types of disrespectful behavior. Dismissive put-downs of patients and nurses and "education by humiliation" or "pimping" of students are widely experienced. This had to change if we were to create the learning and supportive culture that is essential to safety. I became convinced that pervasive disrespect was the core of the culture problem. What could we do about it?

A Group of Leaders

Perhaps if Harvard took the lead, others would follow. If our staid, old, conservative hospitals could come to grips with the problem, others could as well. I raised the question to a number of knowledgeable, respected leaders who I knew at Harvard Medical School (HMS) and its hospitals. To my delight, but not surprise, they were all interested in taking it on. They knew disrespectful conduct was a serious problem, and they responded to the opportunity to do something about it.

In September 2010, I brought them together for dinner at the Harvard Faculty Club for the first meeting:

- *Ron Arky*, Professor of Medicine
- *Jules Dienstag*, Dean for Medical Education
- *Susan Edgman-Levitan*, Executive Director, Stoeckle Center, MGH
- *Dan Federman*, former Dean for Medical Education
- *Ed Hundert*, Director, Center for Teaching and Learning
- *Jeannette Ives-Erickson*, Vice President for Nursing, MGH
- *Gerry Healy*, Professor of Otology and Laryngology
- *Bob Mayer*, Professor of Medicine
- *Gregg Meyer*, Senior Vice President for Quality and Safety, MGH
- *Miles Shore*, Bullard Professor of Psychiatry and Chair, HMS Promotions and Review Board
- *Richard Schwartzstein*, Professor of Medicine, Director of the Academy, HMS
- *Andy Whittemore*, Professor of Surgery and Chief Medical Officer, BWH

I welcomed the group with a blunt statement that the purpose of the meeting was not to *talk* about unprofessional behavior, but to determine if we wanted to *do* something about it. I laid out the scope: disruptive behavior, humiliation of students and nurses, disrespectful treatment of patients, and passive resistance and non-participation in quality improvement. I gave them statistics from surveys of nurses and medical students and read quotes from my students' papers describing episodes of dismissive and demeaning treatment of patients by their doctors.

A great discussion followed: we tolerate disrespect, it is a leadership issue, reform has to come from the top; we have actually rewarded bad behavior, we need a system to deal with it, we should do "360" evaluations of everyone, etc. Members recounted examples of bad conduct and poor support of students and nurses; it was more than just a problem of individual professionalism, as so often described, it was the culture.

We agreed that it was time for action and that a statement from HMS would be powerful. We would meet again.

At the second meeting, we found broad agreement that the problem was severe and prevalent, that leadership is necessary to address the issue, and that we needed a different structure for responding to bad behavior. Our goal would be to develop an institution-wide (all HMS teaching hospitals) program. We would identify structures and processes that need to be put in place to identify and deal with disrespectful conduct of all kinds: i.e., the specifics of what we wanted hospitals to do. We decided to write a white paper laying out the problem and our recommendations and try to get HMS leadership and hospital CEOs on board.

"Champions"

I also convened a second group: frontline safety leaders at each of the teaching hospitals who could advise us on implementation. I dubbed this group of key safety people "Champions" from our QI jargon, i.e., clinical leaders who make things happen. I saw the two groups as symbiotic: the senior, professionalism working group would develop theory and policy, and the frontline leaders would work on the ground-level implementation.

This Champions group, all of whom I knew, and all physicians, included:

- *Bob Truog*, Children's Hospital
- *Sigall Bell*, Beth Israel Deaconess Hospital
- *John Herman*, Mass General Hospital
- *Craig Bunnell*, Dana-Farber Cancer Institute
- *Jo Shapiro*, Brigham and Women's Hospital
- *Elizabeth Gaufberg*, Cambridge Health Alliance
- *Mitch Rein*, North Shore Hospital
- *Les Selbovitz*, Newton Wellesley Hospital
- *Susan Abookire*, Mt Auburn Hospital
- *Luke Sato*, CRICO

As with the senior group, all were eager to participate. I explained the different functions of the two groups: the senior group's mission was to motivate the Dean and the hospital CEOs to develop and implement more effective policies and processes for dealing with disrespectful behavior; we were writing a white paper for that. The Champions' group would develop strategies and plans for implementation. An obvious place for them to start was the current situation regarding codes of conduct. So, in preparation for the first meeting, I asked each of them to send me their hospital's code for dealing with disrespectful behavior.

The Champions first convened in January. The codes were all over the map! Several hospitals didn't even have a code! I thought this would be a great opportunity: we could work together to come up with a universal code that all Harvard hospitals could agree to.

But the group had little interest in that. They weren't sure just what they were interested in, but my various suggestions fell on deaf ears. We spent the first meeting with each person talking about what they were doing in their institutions and agreed to meet again. We met several times over the next year but could never really agree on proceeding in a clear direction. To my great disappointment, in the end the group had no positive impact. But, as we shall see, it did have an unfortunate negative effect.

Meanwhile, the senior working group met monthly over the period of a year and were very active. We wanted the medical school to take the lead here, but that would not be easy. Because of the unusual structure of HMS in which all of the teaching hospitals are fairly autonomous, the Dean was sensitive to their strong sense of independence and not anxious to tell them what to do. We gathered information on codes and practices and outlined the paper. We added several people to the group: deans Maureen Connelly and Gretchen Brodnicki; the Chairman of Faculty Discipline, Paul Russell; and Luke Sato from CRICO, our liability insurer.

Miles Shore and I went to work drafting a white paper that would lay out the various aspects of disrespect, defining the types of behavior and the varied situations where it occurred. We had learned a great deal from our research; the problem was far worse than we had suspected. There was ample evidence: studies documenting the extent to which nurses, students, and doctors were treated badly, plus the trove of patient stories from my students' interviews.

The Problem

Disruptive behavior was what brought us together, and it was the situation crying out most loudly for solution. As noted, most nurses experience shouting, demeaning comments, or humiliation by a physician at some time, many frequently. Similarly, while most of their encounters with physicians are positive, many patients have had a bad experience. Almost all medical students can recount humiliating treatment by their teaching attendings in hospitals.

The most disturbing finding from our review of the literature and pooled experience, however, was not about disruptive behavior, but that lesser types of disrespectful behavior are pervasive and not limited to physicians. While only a few "bad apples" engaged in obvious egregious disruptive behavior, lesser degrees of disrespectful conduct were common.

Passive aggressive behavior is a pervasive form of disrespect, but it is seldom commented on. For example, many physicians have not been enthusiastic about patient safety—they claim to not see the problem in their own practices, and they are too busy to participate in hospital-organized "quality improvement" projects. When asked or required to participate, they act out their resistance passively—by missing or coming late to meetings, by not offering ideas or doing the work, by being slow to carry out their tasks.

Another pervasive aspect of disrespect that is not even recognized by those affected is systemic or *institutionalized* disrespect. This is the disrespect embedded in many of the well-accepted practices that are part of everyday care in hospitals. The most obvious example is working conditions. Research evidence is clear that long hours, sleep deprivation, and excessive workloads cause increased errors. Yet, long hours and heavy workloads are standard operating procedures in health care, especially in teaching hospitals.

If you stop and think about it, requiring doctors and nurses to work under these conditions is the ultimate in disrespect. Not only are you treating them badly, you are *knowingly* putting them in a position where they are more likely to harm their patients. For hospital leaders, administrative or clinical, to do so is unconscionable, yet it is the norm almost everywhere.

A more subtle form of institutionalized disrespect is waiting times. Millions of hours are lost every day in the USA by patients waiting for care. We say, in effect, your time is worth less than my time. We ignore the immense costs, social and fiscal, of keeping people out of work and children out of school. Patients bear the brunt of this form of disrespect, but the inefficiency also exacts its toll from the physicians and employees who also wait.

And it is unnecessary. Operational research has developed methods for "queuing" and task management that virtually eliminate waiting and are well-known; they just need to be implemented. Some hospitals have done that and even eliminated waiting rooms [2]. All hospitals and doctors' offices should.

The evidence of pervasive disrespect in health care is clear, but the literature was remarkably shy of insight into the *causes* of disrespect. For this we had to rely on the insights about general human behavior gathered over the years by psychologists. We did find examples of some very well-thought-out policies and procedures for dealing with egregious behavior, particularly the College of Physicians and Surgeons of Ontario's *Guidebook for Managing Disruptive Physician Behavior* [3].

A Culture of Respect

By March we had completed a first draft, and various members were working on revisions. Jeff Flier, Dean of HMS, had indicated that he would welcome a proposal for a policy on respectful behavior. However, in the end he preferred that we distribute the white paper to Harvard hospitals and not to colleagues on the quad, the formal HMS campus.

The group thought it should also be published in the medical literature, so Miles Shore and I worked with several other members to finish the paper, and in July 2011 we submitted it to Academic Medicine. I was dubious that such a long paper would be published by a journal. Fortunately, the editor recognized its value and accepted it with the proviso that we break it into two papers that were published in the same issue:

A Culture of Respect, Part 1: The Nature and Causes of Disrespectful Behavior by Physicians [4]

The first paper described the dimensions and the extent of the problem of disrespectful behavior.

The numbers are arresting: 95% of nurses have witnessed or received abuse, and 64% reported an episode of verbal abuse at least every 2–3 months. But the number of doctors responsible is small: 5.7% [5]. More than a third of nurses believe disruptive behavior is a cause of nurses leaving an institution [6].

As noted in Chap. 20, abuse of medical students is also common. Dismissive comments or humiliation is experienced by two thirds of students [1, 7, 8]. More than half show signs of burnout, and 14% have symptoms of serious depression. Half of residents are victims of bullying, belittling, and humiliation [9]. Patient surveys show that 13–27% of patients report problems with doctor communication [10]. Patient interviews show the percentage is closer to 50% [11].

The paper then defined the types of disrespectful behavior and their effects and explored the causes of disrespect. We proposed that the slow progress in patient safety results from the dysfunctional culture of health-care institutions, and the root cause of that dysfunctional culture is disrespectful behavior.

Six different forms of disrespect were identified as common in health-care organizations:

1. *Disruptive behavior*, such as angry outbursts, threats, bullying, and the use of profane and abusive language
2. *Humiliating and demeaning treatment of nurses, residents, and students*
3. *Passive-aggressive behavior*, such as blaming others for your failures and making frequent negative comments about the hospital or colleagues
4. *Passive disrespect*, such as being chronically late to meetings, delay in dictating charts, and resistance to following safe practices, such as hand washing
5. *Dismissive treatment of patients*

6. *Systemic disrespect*: practices that are taken for granted, such as long hours and excessive workloads for nurses and residents, long waiting times for patients, and not disclosing and apologizing after harm caused by an error

All of these forms of disrespect create barriers to communication among all parties—doctors, nurses, residents, and patients. Disrespect is a major barrier to efforts to improve patient safety. It undermines the teamwork that is essential to changing systems to improve safety; it saps meaning and satisfaction from work, leading to burnout and low morale. It is particularly damaging to students and patients, especially when they are harmed by a medical error.

We identified both internal (individual) and external (environmental) causes of disrespectful behavior. Internal causes include personal feelings of insecurity and anxiety, depression, narcissism, aggressiveness, and prior victimization. The extent to which these antecedent problems result in disrespectful behavior, however, is largely determined by the external environment.

Key environmental factors that foster disrespect are the hierarchical nature of health-care organizations and a blaming culture. But also important are the long hours, heavy workloads, and "production pressure" to deliver quality care.

A Culture of Respect, Part 2: Creating a Culture of Respect [12]

The main theme of the second paper is that creating a culture of respect is the core of the broader cultural transformation that is needed to create a culture of safety in health care. The responsibility for creating a culture of respect falls squarely on the shoulders of the organization's leader "because only he or she can set the tone and initiate the processes that lead to change."

We challenged health-care organization CEOs to accomplish five major tasks:

1. *To motivate and inspire* others to take action "and to create a sense of urgency around doing so"

2. *To establish preconditions for a culture of respect* by showing concern for the well-being of faculty and staff by addressing issues of hours and workloads and physical hazards
3. To *establish policies regarding disrespectful behavior,* i.e., *codes of conduct*
4. To *facilitate engagement of frontline workers* by addressing systemic stressors
5. To *create a learning environment* by modeling professional behavior and valuing the learner

The paper then provided extensive and explicit recommendations on creating a code of conduct, drawing on experience from various sources, especially the College of Physicians and Surgeons of Ontario's *Guidebook for Managing Disruptive Physician Behavior* [13]. We emphasized the importance of developing effective means of implementing and enforcing such a code, including enabling safe reporting and responding promptly.

The final section dealt with prevention, which includes education at all levels, the design and use of appropriate performance evaluations, and support of individuals at all levels who work to create a safe environment. Creating transparency, breaking down authoritarianism, learning to work in teams, and creating a "just culture" are all part of the challenge of creating a respectful culture.

A Strange Twist

When we submitted the papers to Academic Medicine in July 2011, I sent a copy to each member of the Champions group knowing they would be interested in what we had learned. To my great surprise, several were upset that they hadn't been included as authors! I thought this was a bit weird, because 6 months earlier I had sent them a draft so they would know what we were doing (presumably the foundation for their work), and we discussed the findings at a Champions meeting. Only one person sent me any comments about it, and no one suggested any edits. Given this prior behavior, it was a mystery to me why any of them would now think they were entitled to authorship.

Clearly, however, there was a major miscommunication that even in retrospect neither Miles nor I nor any of the authors were able to understand. We spent a great deal of time trying to mollify the Champions and resolve differences. Several disagreed substantially with the emphasis of the paper on consequences and response rather than on a supportive culture. They were upset about being left out of a major paper on this subject coming from Harvard—despite the fact they had contributed nothing to it!

Meanwhile, the paper was provisionally accepted, with the usual request that we respond to reviewers' comments. We saw this as an opportunity to ask several of the disaffected to write an additional section in response to the reviewers, in which they could weave in some of their ideas and be legitimately added as authors. I thought this was a good solution.

However, despite the general angst, only two of them volunteered to do this. Unfortunately, instead of writing an additional section, they set about rewriting the whole paper! This would obviously not be acceptable to the editors, but they were insistent. So the whole effort ended in naught. I felt very bad about it—especially since a number of the group were old friends and associates.

Response

The two papers came out in the Academic Medicine in July 2012 and were well received. The earliest most obvious impact in our hospitals was that several tightened up their procedures and fired some of their most outrageous offenders, physicians whom colleagues had complained about for years.

A more impressive tangible result was that Virginia Mason Medical Center (VMMC) took the papers to heart. Nationally recognized as the leader in reducing errors and creating a culture of safety, VMMC was a fertile field in which this seed could germinate. Not only did VMMC upgrade their standards and processes for dealing with disrespectful behavior, they developed a comprehensive continuing education course on respect and required all 5000 of their staff and employees to take it. The course has subsequently been marketed to hundreds of other hospitals worldwide.

It is hard to measure the impact of the papers nationally, but I noticed that the word "respect" began to appear in conversations and writings about quality and safety. More specifically, medical schools and residency programs now routinely survey students and residents about receiving abusive behavior. Questions about how their doctors treated them were added to the post- hospitalization questionnaires that were sent to patients to evaluate their care. The feedback from those surveys puts immense pressure on hospitals, which, perhaps more than anything else, is slowly leading to a more respectful environment.

References

1. National Patient Safety Foundation. Unmet needs: teaching physicians to provide safe patient care. Boston: Lucian Leape Institute at the National Patient Safety Foundation; 2010.
2. Kenney C. Transforming health care: the Virginia Mason Medical Center story. New York: Wiley; 2011.
3. Barer ML, Evans RG, Stoddart GL. Controlling health care costs by direct charges to patients. Toronto: Ontario Economic Council; 1979.
4. Leape L, Shore M, Dienstag J, et al. A culture of respect: I. The nature and causes of disrespectful behavior. Acad Med. 2012;87:845–52.
5. Rosenstein AH, O'Daniel M. A survey of the impact of disruptive behaviors and communication defects on patient safety. Jt Comm J Qual Patient Saf. 2008;34:464–71.
6. Rosenstein AH, Russell H, Lauve R. Disruptive physician behavior contributes to nursing shortage. Study links bad behavior by doctors to nurses leaving the profession. Physician Exec. 2002;28:8–11.
7. Leape L, Fromson JA. Problem doctors: is there a system-level solution? Ann Intern Med. 2006;144:107–15.
8. Kassebaum D, Culer E. On the culture of student abuse in medical school. Acad Med. 1998;73:1149–58.
9. Chadaga AR, Villines D, Krikorian A. Bullying in the American graduate medical education system: a national cross-sectional survey. PLoS One. 2016;11:e0150246.
10. HCAHPS fact sheet (CAHPS hospital survey). AHRQ; 2010. Accessed 29 Mar 2012, at http://www.hcahpsonline.org/files/HCAHPS%20Fact%20 Sheet%202010.pdf.

11. Leape LL. Unpublished data.
12. Leape L, Shore M, Dienstag J, et al. A culture of respect, part 2: creating a culture of respect. Acad Med. 2012;87:853–8.
13. Ontario_College_of_Physicians_and_Surgeons. Guidebook for managing disruptive physician behavior. Toronto; 2008.

Part IV
Creating a Culture of Safety

Chapter 22
Make No Little Plans: The Lucian Leape Institute

Despite encouraging progress in the early years of the patient safety movement, it soon became evident that there were deeper issues that needed to be addressed. We realized that we were not going to make health care safe by making process changes one by one, even powerful changes such as eliminating CLABSI or implementing the surgical checklist.

We needed to fundamentally reimagine the way we think about delivery of health care. Health care needed not just to be improved but to be transformed. A sustainable strategy—probably several strategies—was needed to enable us to deal with the fundamental systemic and behavioral issues that drive unsafe behavior.

Fortunately, as noted in Chap. 5, in 2007 the National Patient Safety Foundation created a mechanism to do that, the *Lucian Leape Institute*, a "think tank" of experts whose leadership roles had given them experience and insights that would enable them to identify the issues and make authoritative recommendations for changes.

The charge to the Institute was to "define strategic paths and calls to action for the field of patient safety and provide vision and context for the many efforts underway within the health care system. Through its Roundtables, it will issue reports that will guide the work of the field and challenge the system to address the issues critical to making the system safer."

© The Author(s) 2021
L. L. Leape, *Making Healthcare Safe*,
https://doi.org/10.1007/978-3-030-71123-8_22

I chaired the Institute. The other initial members were:

- *Don Berwick*, founder and CEO of the Institute for Healthcare Improvement, who brought quality improvement to health care
- *Carolyn Clancy*, Director, Agency for Healthcare Research and Quality, who spearheaded its early work on safety
- *Jim Conway*, Senior VP, Institute for Healthcare Improvement and previous COO of Dana-Farber Cancer Institute, who led its reorganization for safety
- *David Lawrence*, CEO of Kaiser Foundation Health Plan, former Executive Session member, who brought patient safety to Kaiser-Permanente
- *Julianne Morath*, Chief Quality and Safety Officer, Vanderbilt University Medical Center, who led Allina Health's entry into patient safety
- *Dennis O'Leary*, President of the Joint Commission, also a former Executive Session member, who focused the Commission on patient safety
- *Paul Gluck*, immediate past chair of NPSF Board of Directors
- *Diane Pinakiewicz*, President of NPSF

At the first meeting of the Lucian Leape Institute, we had a lively discussion about our purpose and how to most effectively go about strategic planning. After surfacing dozens of ideas, we decided to focus our efforts on core concepts that we believed were foundational to achieving meaningful improvement in patient safety.

They were obviously not the *only* thing needed, but we believed they were essential. Without embracing these concepts, health-care

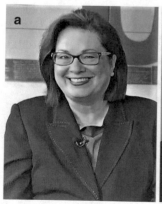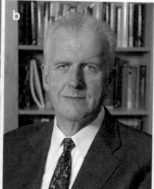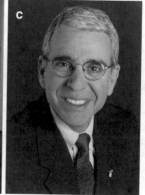

(a) Julie Morath, (b) Jim Conway, and (c) Paul Gluck.

organizations could not mobilize the resources and motivate their workforce to achieve safe care. We identified five concepts: Reforming Medical Education, Integrating Care, Finding Joy and Meaning in Work, Patient Engagement, and Transparency. We called them *Transforming Concepts*.

Each concept requires a change of consciousness to move thinking beyond traditional boundaries, and each implies profound behavioral changes. We wrote a paper, *Transforming health care: a safety imperative*, that explained the transforming concepts, summarized the importance of each, and defined the issues to be resolved [1]. Then we set to work.

Over the next several years, LLI convened a roundtable of national experts and stakeholders, including patient advocates, for each of the five concepts to explore the critical issues, understand them better, and make recommendations for transformative change. To stimulate buy-in and ownership, we made a special effort to include on each panel leaders of organizations for which the issue was especially relevant and who could implement the recommendations. LLI members chaired the roundtables.

The typical roundtable had 25–30 participants and met twice in two-day sessions. We had no trouble recruiting members for each topic; the relevant thought leaders shared our interest and were eager to participate. Prior to convening, we provided participants with a comprehensive literature review on the topic. The discussions were spirited and wide-ranging and concluded with recommendations for health-care organizations and their leaders.

Following each roundtable, the leaders wrote a white paper that combined facts and insights from the literature with the results of the panel discussions to provide a comprehensive account of the topic with specific recommendations for action by health-care providers, leaders, and policy makers. These white papers are available, free of charge from IHI at IHI.org.

The five white papers are summarized below, including for each also a review of progress made since the paper was published and a discussion of remaining challenges. These are verbatim combinations of text taken from two summaries later published by LLI: *Transforming Health Care: A Compendium of Reports from the National Patient Safety Foundation's Lucian Leape Institute*, IHI, 2016 [2], and *Transforming concepts in patient safety: a progress report*. BMJ Quality & Safety, 2018 [3].

Unmet Needs [4]

Teaching Physicians to Provide Safe Patient Care

Workshop Leaders: Dennis O'Leary and Lucian Leape

Health-care delivery continues to be unsafe despite major patient safety improvement efforts over the past decade. The roundtable concluded that substantive improvements in patient safety will be difficult to achieve without major medical education reform at the medical school and residency training program levels. Medical schools must assure that future physicians not only have the requisite knowledge, skills, behaviors, and attitudes to practice competently but also are prepared to play active roles in identifying and resolving patient safety problems. These competencies should become fully developed during the residency training period.

Medical schools today focus principally on providing students with the knowledge and skills they need for the technical practice of medicine but often pay inadequate attention to the shaping of student skills, attitudes, and behaviors that will permit them to function safely and as architects of patient safety improvement in the future. Specifically, medical schools are not doing an adequate job of facilitating student understanding of basic knowledge and the development of skills required for the provision of safe patient care, to wit: systems thinking, problem analysis, application of human factors science, communication skills, patient-centered care, teaming concepts and skills, and dealing with feelings of doubt, fear, and uncertainty with respect to medical errors.

In addition, medical students all too often suffer demeaning experiences at the hands of faculty and residents, a phenomenon that appears to reflect serious shortcomings in the medical school and teaching hospital cultures. Behaviors like these that are disruptive to professional relationships have adverse effects upon students, residents, nurses, colleagues, and even patients. Students frequently tend to emulate these behaviors as they become residents and practicing clinicians, which perpetuates work environments and cultures that are antithetical to the delivery of safe, patient-centered care.

Summary of Recommendations (Table 22.1)

Table 22.1 Key recommendations from *Unmet Needs: Teaching Physicians to Provide Safe Patient Care*

Target of recommendation	Recommendation
Medical school and hospital leaders	Place the highest priority on creating a learning culture that emphasizes patient safety, professionalism, transparency, and valuing the individual learner
	Eliminate hierarchical and authority gradients
	Emphasize that professionalism includes demonstrating mutual respect and non-tolerance of abusive or demeaning behavior
	Declare and enforce a zero-tolerance policy for confirmed egregious disrespectful behavior by faculty, staff, or residents
	Promote the development of interpersonal skills, leadership, teamwork, and collaboration among faculty and staff
	Provide incentives and resources to enhance faculty capabilities to teach and practice patient safety and to be effective role models
	The selection process for admission to medical schools should emphasize attributes that reflect professionalism and orientation to patient safety, such as compassion, empathy, and collaboration
Medical schools	Treat patient safety as a science that encompasses human factors, systems theory, and open communication
	Emphasize the shaping of desired skills, attitudes, and behaviors as set forth in the core competencies defined by the IOM, the American Board of Medical Specialties, and the Accreditation Council for Graduate Medical Education
	The educational experience should be coherent, continuing, and flexible throughout undergraduate medical education, residency and fellowship training, and lifelong continuing education
Accrediting bodies	Amend medical school accreditation requirements and residency program requirements to include expectations for the creation of learning cultures and the development of patient safety-related behavioral traits.
	Survey medical schools to evaluate education priorities for patient safety and the creation of school and hospital cultures that support patient safety

Progress

In recent years, medical school curricula have increasingly included patient safety and safety science, and these concepts have also become more common in education for other clinicians and frontline staff. For example, the American Medical Association's Accelerating Change in Medical Education Consortium brought medical schools together to innovate, develop curricula, and share best practices, including those addressing quality and safety.

The Accreditation Council for Graduate Medical Education Clinical Learning Environment Review (ACGME CLER) program requires medical resident participation in quality and safety learning. Recently, the Association of American Medical Colleges (AAMC) initiated a program to create a shared understanding of Quality Improvement and Patient Safety (QIPS) competencies across the full continuum from medical school to continuing practice.

Other clinical disciplines, particularly nursing, have often pioneered educational pathways, and a concerted effort is underway to emphasize the importance of interprofessional teams. The Quality and Safety Education for Nurses (QSEN) program has focused on enhancing education around safety science in nursing schools for more than a decade. More recently, the National Collaborative for Improving the Clinical Learning Environment (NCICLE) highlighted the "patient safety gap" in the education and training of all clinicians and provided clear recommendations for improvement [3].

To assist health-care students and professionals in building core skills in improvement, safety, and leadership, the Institute for Healthcare Improvement (IHI) developed a web-based interactive educational program called the Open School. More than 650,000 learners have enrolled in the Open School since it opened its virtual doors in 2008.

To address the need for training in postgraduate medical education, in 2012 the NPSF created a course in patient safety and safety science that more than 7000 learners of diverse disciplines have utilized. Several universities have developed graduate education and fellowships in quality and safety, and clinicians, risk managers, pharmacists, executives, and others have pursued these as well as certificate programs and professional certification in patient safety.

Remaining Challenges

Still, opportunity lies ahead for greater consistency in how health professionals learn about patient safety. A 2016 report from ACGME CLER reveals gaps in areas such as feedback on safety reporting and experiential learning, lack of awareness of the range of patient safety issues, and shortage of opportunities for interprofessional system-based improvement efforts. Contributing to this learning gap is a shortage of academic faculty with safety and quality improvement expertise.

Continuing education requirements for attending physicians are highly variable. While some medical specialties require continuing education in patient safety, the American Board of Internal Medicine recently removed it as a requirement from Maintenance of Certification. Health-care organizations would benefit from encouraging study of safety science by all team members, including board members, and operationalizing ways to achieve continuous learning as safety science expands.

As these and other activities gain momentum, the core agenda remains consistent, clear, and urgent: to mainstream the preparation of health professionals' awareness, skills, commitment, and practical training about the scientific pursuit of safer care. Embracing the science of safety in medical education is crucial to the future health and well-being of patients, families, and communities.

Order from Chaos [5]

Accelerating Care Integration

Workshop Leaders: David Lawrence and Richard Bohmer

Lack of care coordination and integration was identified as a major contributor to the frequency of avoidable errors in patient care in the Institute of Medicine (IOM) report *To Err Is Human* (1999). Care integration was presented as the cornerstone for achieving high quality in the subsequent IOM report *Crossing the Quality Chasm* (2001). The Agency for Healthcare Research and Quality (AHRQ) has included care integration and patient safety in its scope of work since early in this decade. Federal government administration arguments for the Patient Protection and Affordable Care Act of 2010 included numerous references to this issue.

Modern care delivery is extraordinarily complex. To protect the patient and avoid errors require a planned, coordinated, and fully integrated approach to care. In addition to the complexity inherent in modern treatment for patients with difficult and often multiple conditions, complexity is found throughout the care experience: in the number of physicians involved, the number of professionals and support personnel required, the multiple venues where care is provided, and the diverse requirements and expectations of patients. As a consequence, the risks of harm also rise unless careful attention is given to the way care is organized and delivered, that is, to the system of care delivery itself. The system must be designed to protect the patient while ensuring that he or she receives the full benefits of the remarkable advances that have occurred over the past century.

And here we arrive at care integration, the planned, thoughtful design of the care process for the benefit and protection of the patient. Unfortunately, physicians and leaders of delivery systems (with notable exceptions such as those at the Mayo Clinic, Geisinger Health System, and Kaiser-Permanente) have been unwilling or unable to embrace greater care integration. As described in *Crossing the Quality Chasm*, most patient care is fragmented and uncoordinated. Where integration has occurred, it is most often structural: assembling piece parts under a single governance umbrella while leaving the underlying care delivery processes largely untouched.

The care delivery system is struggling to escape the straitjacket of physician autonomy and economic independence, a payment system that reinforces fragmentation and independent decision-making, and a regulatory framework that places legal responsibility on the individual professional without corresponding accountability of the team or the system within which that professional works. The medical education system reinforces these expectations and does little to prepare new physicians for the team-based, interdependent work that is required to achieve high-quality and safe care.

Summary of Recommendations (Table 22.2)

Table 22.2 Key recommendations from *Order from Chaos: Accelerating Care Integration*

Target of recommendation	Recommendation
All stakeholders: federal and state governmental agencies, consumer groups	Create mechanisms for developing a shared understanding among public and private stakeholders regarding the link between care integration and patient safety Utilize working groups and public forums, best practices, and patient stories to be catalogued and disseminated
Health-care leaders and practitioners, public	Patients and families must become active participants in process improvement and design and redesign efforts and review organizational performance
Regulatory and accrediting bodies	Create methods of measuring care integration, along with robust assessment and evaluation metrics, and incorporate these measures into public reporting systems
Medical schools, professional societies, nonprofits	Provide education and training for executives, boards, clinicians, and medical students that focus on patient safety and care integration
Researchers, industry	Develop the technology and infrastructure to allow for national spread of organizational and operational expertise to support care integration

Progress

With an increased call for improved coordination of care and focus on patient safety across the care continuum, methods for improving handoffs and communication among teams, providers, and patients are gaining traction. Today the focus on population health and market-specific shifts in payment models serve as incentives for greater care integration and coordination.

Progress has been made to develop systems and structures to encourage and incentivize care integration. Accountable care organizations (ACOs) have brought together groups of health providers to incentivize better quality care at a lower cost. Likewise, the development of the patient-centered medical home (PCMH) aims to reorganize and reinvigorate primary care, and early evidence shows promise in achieving lower costs, improved patient experience, and better care quality.

Other encouraging examples of improved care integration include Project Re-Engineered Discharge (Project RED), the PCORI-funded Project ACHIEVE (Achieving Patient-Centered Care and Optimized Health In Care Transitions by Evaluating the Value of Evidence), and the Johns Hopkins School of Nursing–led Community Aging in Place: Advancing Better Living for Elders (CAPABLE). For example, Project RED developed strategies to improve the hospital discharge process to promote patient safety and has been proven to reduce rehospitalizations and yield high rates of patient satisfaction.

Finally, the increase in employed physicians and continued refinement of the electronic health record have accelerated care integration. Improving interoperability of health information technology has been a major initiative at the federal level to improve information flow across the entire care continuum.

Remaining Challenges

Despite incremental improvement, coordination and integration of care remain difficult, particularly for patients with multiple chronic conditions. Even with a national push toward more integrated care models (perhaps most focused on the development of ACOs), so far results toward safer, more coordinated care have been mixed. Furthermore, care integration issues are compounded for older adults. One study found that the average Medicare beneficiary spent about 17 days in contact with the health-care system through an average of 3.4 different clinicians. Only 55% of these individuals coordinated their care principally with a single primary care physician.

Structural changes alone will not ensure optimal care integration. Strong clinician leadership and patient engagement will be required to further improve care coordination. Involving patients and families in the codesign of care, especially around coordination and care delivered in the home, will help identify unmet needs and educational deficits.

Care integration remains perhaps the most challenging of the transforming concepts because of the fragmentation of the US health-care system. When Americans are asked to reflect on the integration of care from their own experiences, some refer to the term "health-care system" as an oxymoron.

Individuals responsible for coordinating care and helping patients navigate the care system include primary care physicians, specialists, nurses, pharmacists, social workers, and care managers, as well as health plan and delivery system personnel. As care becomes more complex and shared among more providers, it is essential to improve both processes (e.g., teamwork, communication, and patient engagement) and technologies (e.g., EHRs) for patients and providers.

Through the Eyes of the Workforce [6]

Creating Joy, Meaning, and Safer Health Care

Workshop Leaders: Julie Morath and Paul O'Neill

The health-care workforce is composed of well-intentioned, well-prepared people in a variety of roles and clinical disciplines who do their best every day to ensure that patients are well cared for. It is from this mission of caring for people in times of their greatest vulnerability and need that health-care workers find meaning in their work, as well as their experience of joy.

Yet many health-care workers suffer harm—emotional and physical—in the course of providing care. Many are subjected to being bullied, harassed, demeaned, ignored, and, in the most extreme cases, physically assaulted. They are also physically injured by working in conditions of known and preventable environmental risk. In addition, production and cost pressures have reduced complex, intimate, caregiving relationships into a series of demanding tasks performed under severe time constraints. Under these conditions, it is difficult for caregivers to find purpose and joy in their work or to meet the challenge of making health care safe for patients they serve.

Vulnerable Workplaces

The basic precondition of a safe workplace is protection of the physical and psychological safety of the workforce. Both are conspicuously absent or considered optional in many care delivery organizations. The prevalence of physical harm experienced by the health-care workforce is striking, much higher than in other industries. Up to a third of nurses experience back or musculoskeletal injuries in a year, and many have unprotected contact with blood-borne pathogens.

Psychological harm is also common. In many health-care organizations, staff are not treated with respect—or, worse yet, they are routinely treated with disrespect. Emotional abuse, bullying, and even threats of physical assault and learning by humiliation are all often accepted as "normal" conditions of the health-care workplace, creating a culture of fear and intimidation that saps joy and meaning from work.

The absence of cultural norms that create the preconditions of psychological and physical safety obscures meaning of work and drains motivation. The costs of burnout, litigation, lost work hours, employee turnover, and the inability to attract newcomers to caring professions are wasteful and add to the burden of illness. Disrespectful treatment of workers increases the risk of patient injury.

What Can Be Done?

An environment of mutual respect is critical if the workforce is to find joy and meaning in work. In modern health care, teamwork is essential for safe practice, and teamwork is impossible in the absence of mutual respect.

Former CEO of Alcoa Paul O'Neill advises that, to find joy and meaning in their daily work, each person in the workforce must be able to answer affirmatively three questions each day:

1. Am I treated with dignity and respect by everyone?
2. Do I have what I need so I can make a contribution that gives meaning to my life?
3. Am I recognized and thanked for what I do?

Developing Effective Organizations

To create a safe and supportive work environment, health-care organizations must become effective, high-reliability organizations, characterized by continuous learning, improvement, teamwork, and transparency. Effective organizations care for their employees and continuously meet preconditions not subject to annual priority and budget setting. The most fundamental precondition is workforce safety, physical and psychological. The workforce needs to know that their safety is an enduring and non-negotiable priority for the governing board, CEO, and organization.

Knowing that their well-being is a priority enables the workforce to be meaningfully engaged in their work, to be more satisfied, less likely to experience burnout, and to deliver more effective and safer care.

Achieving this vision requires leadership. The governing board, CEO, and organizational leaders create the cultural norms and conditions that produce workforce safety, meaning, and joy. Effective leaders shape safety culture through management practices that demonstrate a priority to safety and compassionately engage the workforce to speak about and report errors, mistakes, and hazards that threaten safety—their own or their patients'. Joy and meaning will be created when the workforce feels valued, safe from harm, and part of the solutions for change.

Summary of Recommendations (Table 22.3)

Table 22.3 Key recommendations from *Through the Eyes of the Workforce: Creating Joy, Meaning, and Safer Health Care*

Target of recommendation	Recommendation
Hospital and health-care leaders, professionals, board members	Develop and embody shared core values of mutual respect and civility; transparency and truth telling; safety of all workers and patients; and alignment and accountability from the boardroom through the front lines
Hospital and health-care leaders, professionals, board members	Adopt the explicit aim to eliminate harm to workforce and patients Recognize and celebrate the work and accomplishments of the work force, regularly and with high visibility
Hospital and health-care leaders, board members, managers	Commit to creating a high-reliability organization (HRO) and demonstrate the discipline to achieve highly reliable performance This will require creating a learning and improvement system and adopting evidence-based management skills for reliability
Hospital and health-care leaders	Establish data capture, database, and performance metrics for improvement and accountability
Government and nonprofit funders	Support industry-wide research to explore issues and conditions in health care that are harming our workforce and patients

Progress

Multiple initiatives are underway to increase awareness of the importance of joy and meaning in work and workforce safety. The National
Academy of Medicine and several health-care professional groups
and insurers, such as the American Association of Critical-Care
Nurses (AACN), the American Nurses Association (ANA Enterprise),
the American Medical Association (AMA), and the Harvard Risk
Management Foundation are addressing the issue of resilience and
burnout.

IHI has developed a framework for increasing joy in work that recommends domains such as reward and recognition, choice and autonomy, camaraderie and teamwork, and physical and psychological
safety. Some have observed that the widely accepted Triple Aim
should be expanded to include workforce safety and joy and meaning
in work—the Quadruple Aim.

Regarding health-care workforce physical safety, noteworthy
efforts are proceeding. With the support of the Centers for Medicare
& Medicaid Services (CMS), the US Occupational Safety and Health
Administration recently launched an initiative to encourage hospitals
and health-care facilities to implement safety and health management
systems to prevent injuries among their workforce and patients.
Similarly, the Joint Commission has provided detailed reports and
tools for improving workforce safety and reducing workplace
violence.

Remaining Challenges

Despite these efforts, according to one recent study, more than half of
US physicians suffer from burnout. Among critical-care nurses,
25%–33% have symptoms of severe burnout syndrome. Not only do
physicians have higher rates of burnout than the general public, but
they also suffer higher rates of depression and suicide. The Covid
pandemic has substantially increased all of these problems. The
effects of psychological, emotional, and physical harm to the workforce surface in the form of litigation, lost work hours, employee turnover, and inability to attract newcomers to caring professions. With
health-care   reform,   pay-for-performance,   the   introduction   of

electronic health records, and other innovations, health-care workers spend less time directly caring for patients—further draining energy, meaning, and joy.

Compounding the issue, a recent survey found that only 23% of hospital boards review workplace safety dashboards. Our health-care workforce is endangered, and without a healthy, engaged, and supported workforce, safer patient care will remain elusive.

Safety Is Personal [7]

Partnering with Patients and Families for the Safest Care

Workshop Leaders: Susan Edgman-Levitan and James Conway

Receiving safe care is definitely a personal experience. The harm to patients resulting from medical errors at the most vulnerable moments of their lives is a profoundly intimate experience for everyone involved. Clinicians and staff are also deeply affected when they are involved in an adverse event and frequently suffer shame, guilt, fear, and long-lasting depression.

But ensuring safety can also be shared and rewarding. The insights and perspectives of both those who experience care at its best and those who experience it at its worst can help health-care leaders, clinicians, and staff at every level make the improvements needed to create a safer and more patient-centered system.

Engaging patients and families in improving health-care safety means creating effective partnerships between those who provide care and those who receive it—at every level, including individual clinical encounters, safety committees, executive suites, boardrooms, research teams, and national policy-setting bodies. Increasing engagement through effective partnerships can yield many benefits, both in the form of improved health and outcomes for individuals and in safer and more productive work environments for health-care professionals.

Patients, families, and their advocates increasingly understand the wisdom of this partnership. Too often, standing in the way is the health-care system itself—whether by intention or not—because of its fragmentation, paternalistic professional culture, abundance of poor process design, and lack of experience on the part of health-care leaders and clinicians with practical methods of engaging patients in the safety enterprise.

While patients and families can play a critical role in preventing medical errors and reducing harm, the responsibility for safe care lies primarily with the leaders of health-care organizations and the clinicians and staff who deliver care. Many of the barriers to engagement faced by patients and families—such as lack of access to their health records, intimidation, fear of retribution, and lack of easy-to-understand tools and checklists for enhancing safe care—can only be overcome if leaders and clinicians support patients and families to become more confident and effective in their interactions with health-care providers. Many of the tools necessary to do this already exist, but the system must also provide the education and training needed by professionals and patients alike to become more effective partners.

Summary of Recommendations (Table 22.4)

Progress

With the increasing use of decision aids, patient portals, OpenNotes, care engagement plans, and the spread of Patient and Family Advisory Councils (PFACs), health-care leaders and clinicians are beginning to understand the power of engaging patients and families as integral partners. The OpenNotes program has demonstrated that patients can contribute to preventing or mitigating errors.

Patient experience data is being used more widely and effectively. Mandates from CMS, the National Committee for Quality Assurance (NCQA), and other payers for use and improvement of Consumer Assessment of Healthcare Providers and Systems (CAHPS) patient experience survey data are linked to improved performance and outcomes.

Health-care systems, hospitals, and ambulatory practices are also beginning to incorporate patient preferences into care design by

Table 22.4 Key recommendations from *Safety Is Personal: Partnering with Patients and Families for the Safest Care*

Target of recommendation	Recommendation
Leaders of health systems	Establish patient and family engagement as a core value by involving patients and families as equal partners in all organizational activities. Educate and train clinicians and staff to be effective partners; and partner with patient advocacy groups and community organizations to increase public awareness and engagement
Health-care clinicians and staff	Support patients and families to engage effectively in their own care by providing the information, training, and tools they need to manage their health conditions according to their expressed wishes Engage patients as equal partners in safety improvements and care design Support patients and families when things go wrong
Health-care policy makers	Involve patients in all policy-making committees and programs Develop, implement, and report safety metrics that foster accountability and transparency Engage patients in setting and implementing the research agenda
Patients and families and the public	Ask questions about their care and understand their medicines and care plans. They should also be instructed in basic safety steps: repeating back instructions and information to clinicians in their own words; bringing a friend or family member to all appointments; and understanding who is in charge of their care

including patients and their families as active participants in codesign and research studies funded by the Patient-Centered Outcomes Research Institute (PCORI). The internationally observed "What Matters to You?" Day aims to encourage meaningful conversations between patients, families, and providers.

Patient and family perspectives are valuable in many arenas, from design of the physical environment and care coordination plans to reporting safety concerns and participation in root cause analyses. Patient engagement should be authentic and take place across the continuum of care from the bedside to the boardroom to national policy committees. The newly established Patient Experience Policy Forum affiliated with the Beryl Institute is advocating for patient and family partnerships in codesign and policy making nationally.

Remaining Challenges

While some exemplary organizations are fully engaging patients in the care process, ample opportunities for improvement remain. Many organizations lack effective PFACs and have not devoted resources to train staff in shared decision-making practices or to offer evidence-based decision aids. The current fee-for-service payment system does not encourage clinicians to spend the time needed to communicate with patients nor to elicit their preferences.

Many organizations still lack process improvement skills to support integrating better communication into clinical workflows. As care shifts from inpatient to ambulatory and home care settings, patients and families are becoming more responsible for delivering their own care. However, they may not be well equipped to manage complicated medication regimens, activities of daily living, medical devices, or infection control procedures.

Overwhelming evidence indicates that collecting patient feedback and including patients as equal partners in their care support improvement in both patient experience of care and clinical outcomes. Opportunities remain to partner with patients, families, and communities to accelerate improvement in education, patient satisfaction, and quality of care.

Shining a Light [8]

Safer Health Care Through Transparency

Workshop Leaders: Gary Kaplan and Robert Wachter

During the course of health care's patient safety and quality movements, the impact of transparency—the free, uninhibited flow of information that is open to the scrutiny of others—has been far more positive than many had anticipated, and the harms of transparency have been far fewer than many had feared. Yet important obstacles to transparency remain, ranging from concerns that individuals and organizations will be treated unfairly after being transparent to more practical matters related to identifying appropriate measures on which to be transparent and creating an infrastructure for reporting and disseminating the lessons learned from others' data.

To address the issue of transparency in the context of patient safety, the National Patient Safety Foundation's Lucian Leape Institute held two roundtable discussions involving a wide variety of stakeholders representing myriad perspectives. In the discussions and in this report, the choice was made to focus on four domains of transparency:

- Transparency between clinicians and patients (illustrated by disclosure after medical errors)
- Transparency among clinicians themselves (illustrated by peer review and other mechanisms to share information within health-care delivery organizations)
- Transparency of health-care organizations with one another (illustrated by regional or national collaboratives)
- Transparency of both clinicians and organizations with the public (illustrated by public reporting of quality and safety data)

One key insight was the degree to which these four domains are interrelated. For example, creating environments in which clinicians are open and honest with each other about their errors within organizations (which can lead to important system changes to prevent future errors) can be thwarted if these clinicians believe they will be treated unfairly should the same errors be publicly disclosed. These tensions cannot be wished away; instead, they must be forthrightly addressed by institutional and policy leaders.

In this report, the NPSF Lucian Leape Institute comes down strongly on the side of transparency in all four domains. The consensus of the roundtable discussants and the Institute is that the evidence supports the premise that greater transparency throughout the system is not only ethically correct but will lead to improved outcomes, fewer errors, more satisfied patients, and lower costs. The mechanisms for these improvements are several and include the ability of transparency to support accountability, stimulate improvements in quality and safety, promote trust and ethical behavior, and facilitate patient choice.

In the report, more than three dozen specific recommendations are offered to individual clinicians, leaders of health-care delivery organizations (e.g., CEOs, board members), and policy makers.

If transparency were a medication, it would be a blockbuster, with billions of dollars in sales and accolades the world over. While it is crucial to be mindful of the obstacles to transparency and the tensions—and the fact that many stakeholders benefit from our current largely nontransparent system—our review convinces us that a health-care system that embraces transparency across the four domains will be one that produces safer care, better outcomes, and more trust among all of the involved parties. Notwithstanding the potential rewards, making this happen will depend on powerful, courageous leadership and an underlying culture of safety.

Summary of Recommendations (Table 22.5)

Progress

Today, the call for greater transparency in health care is growing louder. Consumers have begun to post reviews of their physicians, care teams, and health-care organizations on online review platforms. Moreover, some health-care systems are now collecting and posting information from patient experience surveys at the service or physician level. Recently, several health systems have begun to provide forums for free-response comments online, often with positive results.

The 2005 Patient Safety and Quality Improvement Act and the rise of patient safety organizations (PSOs) have facilitated increased transparency among clinicians and health-care organizations. Additionally, collaboratives like Solutions for Patient Safety (SPS), a network of more than 130 children's hospitals working together to eliminate serious harm, have shown compelling evidence that sharing data, successes, and failures can markedly accelerate learning and improvement.

Health care is also seeing greater transparency between patients and clinicians in the aftermath of adverse events. A growing number of communication and resolution programs have been established, fueled by growing evidence that prompt disclosure, honesty, and

Table 22.5 Key recommendations from *Shining a Light: Safer Health Care Through Transparency*

Target of recommendation	Recommendation
All stakeholders	Ensure disclosure of conflicts of interest, and provide patients with reliable information in a form that is useful to them Create organizational cultures that support transparency, shared learning, and core competencies regarding communication with patients and families, other clinicians, and the public
Leaders and boards	Prioritize transparency and safety, and frequently review comprehensive safety performance data Link hiring, firing, promotion, and compensation to results in cultural transformation and transparency
Governmental agencies	Develop data sources for collection of safety data, improve standards and training materials for core competencies, and develop an all-payer database and robust medical device registries
Clinicians	Inform patients of clinician's experience, conflicts of interest, and role in care, and provide patients with a full description of all the alternatives for tests and treatments and the pros and cons for each Provide patients with full information about all planned tests and treatments
Hospitals and health systems	Provide patients with full access to their medical records, and include patients and family members in interdisciplinary bedside rounds
Hospitals and health systems, health professionals	Provide patients and families with full information about any harm resulting from treatment, followed by apology and fair resolution Provide patients and clinicians support when they are involved in an incident. Include patients/family members in event reporting and in root cause analysis
Hospital and health leaders	Create a safe, supportive culture for caregivers to be transparent and accountable to each other Create multidisciplinary processes and forms for reporting, analyzing, and sharing data Create processes to hold individuals accountable for risky or disruptive behavior
Health-care organizations, hospital associations, PSOs	Have clear mechanisms for sharing and adopting best practices, for example, by participating in state and regional collaboratives
Hospitals and health-care organizations	Report and publicly display measures used to monitor quality and safety, and clearly communicate to the public about performance

apology following patient injury can decrease medical malpractice liability and improve the satisfaction of all parties. Toolkits are now available to promote such programs.

Remaining Challenges

Many challenges to achieving full transparency remain. A recent survey found that less than 40% of quality and safety leaders rated their board's understanding of disclosure and apology as "high," and even fewer felt their boards had a comprehensive understanding of safety concepts related to transparency about error and harm. Transparency within organizations and between providers requires creating an environment of trust as well as improving technology and processes to ensure they are efficient and effective and promote regular open and honest communication and data sharing.

Transparency with the public is equally challenging. Hospital and clinician concerns about litigation; reputational costs; and the accuracy, interpretability, and comprehensiveness of safety metrics need to be addressed. Additionally, national rating systems and websites, including Leapfrog and *U.S. News & World Report*, share few common scores and often generate more confusion than clarity. For example, as of 2015 no hospital was rated as a high performer by all four major national US rating systems. In the future, data must be understandable and actionable for both patients and provider organizations.

As more organizations publicly share their quality, safety, and patient experience data, transparency will be increasingly demanded by all stakeholders. To benefit patients as well as care providers, organizations will need to prepare their boards, clinicians, and staff for a more transparent health-care system. Transparency at these levels will eventually facilitate decision-making about where to receive care and where to work, but a long road lies ahead to make this comparable and uniform across all health entities.

The last of the five white papers was published in 2015. Printed copies of all of them were circulated widely to CEOs and patient safety leaders of schools and health-care organizations, patient safety specialists, and members of the roundtables, who you will recall included individuals and leaders of organizations that could implement the recommendations.

While all of the reports were well-received, it is impossible to know their impact. Implementing the recommendations requires strong leadership and major cultural changes. Stimulating those changes, of course, is what we were trying to do with the white papers by providing the evidence, the arguments, and the tools for change. Some minds were undoubtedly changed. The foundation was laid for the transformations needed to make health care safe.

Transforming Health Care: A Compendium

While the white papers got good reviews and wide circulation, we were well aware that their lengths would be barriers to reading them for many who would benefit from them. So, when the last of the five white papers was finished in 2015, we wrote a compendium that brought together the executive summary and recommendations for each of the five topics, plus additional recommendations for getting started on making the changes: *Transforming Health Care: A Compendium of Reports from the National Patient Safety Foundation's Lucian Leape Institute* [2].

Our hope was that this 30-page document would not only make some of the many lessons and critical insights we had gathered more accessible, but that it would also stimulate readers to read the original monographs. Like the white papers, *Transforming Health Care: A Compendium* is available free on the IHI website.

Members

Since its inception, the membership of the Institute has changed as new members were added and others retired. Early on, we invited patient advocate *Susan Edgman-Levitan*, Executive Director of the John D. Stoeckle Center for Primary Care Innovation at the MGH to join us. To bring in outside perspectives, we were fortunate to attract *Paul O'Neill*, former CEO of Alcoa and 72nd United States Secretary of the Treasury, and *James Guest*, head of Consumers Union. *Janet Corrigan*, former IOM staff director for *To Err is Human* joined us shortly thereafter, as did *Robert M. Wachter*, founder of the hospitalist specialty and Associate Chair Department of Medicine, UCSF, and *Charles Vincent*, UK leader of patient safety research of the University of Oxford.

Later additions included *Amy Edmondson*, Professor at Harvard Business School; *Sue Sheridan*, Director of Patient Engagement, Patient-Centered Outcomes Research Institute; *David Michaels*, former Head of the Occupational Safety and Health Administration; *Gregg Meyer*, Chief Clinical Officer Of Mass General Brigham; and *Joanne Disch*, former Chair of the Board of Advocate-Aurora Health System.

In 2014, *Tejal Gandhi* became president of the Institute when Diane Pinakiewicz retired. *Gary Kaplan*, CEO of Virginia Mason Medical Center, joined LLI when he stepped down as chair of the Board of NPSF. He took over as chair of the Institute when I retired in 2015.

In addition to the five white papers, LLI pursued a number of other strategic efforts to motivate change for patient safety. From the beginning, the annual fund-raising gala had a major educational component. Prior to the evening social event, we presented a full afternoon symposium that provided a variety of unique learning opportunities for attendees, such as an open forum where they could hear presentations and question LLI members and breakout sessions on specific patient safety topics. The evening program featured an address by a world-renowned safety expert.

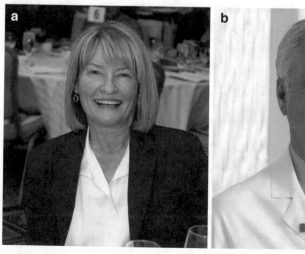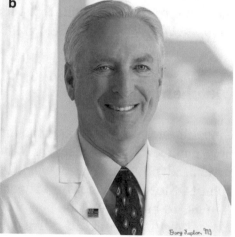

(**a**) Susan Edgman-Levitan and (**b**) Gary Kaplan.

The Institute held a fund-raising gala each year, which included an afternoon educational program conducted by the members and an evening banquet with a featured celebrity speaker. These were highly successful events attracting several hundred attendees each year.

LLI members also participated as faculty in the leadership course and other activities at the annual NPSF Congress. A highly popular feature was the annual LLI panel where several members discussed a current patient safety topic.

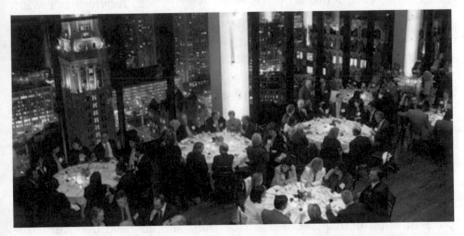

LLI Gala. Source: National Patient Safety Foundation (now Institute for Healthcare Improvement).

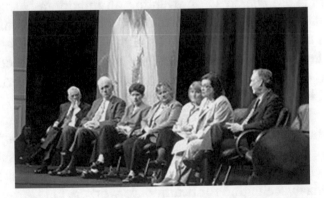

LLI Panel. From left to right: Paul O'Neill, Jim Conway, Carolyn Clancy, Pam Thompson, Susan Edgman-Levitan, Julie Morath, Gary Kaplan. (Source: National Patient Safety Foundation (now Institute for Healthcare Improvement).

Later Work

The "Must Do" List

As the concept of responding to errors by treating them as systems problems instead of blaming individuals became widely accepted, some applied the idea to all failures, and the term "no-blame" culture emerged. This misconception was countered by the definition and promotion of the "Just Culture" as defined by Reason and David Marx, who distinguished error from negligence, reckless behavior, and intentional rule violations [9, 10].

Rule violations can be tricky, since there are times when a non-standard response is required in an individual situation. These should be dealt with on an individual basis. But most violations are not in that category; they result from individual preferences, inconvenience, or resistance to change. A fair and just culture demands that such individual violators be held accountable. Unfortunately, health-care organizations varied widely in which practices they placed in this category and how they responded to violations. Few consistently enforced meaningful sanctions.

Members of LLI were of a single mind that certain safe practices were of such undisputed value that they should be universally followed and that sanctions should be applied to violators, i.e., some failures are truly "blameworthy." The practices in this category are those that (1) are *effective* at preventing an important harm, (2) have substantial *impact*, (3) are *feasible* to comply with and audit, and (4) have been accepted as a *standard* by the NQF and professional consensus. These are safety practices that have sufficiently compelling supportive evidence that clinicians should not have the right of an individual veto. We called them "Must Do" practices.

These concepts were laid out by Bob Wachter in a paper on the Health Affairs Blog, *The 'Must Do' List: Certain Patient Safety Rules Should Not Be Elective*, that provided the rationale for this approach. It identified two practices that currently met the criteria: hand hygiene and influenza vaccination for health-care workers [11].

We called on health-care organizations to expect 100 percent adherence to these practices, to sanction violators, and to be willing to terminate clinicians for deliberate and repeated noncompliance with either of these practices. We recommended that expectation of universal compliance with required practices be included in bylaws and clinician compacts. We also called on the Joint Commission and CMS and other regulators and accreditors to adopt these standards.

Financial Costs of Patient Safety

One of the arguments given by health-care organizations for not moving ahead more aggressively to improve patient safety was that they could not afford it, that implementing new practices costs more than they save. As measurement of adverse events began to take hold, however, research showed that the costs of the additional care and prolonged hospital stays caused by preventable injuries are substantial. The additional cost has been estimated at $16–18 billion annually [12] but is probably considerably higher because of underreporting. The cost of hospital-acquired infections alone has been estimated as more than $10 billion a year [13].

Hospitals were able to absorb these costs because they could bill for additional days and services caused by the injury. That began to change during the Obama Administration with the move toward value-based purchasing. Under bundled and capitated payment programs, the marginal costs of treating injuries are not compensated, eroding hospital margins. Suddenly reducing those harms became more attractive.

LLI decided to write a paper to encourage purchasers to promote safety through financial incentives and identify what further steps could be taken to strengthen marketplace incentives. In *On the safe side: the move to value-based payment models could mean improvements in patient safety*, Corrigan et al. pointed the way [14]. In addition to the direct benefit to patients from reducing adverse events, creating a safe environment enhances workplace productivity, morale, and retention. In the competitive marketplace, improved safety enhances the system's reputation and ability to increase market share. Malpractice costs will decline.

We called on executives to increase awareness of the costs by including estimates of the direct and indirect expenses associated with medical errors in financial statements shared with trustees, leadership, staff, and the public and to ensure that a portion of their organizations' capital budgets are allocated for investments in safety such as barcoding. When the financial consequences of unsafe care are accounted for, it is clear that investing in patient safety is both the right thing to do and the profitable thing to do.

Collaboration with American College of Healthcare Executives

As health-care organizations gained experience with changing systems, it became increasingly clear that more extensive culture changes were needed, and this required strong leadership. LLI began to look for strategies to engage and motivate health-care systems leaders.

In 2015, LLI approached the American College of Healthcare Executives (ACHE) regarding a joint effort. The timing was fortuitous. Under new leadership, ACHE was seeking to establish itself as a thought leader in the executive space. We formed a partnership to sponsor two roundtables on leading a culture of safety, co-chaired by leaders of the two organizations.

The participants in these roundtables, held in 2016, included CEOs and patient safety officers from a number of hospitals and systems, large and small, academics, and leaders of professional organizations, such as the AONE, AHA, ANA, and IHI, and leadership consulting organizations.

The work of the roundtables was summarized with recommendations in *Leading a Culture of Safety: A Blueprint for Success*, published jointly by ACHE and LLI [15]. This is probably the most comprehensive and useful guide for creating a culture of safety. It is described in more detail in the next chapter.

Since 2015, the end of the period of this history, NPSF merged with IHI, which committed to continuing support of LLI. Major LLI initiatives since then include:

- Partnering with NORC at the University of Chicago to conduct a survey of American's experience with medical errors and views on patient safety [16].
- *Transforming concepts in patient safety*: a report on progress in each of the five areas since they were formulated in 2009 [3].
- Framework for Effective Board Governance of Health System Quality [17].
- The Salzburg Statement on Moving Measurement into Action: Global Principles for Measuring Patient Safety [18].

Conclusion

How much impact the white papers and other LLI initiatives have had on making health care safer is impossible to know. The roundtables for the five transforming concepts and the one engaging leaders with ACHE were highly motivating for the participants. These key organizational and policy leaders—the "movers and shakers"—were enthusiastic participants, and the discussions clearly advanced thinking about each of the issues in practical and actionable ways.

The roundtables and white papers also appear to have significantly increased awareness of the complex issues in patient safety and deepened understanding of these issues for many other leaders in health care. They truly changed the conversation and helped put patient safety on everyone's agenda. To that extent, the Institute has made great progress in meeting its charge, to "define strategic paths and calls to action for the field of patient safety."

References

1. Leape L, Berwick D, Clancy C, et al. Transforming healthcare: a safety imperative. Qual Saf Health Care. 2009;18(6):424–8.
2. National Patient Safety Foundation's Lucian Leape Institute. Transforming health care: a compendium of reports from the NPSF Lucian Leape Institute. Boston: National Patient Safety Foundation; 2016.
3. Gandhi TK, Kaplan GS, Leape L, et al. Transforming concepts in patient safety: a progress report. BMJ Qual Saf. 2018;27(12):1019–26.
4. National Patient Safety Foundation. Unmet needs: teaching physicians to provide safe patient care. Boston; 2010.
5. Lucian Leape Institute. Order from Chaos: accelerating care integration. Boston: National Patient Safety Foundation; 2012.
6. Lucian Leape Institute. Through the eyes of the workforce: creating joy, meaning, and safer health care. Boston: National Patient Safety Foundation; 2013.
7. National Patient Safety Foundation's Lucian Leape Institute. Safety is personal: partnering with patients and families for the safest care. Boston: National Patient Safety Foundation; 2014.
8. National Patient Safety Foundation's Lucian Leape Institute. Shining a light: safer health care through transparency. Boston: National Patient Safety Foundation; 2015.
9. Reason JT. Managing the risks of organizational accidents. Aldershot, Hants; Brookfield: Ashgate; 1997.
10. Marx D. Patient safety and the "just culture": a primer for health care executives. New York. 17 Apr 17, 2001.

11. Wachter RM. The 'Must Do' list: certain patient safety rules should not be elective. In. *Health Affairs Blog*. Vol 2020: Health Affairs; 20 Aug 2015.
12. U.S. Department of Health and Human Services. New HHS data shows major strides made in patient safety, leading to improved care and savings. 7 May 2014.
13. Zimlichman E, Henderson D, Tamir O, et al. Health care-associated infections: a meta-analysis of costs and financial impact on the US health care system. JAMA Intern Med. 2013;173(22):2039–46.
14. Corrigan JM, Wakeam E, Gandhi TK, Leape LL. On the safe side: the move to value-based payment models could mean improvements in patient safety. Healthc Financ Manage. 2015;69(8):94.
15. American College of Healthcare Executives and IHI/NPSF Lucian Leape Institute. Leading a culture of safety: a blueprint for success. Boston: American College of Healthcare Executives and Institute for Healthcare Improvement; 2017.
16. NORC at the University of Chicago and IHI/NPSF Lucian Leape Institute. Americans' experiences with medical errors and views on patient safety. Cambridge: Institute for Healthcare Improvement and NORC at the University of Chicago; 2017.
17. Daley Ullem E, Gandhi TK, Mate K, Whittington J, Renton M, Huebner J. Framework for Effective Board Governance of Health System Quality. IHI White Paper. Boston: Institute for Healthcare Improvement; 2018.
18. Salzburg Global Seminar & Institute for Healthcare Improvement. The Salzburg statement on moving measurement into action: global principles for measuring patient safety: Institute for Healthcare Improvement and Salzburg Global Seminar; 2019.

Chapter 23
Now the Hard Part: Creating a Culture of Safety

In 2020, the coronavirus pandemic killed 1,800,000 people, 346,000 of them Americans. In that same year, if recent estimates are correct, about the same number died as a result of medical errors, all despite the enormous effort of the past 20 years to eliminate preventable harm, an effort that has involved people at all levels: policy makers, government agencies, oversight bodies, quality improvement organizations, major health-care systems, and thousands of providers and caregivers on the frontline.

Many injuries have been prevented, and thousands of lives have been saved. Fewer people suffer from hospital-acquired infections and medication errors, surgical complications, and falls in the hospital. But the overall number of preventable injuries has hardly budged. The relentless advances in medical science and the constantly changing demands of the environments in which we deliver care create new opportunities for harm faster than we can keep up.

We have learned a great deal. Driven by the concept that the cause of errors and unintended harm is not bad people, but bad systems, we have been engaged in an immense experiment testing myriad ways to make those systems changes. It has truly been a paradigm shift. Early efforts focused on changing processes at the level of the care unit or hospital. These were initially ad hoc responses to local problems, but with time an impressive repertoire has been developed of standardized practices of proven effectiveness that can be widely adopted (see Chap. 11).

© The Author(s) 2021
L. L. Leape, *Making Healthcare Safe*,
https://doi.org/10.1007/978-3-030-71123-8_23

Several large systems, such as the Veterans Health Administration, Ascension, Kaiser-Permanente, and others, expanded the use of these proven practices to all of their hospitals and clinics. Collaboratives have been developed that brought together quality improvement teams from a region or nationally to work together to implement a practice. Some of these were spectacularly successful, virtually eliminating a major threat in those hospitals [1].

Despite these impressive successes, the painful fact is that with few exceptions (such as two-factor identification of patients, barcoding of medications, and perhaps hand hygiene), most of this awesome array of standardized effective practices has not been adopted by the majority of providers and health-care organizations. Health care is still stunningly unsafe.

But even if the adoption problem could be solved, relying on universal implementation of specific practices is not likely to be an effective strategy for achieving safe health care. The potential number required must be in the thousands, and the complexities of health care ensure that new hazards will constantly arise for which there are no known practices.

If the experience of other industries that have succeeded in becoming safe is a guide, it will require much more than changing our practices to prevent specific harms. It will require changing our culture. A change that was called for in the earliest writings on patient safety [2] and in the legendary IOM report [3].

What are we talking about? What is culture, and what is the culture change that is required?

What Is Culture?

The word culture has been used, abused, and misused a great deal in the health-care literature. A major disagreement, especially in the UK, centers on whether the culture of a group should be defined in terms of its attitudes, assumptions, values, and beliefs or in terms of its actions, "how we do things around here." Is culture who we *are* or what we *do*? I believe the evidence is clear that it is both – and that each determines the other, which is the point of this chapter.

For example, from time immemorial, a well-established espoused value and assumption about physician behavior was that the physician had the sole authority to make treatment decisions, irrespective of external guidelines or internal contrary advice. The result – the practice – was deference to their authority. When that practice has been changed, when a hospital adopts adherence to standards as a condition of practice, not only does the "way we do things" change, so do, gradually, the attitudes and the values of the culture overall.

In anthropology, culture refers to social behavior in different societies or the knowledge, beliefs, and customs of their members expressed in their traditions, mythology, or religion. Nation-states pride themselves on their cultures, their traditions, their "solidarity" (or lack of it), and their particular religious commitment. We also speak of culture as a term of human refinement to differentiate elite from others.

Within societies we speak of the culture of subgroups, such as the military, medicine, "hippies," or the culture of a firm such as IBM or Apple. We note regional cultures such as those of the South or Midwest. In all these contexts, culture reflects the deep shared values and assumptions that guide us in what we should and should not do. Those values are expressed in behavior, "how we do things around here."

When we think of "how we do things around here" in health care, the focus is not just on patient care and the provider-patient interface but also includes the relationships and interactions of all who work in the care delivery setting. Individual medical specialties, nursing, pharmacy, etc. have strong subcultures, but it is predominantly the *organizational culture* of the hospital or clinic that determines how patients are cared for.

Most of what we know about organizational culture comes from studies of other industries. The work of Edgar Schein is preeminent [4]. Schein notes that three elements define an organization's culture: its shared *assumptions*; its *espoused values*, i.e., what a group ideally wants to be and wishes to present itself to the public; and the day-to-day *behaviors*. Culture includes everything we do in an organization; it makes sense of what we do, it provides stability.

The shared assumptions run deep. They are the "truth" as perceived by the organization's members: their beliefs about human nature, such as whether people are intrinsically self-motivated or motivated by money, their perceptions of reality, and their concept of mission. In health care, shared assumptions include a commitment to responding to emergencies and putting the patient's interest first. They are the unwritten rules.

Espoused values include such things as individualism, respect for authority, and working hard. Behaviors are the visible manifestations of the culture, the rituals and how we treat one another, labelled by Schein as "artifacts" [4]. Others have used the term *safety climate* to refer to these expressions of the culture.

Schein summarizes this in a definition of culture that is widely accepted as capturing the essential aspects: "A pattern of shared basic assumptions that was learned by a group as it solved its problems of external adaptation and internal integration, that has worked well enough to be considered valid and, therefore, to be taught to new members as the correct way to perceive, think, and feel in relation to those problems" [4].

In large organizations such as hospitals, the individual units, services, and divisions also have their own cultures. These subcultures share some of the organization's values and assumptions, but not necessarily all, with the result that members of one unit may engage in behaviors that differ substantially from those in another. For example, when a nurse makes an error, whether the unit's nursing culture is supportive or blaming affects whether they will report the error so it becomes known and can be investigated. The culture in the ICU may be very different from that in the emergency room or from another ICU down the hall.

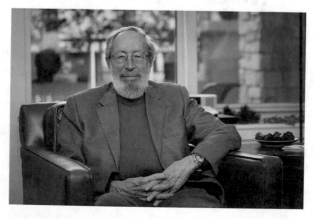

Edgar Schein. (All rights reserved)

A Culture of Safety

What is a *culture of safety*? The term was first used by the International Nuclear Safety Advisory Group report following the 1986 disaster at the Chernobyl Nuclear Power Plant, the cause of which was attributed to a breakdown in the organization's safety culture [5, 6].

A useful definition was later put forth by the UK Health and Safety Commission:

> The safety culture of an organization is the product of the individual and group values, attitudes, competencies and patterns of behavior that determine the commitment to, and the style and proficiency of, an organization's health and safety programs. Organizations with a positive safety culture are characterized by communications founded on mutual trust, by shared perceptions of the importance of safety, and by confidence in the efficacy of preventive measures [7].

One of the earliest and most respected students of organizational culture, James Reason, of the University of Manchester, UK, identified five components that characterize a culture of safety [8]. It must be:

- An *informed culture*: It needs data about incidents and near misses.
- A *reporting culture*: Workers must feel it is safe to report and that it makes a difference.
- A *just culture*: People are rewarded for providing essential safety information, but deliberate breaking of the rules is not tolerated.
- A *flexible culture*: The organization can reconfigure itself in response to a new danger, such as moving from hierarchical structure to a flattened structure as needed.
- A *learning culture*: It is able to draw the right conclusions from its information system and has the will to implement major reforms when needed.

One follows from another. An informed culture can only be built on the foundations of a reporting culture. This, in turn, depends upon establishing a just culture. Flexibility and learning are only possible if the other components are established. But none of this is possible without openness and trust.

As Schein points out, a culture of safety can only exist within the broader culture of a health-care organization that is committed to providing patients with the experience of high-quality effective care, delivered efficiently by valued and engaged workers. While in other industries the safety focus is on *workers*, in health care it is primarily on the patient, but to succeed it must also include worker safety.

Characteristics of a Safe Culture

Unfortunately, few health-care organizations have seriously striven to become a safe culture. What should it look like? What are the characteristics of a safe culture in health care?

At the *organizational* level, in a culture of safety everyone shares a commitment to the goal of zero harm and to the continuing improvement and innovation that are required to get there – to the belief that anything is possible. There is a sense of individual responsibility at every level, that safety is everyone's job. Leaders exemplify these commitments and motivate others to share them. Their sincerity of purpose, consistency, and transparency inspire trust.

The individual is valued, and every voice is heard. Leaders seek to follow the advice of Paul O'Neill, the highly successful CEO of Alcoa, who taught that every worker, every day, should come to work feeling they are respected regardless of rank or expertise, supported to do their work well, and appreciated for what they contribute.

At the *operational* level, in a culture of safety people work in teams and are open and trusting of one another. They share the mission of providing care that is free of harm. There is a commitment to standard work, i.e., finding the best way to do something and everyone doing it, yet they are open to changing it to make it better. Innovation and improvement are part of everyday work and are everyone's responsibility. They give meaning to work. Patients are fully engaged as partners in their care and in improvement.

At the *individual* level, in a safe culture, workers feel valued and supported. Their deep sense of individual responsibility for safety is expressed not only by being careful but by being alert and looking for hazards, "accidents waiting to happen." Errors, harms, near misses, and hazards are promptly reported because they know they will be taken seriously, promptly investigated, and acted upon.

A culture of safety is a *learning culture*. It is an environment where everyone is aware of how far their work falls short of what it could be and is committed to improve. A learning culture is characterized by its members' ability to self-reflect and identify strengths and defects [9]. People pay attention, notice problems, and reflect on them. Problems are analyzed, and solutions are imagined and created. Changes are implemented.

Schein emphasizes that a learning culture is based on positive assumptions about human nature: that human nature is good and that people will learn if it is psychologically safe to do so. There is commitment to learning to learn, to truth as discovered by inquiry, to full and open communication, to systems thinking [4]. A learning culture is based on trust, transparency, and reliability.

A Just Culture

A culture of safety is also a *fair and just culture*. What does this mean? From the beginning, the fundamental aim of the patient safety movement has been to shift the focus from the individual to the system when things go wrong. Some (not your author) have referred to this as a "no-blame" approach. For the vast majority of iatrogenic harms, probably 90% or more, this is appropriate. The harm was unintentional and resulted from poor system design. The caregiver is truly the "second victim."

But some errors and some injuries are caused by intentional acts. For these a no-blame approach is inappropriate.

If the individual intended to cause harm, the act is assault and should be dealt with by the legal system. Fortunately, assault is exceedingly rare in health care (serial murders, etc.). The much more common intentional act is *rule breaking* in which the caregiver does not intend harm, but deliberately fails to follow a standard procedure.

This form of violation is actually quite common. Because of time and workload pressures, nurses and doctors often "cut corners" to get their patients taken care of, especially if the rule doesn't make sense, doesn't seem to apply in this case, or prevents them from getting their work done. But even if the act seemed justified, the caregiver will feel ashamed if it harms the patient because they will realize they have "done something wrong."

These cases should be carefully investigated. If the broken rule is a bad rule, or unworkable, it should be changed, by a process that involves all stakeholders. If the existing rule is good and necessary, education may be necessary; if time pressures or workloads are the issue, these should be addressed. On the other hand, if a violation results just from the caregiver's personal preference or convenience, discipline may be indicated, especially if there is a pattern of such behavior.

Seeing that indefensible repeated violations have consequences is important for co-workers in two ways. They see that justice is done – the person didn't "get away with it" – and it reinforces their own rule-abiding behavior. A just culture is the necessary balance to a systems approach [8, 10].

The term safety culture is sometimes confused with safety *climate*, which is its outward manifestation – its visible evidence, or "artifacts" as Schein puts it. Safety climate more appropriately refers to the *perception* of the culture, what people think about themselves and "what we do around here." It is what we measure when we attempt to measure safety culture [11].

High-Reliability Organizations

Much has been written about *high-reliability organizations* (*HRO*) and whether they are the model for a safe culture. The concept is based on a series of studies in the early 1990s by Roberts and colleagues of highly hazardous industries, such as aviation and nuclear power, that had succeeded in becoming extremely safe [12]. While it is true that, unlike health care, these industries had strong business cases for safety – they would be out of business if unsafe – the fact is that they are amazingly successful.

Weick and Sutcliffe identified five characteristics that account for the success of HRO, which they label *collective mindfulness*: (1) preoccupation with failure, the continual looking for and reporting of hazards; (2) reluctance to simplify, not accepting the obvious explanation for a failure; (3) sensitivity to operations, paying attention to issues at the frontline; (4) commitment to resilience, the ability to detect errors, react, and recover; and (5) deference to expertise, the flattening of the hierarchy in an emergency so that the most qualified person is in charge, regardless of seniority [13].

Collective mindfulness leads to the essential behavior for safety, which is that everyone understands that even small failures can lead to catastrophic outcomes and accepts responsibility both for identifying hazards early and for correcting them before harm occurs [13].

In other industries, HROs have achieved a culture of safety and enviable outcomes. The idea of applying these principles to health care is attractive [14]. Certainly these characteristics of structure, attitude, and expertise need to be part of the changes in quality of care and experience that make health care safe.

The originator of the concept of HROs, Karlene Roberts, also attributes much of their success to the emphasis on *relational* aspects of the culture: interpersonal responsibility, person-centeredness, being supportive of co-workers, friendliness, openness in personal relations, creativity, credibility, interpersonal trust, and resiliency [12, 15].

The Problem

Most health-care organizations fall woefully short of achieving a culture of safety. With just a few exceptions, hospitals and health-care systems, including some of the most highly regarded academic health centers, have settled for implementing some safe practices; the culture is unchanged.

In a safe culture, there is a strong commitment to the goal of zero harm and to the continuing improvement and innovation that is required to get there. In health care, safety is too often an afterthought or at best a distant second fiddle to the bottom line. There is no sense of commitment, no goal of zero harm. Deliberate unsafe care is often tolerated, especially among big earners.

In a safe culture, safety information systems collect data on incidents and near misses. Reporting of adverse events or hazards is encouraged and leads to investigation, analysis, and, where possible, redesign of a process or system to eliminate the risk. In health care, many institutions have established reporting system and a process for root cause analysis of events to meet accreditation requirements, but their use is often perfunctory. Now 25 years after hospitals were urged to stop blaming people for errors, nearly half of nurses surveyed by the Joint Commission say they do not report errors because of fear that they or a colleague will be punished.

In a safe culture, workers feel valued, supported, and empowered. They have a sense of ownership, of responsibility, to prevent harm and work well in teams. Sadly, in health care this sense of responsibility and empowerment has long been inhibited by a hierarchical system that devalues their contributions and makes working in teams difficult. It is a culture of low expectations and low accountability.

Why Changing Culture Is so Hard to Do

Creating a safe culture is the key part of the transformation that a health-care organization must undergo overall to reliably provide a patient experience of high-quality, effective, and efficient care. Under the best of circumstances, these are difficult changes to carry off, but health care also offers a staggering array of barriers to change.

The first has been *resistance* by the key members of the workforce: physicians. Products of an educational system that traditionally emphasized personal responsibility for patient care, many viewed standardization as a threat to their independence and personal judgment. Giving up control and sharing responsibility by working in teams were hard to do.

Fortunately, that has begun to change. Younger physicians have learned the importance of quality improvement and are amenable to working in teams. They "get it" and now constitute a significant majority of physicians.

The second major barrier to change is an incredibly complicated demand/incentive *payment system* that compels hospitals – i.e., doctors and nurses – to document that they meet quality and volume requirements. The result is an extensive, and, for caregivers, depressing, set of demands on their time that compete directly with their primary mission of taking care of patients.

This oppressive payment system is the product of two forces that changed dramatically in the past several decades: the ability to measure safety and quality and the rising cost of care.

Twenty years ago, as the quality and safety movement was gaining steam, many complained about the paucity of good measures. For safety, what were the errors and systems failures we should focus on? For quality, the IOM called for care that was safe, efficient, timely, patient-centered, efficient, and equitable [16]. But, again, how would we know? Well, in the past 20 years we've developed methods for measuring all of these. More are needed, but thanks to an impressive effort by quality and safety researchers we can now measure quite a bit.

The other major driver of demand/incentive payment changes is *costs*, which have risen dramatically since the middle of the twentieth century primarily as the result of awesome improvements in diagnosis and treatment that have been heavily weighted toward expensive technologies. Magnetic resonance imaging, PET scans, and surgical robots, for example, cost health care millions of dollars a year. A new "miracle" drug may cost hundreds of thousands of dollars a year for a single patient.

Facing the need to contain costs, payers and regulators seized on available measures to assess performance and used them for accreditation and for value-based financial incentives. Lowered reimbursement rates force physicians to see more patients (production pressure).

A particularly painful example for physicians resulted from the generous incentives provided by the government for adoption of the electronic health record (EHR). When computerized records were being developed, many of us were enthusiastic about their potential to improve the quality of care, such as by reducing medication errors and making standardized clinical information available. A number of private companies rose to the opportunity, each with its own product, most of them built around systems they already had for billing and financial management. Not only were these clumsy, inefficient, and non-user-friendly, they were proprietary and thus would not communicate with one another.

Finally, the government stepped in—not to regulate and standardize systems as many of us had hoped, but to promote their use through a massive subsidy for the implementation of these mostly proprietary systems by hospitals and physicians. Because most of these EHRs are poorly designed, the result has been a huge increase in the time that physicians must spend in documentation.

The resulting burdens of using the EHR, increased production pressure, and loss of control are widely considered to be major factors in the dissatisfaction and burnout that has become increasingly common among health workers. We have created an environment where many nurses, doctors, and allied health staff are too exhausted, too disillusioned, and too burned out to have the interest or the energy to engage in efforts to change. There is little time for reflection, improvement, or preventing errors.

In addition to physician resistance and perverse payment incentives, a third barrier to creating a culture of safety stems from *financial threats to institutional survival.* In our predominantly fee-for-service system, economic survival of a hospital depends on the number of services provided and how much they are paid for them. To control costs, government payments—Medicare and Medicaid— are below market for virtually all services. Commercial insurance companies pay much better—sometimes multiples of Medicare reimbursement. They also negotiate rates with hospitals.

In this system, large hospitals increase their income by attracting more patients through providing ever more sophisticated and expensive treatments. Although they have many Medicare patients, large hospitals receive the major share of their income from commercial insurers with whom they negotiate rates.

Smaller hospitals lose on both counts. They are unable to attract more patients with increased services, and they lack the clout to negotiate higher rates with insurance companies. Safety net hospitals, formerly city hospitals for the indigent, and rural hospitals fare even worse. They depend almost totally on local government support and Medicaid, both at "bare-bones" levels.

In all hospitals, the CEO is under constant financial pressure— beholden to "the bottom line." The large expensive hospitals, like other corporations, vie for increased market share by providing additional services. If they become the dominant provider in a region, they can exercise monopoly power and can raise their prices. While technically "not for profit," they generate large profits, which they use to expand their services and to increase the pay of their physicians and, especially, their CEOs. According to Forbes, in 2019 the top 13 nonprofit hospitals and systems paid their CEOS between $five million and $21.6 million; the next 61 paid CEOs between $1 and five million [17].

The fourth barrier to changing culture, compounding all the others, is the incredibly *complex nature* of health care. No other industry comes close. The client—the patient—may suffer from an almost infinite number and variety of diseases. In addition, patients also vary widely in what they bring to the therapeutic encounter in terms of genetic makeup, physical and mental health, and the effect of the living environment where they receive most of their care.

Matching the number and variety of diseases is an incredible number and variety of treatments, using modalities as varied as chemicals (drugs), electromagnetic waves, surgery, robots, and computers. Compounding this is a lack of standardization of use. Each form of treatment can be—and often is—employed according to the judgment, or whim, of the provider. The result is an almost infinite number of ways things can go wrong [18].

Finally, those who *provide* care are a diverse group. In addition to doctors, nurses, and pharmacists, many other workers, such as therapists, aides, clerical staff, and support staff, are essential personnel who make a hospital work. There are 180 specialties and subspecialties in medicine alone, each with its unique knowledge, skills, and approach to patient care.

The complexity of health care and the formidable array of regulatory and financial forces impacting it are awesome. Changing the culture will require that these interests be aligned and that public-private partnerships be developed. But what, exactly, do we want a hospital to do? We have a clear idea of what a culture of safety looks like. How do we get there?

How to Do It

How do we transform the dysfunctional cultures of health-care organizations into cultures of safety? How do we motivate CEOs to make safety a priority, take responsibility for making it happen, inspire others to join the cause, and create an environment of transparency, respect, and personal responsibility?

The leading thought leaders in patient safety have described visions of what a safe culture should be but often have been humble about providing advice on how to get there.

Reason speaks of "engineering" a safe culture in general, not specifically in health care. He describes the critical subcomponents: a reporting culture, a just culture, a flexible culture, and a learning culture. He notes that a safety culture is far more than the sum of its parts, that the rest is "up to the organizational chemistry" [8]. How to create that chemistry is left unanswered.

Likewise, Vincent describes the ingredients in a safety culture and notes that the evidence from studies such as those of Singer [19] shows that a better safety climate is associated with fewer adverse events. But he, too, shies away from prescribing how to achieve a safe culture [7].

However, in their perceptive and influential book, *Safer Healthcare: Strategies for the Real World*, Vincent and Amalberti provide a prescription for achieving safe care that would, in fact, require significant culture change [20]. They observe that the approach to improving patient safety has been too limited, focusing primarily on hospital care and too little on primary care and home care, and that the method used was the same in all settings: improvement of a core issue in a narrow time scale with a specific process change such as the surgical checklist or CLABSI protocol.

They call for a much broader approach using five safety strategies:

1. *Safety as Best Practice*: aspire to standards—reducing specific harms and improving clinical processes, such as the CLABSI protocol and the surgical checklist
2. *Improvement of Healthcare Processes and Systems*: intervening to support individuals and teams, improving working conditions and organizational practices, such as improved handovers, use of daily goals and huddles, and barcoding of medications
3. *Risk Control*: placing restrictions on performance, demand, or working conditions, such as regulations governing radiation therapy, closing unsafe facilities, and limiting individual licenses or privileges
4. *Improving Capacity for Monitoring, Adaptation, and Response*, such as briefings and debriefings, safe reporting, family engagement, and emergency planning
5. *Mitigation*: planning for potential harm and recovery, such as providing patient and peer support after harm

They then show how these five strategies can be used in three settings: hospital, home, and primary care. The specific issue of changing the culture to enable implementation of these strategies is not addressed, however.

Shanafelt et al. are more prescriptive [21]. They describe the steps that must be taken to change the culture of medicine: create psychological safety for people to learn new things, identify collaborative strategies for physicians and leaders to gain experience with new modes of working, and provide resources and formal training, advisors, and coaching. They emphasize that the leader must be convinced of the need to change and spearhead and support the initiatives. Individuals who are the targets of the change must be involved in the process [21].

IHI/Safe and Reliable Healthcare Framework In 2017, the IHI and Safe and Reliable Healthcare jointly published *A Framework for Safe, Reliable, and Effective Care* [9]. The authors, Allan Frankel, cofounder of Safe and Reliable Healthcare, and Carol Haraden, Frank Federico, and Jennifer Lenoci-Edwards, of IHI, propose that achieving safe and reliable care requires attention to three domains: leadership, culture, and the learning system.

The paper provides direction to health-care organizations on the key strategic, clinical, operational, and cultural components involved with each and how they interact. It provides definitions and implementation strategies for nine foundational components: leadership, psychological safety, accountability, teamwork and communication, negotiation, transparency, reliability, improvement and measurement, and continuous learning.

Each of the nine components is described with specific major points, followed by a section, Moving from Concept to Reality, which describes the steps to implementing the ideas in daily practice. For example, the Framework uses Edmondson's definition of psychological safety [22]:

- Anyone can ask questions without looking stupid.
- Anyone can ask for feedback without looking incompetent.
- Anyone can be respectfully critical without appearing negative.
- Anyone can suggest innovative ideas without being perceived as disruptive.

It then gives advice on how to achieve psychological safety, such as coaching, huddles, solicitation of ideas, and providing feedback to suggestions. As the authors suggest, the report provides a framework for thinking about patient safety; training, guidance, and support are also needed. It is not a blueprint or detailed plan.

ACHE/LLI Leading a Culture of Safety   That blueprint is provided for the key element for culture change, leadership, by another publication in 2017, *Leading a Culture of Safety: A Blueprint for Success*, jointly published by the American College of Healthcare Executives and the Lucian Leape Institute [23]. The most detailed and prescriptive advice published so far, its central theme is that leaders create safety. The product of two roundtables of those who have led and those who have studied successful transformations, the document is "an evidence-based, practical resource with tools and proven strategies to assist (leaders) in creating a culture of safety" [23].

The mission is clearly stated up front: "It is both the obligation and the privilege of every healthcare CEO to create and represent a compelling vision for a culture of safety: a culture in which mistakes are acknowledged and lead to sustainable, positive change; respectful and inclusive behaviors are instinctive and serve as the behavioral norms for the organization; and the physical and psychological safety of patients and the workforce is both highly valued and ardently protected.... The elimination of harm to our patients and workforce is our foremost moral and ethical obligation" [23].

The document addresses both "foundational" elements—what is needed to establish a culture of safety—and "sustaining" elements, what is needed to make it permanent. It describes in detail the many elements of both strategy and tactics that are needed to accomplish the objectives. These are organized into six leadership domains that require CEO focus and dedication:

1. *Establish a compelling vision for safety.* An organization's vision reflects priorities that, when aligned with its mission, establish a strong foundation for the work of the organization.
2. *Build trust, respect, and inclusion.* Establishing trust, showing respect, and promoting inclusion—and demonstrating these principles throughout the organization and with patients and families—are essential to a leader's ability to create and sustain a culture of safety.
3. *Select, develop, and engage your Board.* CEOs are responsible for ensuring the education of their Board members on foundational safety science.

4. *Prioritize safety in the selection and development of leaders.* Include accountability for safety as part of the leadership development strategy for the organization. In addition, identify physicians, nurses, and other clinical leaders as safety champions.
5. *Lead and reward a just culture.* Workers must be empowered and unafraid to voice concerns about threats to patient and workforce safety.
6. *Establish organizational behavior expectations.* These include transparency, effective teamwork, active communication, civility, and direct and timely feedback.

Leading a Culture of Safety is a landmark publication. It is by far the most comprehensive exposition of what is needed to achieve a safe culture in health care. It is a blueprint constructed by the most respected leaders in the field that makes a clear and powerful statement that the trust and openness needed to achieve a safe culture start at the top.

Examples of Success

A handful of health-care organizations have succeeded in changing their cultures. Several are worth examining for lessons learned.

Virginia Mason Medical Center

In 2000, Virginia Mason Medical Center (VMMC) in Seattle was in trouble. It was losing money, and it became apparent that the old model based on professional excellence was insufficient. The Board and top management had all read the IOM reports and realized that they too had quality and safety problems and inefficiencies. The Board asked, "if we are so focused on patients, why are all the systems built around the doctors?" Agreeing, Gary Kaplan, the new CEO, proposed to change from a physician-driven organization focused on volume to a patient-oriented organization based on quality of care. The Board gave him full support.

Kaplan and his senior management team spent the next year looking unsuccessfully for a health-care management system to achieve this goal. They then accidentally met John Black, a former Boeing executive, who told them of the impact of implementing the management system Lean. They visited businesses in the USA that used Lean and decided it was what they needed.

Lean is derived from the Toyota Production System that was developed in the 1930s when Toyota began producing automobiles [24]. It is founded on the concept of continuous and incremental improvements of product and process and eliminating waste. It is "a way to do more and more with less and less - less human effort, less equipment, less time, and less space - while coming closer and closer to providing customers exactly what they want" [25].

Lean is based on five key principles:

1. *Value*: Specify the value desired by the customer.
2. *Value Stream*: Identify the *value stream* (*the steps in a process*) that provides value for each product, and challenge all of the wasted steps.
3. *Flow*: Make the product flow continuously through the remaining value-added steps.
4. *Pull*: Introduce pull between all steps where continuous flow is possible.
5. *Perfection*: Manage toward perfection so that the number of steps and the amount of time and information needed to serve the customer continually fall [26].

Persuaded by Black and Carolyn Corvi, who had led dramatic improvements in the production of the 737 aircraft, Kaplan took his senior executive team to Japan to study the Toyota Production System. They were profoundly moved. Workers and managers worked in harmony to produce a flawless product, an automobile. Kaplan's team could see that these methods could be adapted to health care. They came home determined to develop a Virginia Mason Production System (VMPS).

Aren't You Ashamed?   One experience at Toyota struck home with particular force. A *sensei* (teacher) reviewing a VMMC floor plan with the team asked what a certain area was. A waiting room, they said. "Who waits there?" Patients. "For whom?" The doctor. The sensei then found that there were 100 waiting rooms at VMMC and that patients waited on average 45 minutes for a doctor. "Aren't you ashamed?" he said [27]. Suddenly the team understood what "patient first" meant.

Back home, selling VMPS to the staff was another matter. While many—particularly the younger ones who had embraced quality improvement—were supportive, some of the senior staff, including some department chairmen, were not. They rebelled, objected, and in some cases resigned. Education about the new system and training leaders took a year or more, but it was imperative, and the investment of time proved worthwhile.

The changes proposed were indeed monumental. It took several years to implement them, and the work is never done. Four features drove the transformation:

1. A *shared vision* outlined within a strategic plan that places the *Patient First* in everything, always. The strategic plan evolved into a "pyramid" figure with the patient at the top; under that, the vision and the mission; and then the values teamwork, integrity, excellence, and service.
2. *Alignment* of mission and values from the board down. Alignment means all parties share common focus, common goal, common language, and common culture. The "pyramid" facilitates alignment—there is no ambiguity that the patient's interest is always first.

   A key instrument for achieving alignment is the *compact*, an agreement between the organization and physicians that made explicit the reciprocal obligations of both. It took a year to develop. Additional compacts were developed for leaders and for board members.
3. A single improvement *method*—VMPS—that enables continuing improvements in quality, safety, access, efficiency, and affordability, every day at every level of the organization.
4. A culture predicated on deep respect for people and continuous improvement. Two aspects are fundamental: *respect*, meaning every voice is not only heard, but listened to, and *teamwork* that stimulates personal and professional growth and performance.

The transformations of the VMPS were many and profound. They have been extensively documented and explained in several books that are well worth reading [27–29].

Here are a few examples:

Standard Work   A challenge for physicians was the concept of standard work, a cornerstone of innovation in Lean. Reducing variability ensures quality while making it easier to identify and deal with necessary exceptions. Standard work means that all have the obligation to follow a process that is defined by consensus among stakeholders as the most effective and safest. Embracing this concept was an essential first step in establishing the new culture. Over the years, VMMC developed over 70 "must do" processes.

Kaizen Promotion Office (KPO)   "Kaizen" is Japanese for continuous incremental improvement. It assumes that frontline workers are the source of ideas of how to remove waste and improve processes but lack the expertise to develop the new processes. Expert help is needed. At VMMC, the KPO provides that help. The KPO was a clear signal that VMMC was serious about VMPS.

Rapid Process Improvement Workshops (RPIW)   One of the earliest innovations introduced was the Rapid Process Improvement Workshop. This is an intensely serious effort to address a defined quality or flow problem. Trained and certified Workshop leaders convene a team of stakeholders and KPO experts to work full time for 5 days to analyze a problem, identify waste, define the value stream, and reengineer the process. Stretch goals are set—typically 50% for operational issues, 100% for safety.

Examples of innovation from RPIWs include eliminating the waiting rooms in outpatient clinics, cutting triage time in the ER in half, and the institution of Saturday hours. A powerful example was redesigning the cancer center, which took multiple RPIWs.

When VMMC decided to move the cancer center to a large floor with windows all around the periphery, the doctors assumed that is where their offices would be. Not so. If VMMC was serious about putting the patient's interest first, they would go to the patients. And so it was, with the doctors and nurses having their offices and common areas internally.

Not only did the patients get the nice rooms, they could stay there. Analysis of the "value stream" showed that cancer patients typically spent hours walking all over the hospital to see multiple specialists;

get X-rays, lab tests; etc., in addition to lying in bed for hours for intravenous infusion. The fix? A truly radical idea: let them stay in the room and have everyone come to them. Result: the duration of patient visits fell by 50%, patient satisfaction rose to 95%, and VMMC took care of 1100 more patients a year with no increase in staff [27].

Patient Safety Alerts (PSA) Safe and frequent reporting of errors, adverse events, near misses, and hazards is essential to improvement. You can't fix something you don't know about. VMMC labelled them Patient Safety Alerts (PSA) and patterned the response after Toyota's "Stop the Line." Mishaps were no longer "events" to be reported and perhaps evaluated, they were real-time indicators of failure and harm and got immediate attention.

Two features distinguish the PSA system from the usual reporting system: everyone is empowered and obligated to report them in real time, and every report leads to a response. The response may be immediate, stopping a treatment to correct or understand an error or near miss, or urgent root cause analysis, or as an agenda item for improvement. The PSA system enables the frontline worker to directly engage leadership in a collaborative relationship. It is also tangible evidence of the institution's commitment to the target of perfection.

Since its inception in 2002, the PSA system has resulted in 100,000 reports that led to responses and changes that over time dramatically reduced the rate of adverse events and "near misses." Risk-adjusted mortality declined, as did liability costs.

Patient Safety as a Primary Goal In 2004, Mary McClinton died at VMMC during a radiological procedure as a result of accidental intravenous injection of an antiseptic, chlorhexidine, instead of contrast material. The hospital was devastated. Unequivocally committed to transparency, Kaplan went public, explained what happened, and apologized. The newspapers remarked on how unusual his transparency was (and, sadly, still is).

Mary McClinton's death had a profound impact on the hospital staff. In the previous two years, they had made great strides in improving processes and reducing errors. How could this happen? Clearly, they still had a long way to go to achieve harm-free care. But the experience with improving quality and the development of a culture of openness and trust gave them confidence to proceed. The response was quick and decisive: patient safety would not just be part of the transformation, it would become its overarching goal. Prevention of harm would be the core focus for the next several years.

Respect for People In 2011, after a decade of incredibly successful cultural transformation, a routine survey showed that, like other health-care organizations, nearly half of employees still did not feel safe in speaking up about a personal mistake. Lynne Chafez, General Counsel and leader of the changes at VMMC, asked me to come out and consult with them.

We had just written our papers on respect (Chap. 21), so I shared our discovery of the unrecognized subtle forms of disrespect that are pervasive in health care. It fell on fertile ground. They listened, and they responded by developing the Respect for People program as a major safety goal. VMMC developed an educational course on respect that was required for all 5000 of their staff. The approach has subsequently been adopted by hundreds of other hospitals worldwide. It identified ten foundational behaviors expected of everyone working at VMMC. They speak volumes about the kind of culture it strives to be (Box 23.1).

Box 23.1 Respect for People
Foundational behaviors

1. Listen to understand
2. Keep your promises
3. Be encouraging
4. Connect with others
5. Express gratitude
6. Share information
7. Speak up
8. Walk in their shoes
9. Grow and develop
10. Be a team player

Adapted from Ref. [28].

Secrets of Success

The transformation of VMMC was a profound and dramatic culture change. It was challenging, it was threatening, and it never stops. Reflecting on 18 years of progress, Gary Kaplan identified four key transformations that led to successful culture change:

First, *Board and governance engagement.* Members of the board are responsible for governance, not just to attend meetings and leave quality to the doctors, but as partners to achieve it. Board members are trained in VMPS, and, like all senior leaders, every member of the Board is required to go to Japan at least once in their first term. They undergo regular self-evaluation as a board and as individuals.

The Board is seriously involved in ensuring patient respect and care. Patient care failures and successes are presented at every meeting, sometimes by the patient in person. The Board reviews every red PSA (an event that has harmed a patient or has the potential to) and must sign off on the prevention plan before it is implemented.

Clearly, it is a very different kind of board from those of most health-care organizations. Members are neither appointed by CEO nor beholden to him. They are chosen for their expertise, literacy and commitment, not their status in the community or largess. They bring curiosity, active engagement and dissent in open meetings, and, as defined in their compact, relentless commitment to the strategic plan. Outside experts such as Julie Morath and Gregg Meyer are included on the oversight committee.

Second, Kaplan believes *changing minds of leadership* is crucial. All members of the "C-suite"—including legal counsel and the CFO—have to become champions to support middle management. Trust, alignment, and workers' sense of value depend on leadership. Trust comes from leaders being vulnerable in the sense of being willing to admit mistakes and take advice from others. Alignment depends on leaders who are value-driven, embrace the mission and the strategic plan, and have clarity about purpose. Alignment to purpose and respect for people gives workers passion about their work and meaning to their lives.

Continuing development of new leaders is the key to sustainability. VMMC has an active program to continually identify, develop, and formally train leaders at all levels. One or two people are always prepared to step up when someone leaves.

The third critical transformation is *transparency*—truth telling—shining a light on mistakes. Transparency creates the culture that makes reporting work; it reveals behaviors that are not consistent with *patient first*. It ensures open and honest communication with patients when things go wrong. A culture of transparency revealed the problem of disrespect. External transparency, as in the McClinton's, builds trust with the public.

Finally, the fourth transformation is the centerpiece *respect for people*, listening and responding to staff concerns and holding all accountable for respectful conduct with one another and with patients.

VMMC is a model of the transformation needed for a health-care organization to develop a culture of safety. Safety is an organizing principle of its daily work, a pillar supporting its mission to provide high-quality effective care. Zero harm is the goal, safety is everyone's responsibility, and innovation and improvement are part of everyday work. Not surprisingly, year after year, VMMC has been named as one of the top hospitals in the nation by Leapfrog. Hundreds of health-care organizations have come to VMMC to learn how to transform. May they all succeed.

Cincinnati Children's Hospital

When Jim Anderson took over as CEO at Cincinnati Children's Hospital (CCH) in 1997, he found a hospital that, like most academic institutions of the time, prided itself on its research excellence and assumed that its patient care was excellent as well. Anderson was not so sure. Having been CEO of a manufacturing firm, he knew something about quality improvement, and he knew CCH could do better. Lee Carter, the new board chair agreed. He was especially interested in increasing the focus on patients and families.

In 1999, they initiated a strategic planning process that asked their various communities about challenges over the next 3–5 years. One of the groups said that despite having great physicians and nurses, the institution did not provide an environment for the best delivery of that care.

There was more disturbing news. CCH had just joined the Cystic Fibrosis Foundation (CFF) National Quality Initiative, a collaborative with other hospitals to improve the care of cystic fibrosis patients. When they received comparative feedback of baseline data of measures of nutrition and pulmonary function, they were shocked to find that CCH was not only not in the top 10 as they expected, but its results were below the national average.

From his business experience, Anderson knew that fixing quality problems was not only the right thing to do, but that the savings more than offset the costs, making also a compelling business case. Poor quality came from inept management. Carter agreed. They could do better.

The release of the IOM report, *To Err is Human*, provided additional impetus. Quality and safety were compelling issues they needed to address. CCH's new 5-year strategic plan made a commitment to dramatically transform the way they delivered health care. Uma Kotagal, who had led earlier performance efforts, was put in charge.

Lee Carter's comment was memorable: "Well, if we are not the best, we can certainly be the best at getting better, and then we *will* be the best." He established and chaired the Board Patient Care Committee, composed of doctors, nurses, business people, board members, and members of the community.

In the middle of the strategic planning process came the opportunity to apply for a Pursuing Perfection grant from the Robert Wood Johnson Foundation (RWJF) (see Chap. 6 for program details). CCH competed against over 200 hospitals and was one of only four chosen. They would focus on one evidence-based practice, bronchiolitis, and one chronic condition, cystic fibrosis, which they knew from the national quality initiative they needed to work on. After a struggle with CFF, they obtained the name of the hospital that was the national leader in cystic fibrosis care and sent a team to learn from them how to improve their care of these patients.

A core requirement of the RWJF grant was transparency and patient engagement. The Foundation funded and helped produce a video of CCH parents of patients with cystic fibrosis who volunteered to describe their experiences. The film was devastating. It depicted multiple errors in the care they were receiving. Anderson showed it to the Board Patient Care Committee. They were speechless, except for the doctors or nurses who said, "Of course, that's how the system works." Anderson and Kotagal had their work cut out for them.

Participating in Pursuing Perfection had a powerful impact on CCH. While it yielded impressive successes, it also revealed how far they had to go to build capacity to make widespread change. Kotagal realized that people didn't know how to make change. They needed to be trained. She sent key staff to take Brent James' QI course in Salt Lake City.

A central feature of the reorganization was the establishment of clinical systems improvement (CSI) teams consisting of a physician leader, a nurse leader, and executive for each of five domains: inpatient, outpatient, perioperative, home health, and emergency. These CSI teams were responsible for major issues such as flow, safety, and patient experience. They worked with and sponsored unit teams headed by a physician leader and the nurse manager to test patient safety initiatives. All were required to take the course on leadership and capability development.

A robust measurement system was developed to document outcomes, and within each domain influential physicians and nurses formed improvement teams for key negative outcomes such as ventilator-associated pneumonia, catheter-associated bloodstream infections, surgical site infections, and adverse drug events. A senior leader was assigned as champion for each team. Families were involved as members of the teams. Stretch goals were set and met.

Significant improvements occurred and were sustained. As they increased QI capability and developed knowledge of reliability design, they were able to further improve and simultaneously carry out dozens of improvements and build systems capable of 95–99% reliability.

Nonetheless, in 2005 the organization realized its rate of sentinel or serious safety events (SSE) was still high. With the help of consultants, it decided to change the safety management system to apply HRO concepts. They developed five key drivers to achieve a goal of reducing the SSE rate by 80% over 3 years:

1. Restructured governance for patient safety
2. Developing a highly reliable error prevention system
3. A transparent culture of continuous learning

4. State-of-the-art detection and cause analysis system
5. Focused intervention on perioperative processes and culture

Senior leaders adopted Patient Safety as the core value of the organization, and a commitment was made to change the culture by changing behavior. All frontline staff were trained on key safety behaviors, reinforced daily via safety coaches. An organization-wide focus on "Days since the last SSE" continuously gave a sense of wariness and unease. SSE were reduced by 65% in 3 years.

A rigorous root cause analysis process was implemented, overseen by the legal department to ensure that it was a trusted process that everyone could believe in. Senior executives were accountable to make sure it happened in timely way. They took ownership of the problem. This led the staff to have confidence in the process and accept transparency.

In 2005, Cincinnati Children's Hospital, now called Cincinnati Children's Hospital Medical Center (CCHMC), partnered with the other children's hospitals in Ohio and the Ohio Children's Hospital Association to improve safety. The first effort was implementation of medical response teams in all of the hospitals. Cardiopulmonary arrests outside of intensive care units were reduced by 46%. As Kotagal's successor, Steve Muething, recalled, this was a "game changer" for CCHMC: they realized that they could improve better and have more influence by working with others.

Under the leadership of Muething and the new CEO, Michael Fisher, and with funding from CMS and private industry, CCHMC joined the other Ohio children's hospitals in 2009 to formalize this collaboration for safety as the Ohio Children's Hospitals' Solutions for Patient Safety network. Hospital personnel were trained in the Model for Improvement and shared lessons learned with one another. ADEs were subsequently reduced by 50% and SSIs in high-risk children by 60% in all eight hospitals.

In 2012, 25 hospitals across the nation joined the initial 8 Ohio hospitals to form Solutions for Patient Safety (SPS), a network that eventually grew to 142 children's hospitals collaborating to reduce serious patient harm. From 2011 to 2018, hospitals in the SPS reduced their adverse drug events by 74%, catheter-associated urinary infections by 50%, falls by 75%, and pressure ulcers by 27%.

Kotagal and Muething attribute CCHMC's success to six factors:

1. *Alignment and commitment.* From the beginning, Anderson, Carter, and Kotagal were clear and unambiguous about the focus and led the board, senior leaders, and CSI chairs to share a deep commitment to zero serious harm, leadership improvement, and partnerships between physicians and nurses and between leaders and researchers.
2. *Structure for change and integration.* The creation of Clinical System Improvement teams of top leaders for each of the major delivery systems gave coherence and clear responsibility for major changes to improve flow, processes, and patient experience. They worked with unit teams led by trained physician and nurse leaders who carried out specific projects, aligning macro-, meso-, and microsystem structure across the entire system. Patient safety and staff safety were integrated.
3. *Capability and capacity for change.* From the beginning, the organization invested deeply in training in the science of improvement and in the infrastructure support, analytics, and operational research needed to create good visibility of data, response, and action.
4. *Creation of a culture of continuous learning.* Creation of psychological safety, the opportunities for constant improvement, and training in leadership and quality improvement created an environment where learning is part of everyday life.
5. *Respect for the Science.* The belief in the scientific approach enabled the organization to be rational and logical and attract very bright people with a passion to do well by children.
6. *Transparency.* A culture where it is normal and expected that people will surface, address, and ultimately solve issues/problems every day at all levels, especially when things go wrong, is the foundation of trust. Adverse events were promptly acknowledged to the staff, patients, and the public, thoroughly investigated, and the results fed back to the family and to the clinical staff for improvement.

Cincinnati Children's Hospital Medical Center has truly created a culture of safety. It has developed, and continues to refine, a sustainable model of collaborative patient and staff engagement in continuing improvement that has dramatically reduced harm for its patients. It has stimulated other children's hospitals to change their cultures and collaborated with them to do so. They are an impressive model.

Denver Health

Denver Health (DH) is an example of an apparently impressive culture change that turned out to be illusory. Denver Health is the principal safety-net provider in Colorado, providing health care for nearly a third of Denver's population, 46% of whom are uninsured. In 2004, under the leadership of its CEO, Patricia Gabow, MD, and with a grant from AHRQ, DH began a major initiative to transform the way it delivered care, centered on five "Rights":

- Right People: a workforce committed to customer service and quality
- Right Environment: appropriate patient and work spaces
- Right Reward for employees who demonstrate customer-oriented behaviors
- Right Communication and Culture
- Right Process: application of Lean to eliminate waste

Gabow created a new department to take responsibility for patient safety and quality and focus on processes to improve care. Programs were created to manage high-risk and high-opportunity clinical situations, such as failure to rescue, use of antibiotics, CLABSI, etc. Systems were implemented to reduce variability in patient care processes and outcomes. The initiative was supported by a sophisticated electronic health record that provided order entry and decision support in addition to data for research and quality improvement [30].

Like VMMC, Denver Health developed an intensive approach to process change, the Rapid Improvement Event (RIE), a four-day group session focused on an identified problem to develop a method to remove it. Rapid improvement events resulted in marked advances in diabetes care, anticoagulation management, venous thromboembolism prophylaxis, and cancer screening rates.

In its first 4 years, DH estimated that it also gained $42 million in financial benefit due to reduced waste. In 2009, it had the lowest observed/expected aggregate mortality ratio among 106 academic health centers in the University HealthSystem Consortium. Denver Health was hailed as an impressive example of rapid and effective culture change.

Gabow retired in 2012, having received numerous awards and honors for her impressive work at transforming a health-care organization. In 2014, she told her story in *The Lean Prescription: Powerful Medicine for Our Ailing Healthcare System*, which she wrote with Philip Goodman [31].

Then it came undone. Gabow was succeeded by Arthur Gonzales, who quickly undid many of Gabow's changes in response to financial pressures associated with the Affordable Care Act. His leadership style alienated physicians and led to resignations of a number of physicians, including all of the chairs of the major departments. Gonzales was later replaced by Robin Wittenstein.

The rapid reversal of the culture at Denver Health illustrates the difficulty of making real culture change that is sustainable. The impressive transformations implemented by Gabow were evidently not institutionalized well enough among the executive leaders, employees, and middle managers to withstand a change of top leadership. The culture really didn't change. And one can infer that the board was not totally engaged in the transformation and lacked continuity of purpose, or it would not have hired a CEO who put financial goals over safety.

Safe and Reliable Health Care

On a national scale, the most comprehensive effort to date to change culture by developing organizational capacity and capability is a proprietary effort developed by Safe and Reliable Healthcare (S&R), the consulting firm established by Allan Frankel and Michael Leonard, two highly respected physicians who have devoted their professional careers to improving patient safety. Frankel was for years the chief patient safety officer for Partners Healthcare in Boston and on the faculty at IHI. Leonard was for many years the chief safety officer at Kaiser-Permanente.

S&R trains a health-care organization's leadership and its personnel to create and sustain the environment for safe care. The focus of the S&R method is to give frontline personnel *voice* and a *sense of community*. Voice, or agency, means that everyone feels safe to speak up and that their voice is heard and respected and influences what takes place. Community means that everyone feels that their co-workers care about them. The S&R approach changes the structure of the management of the delivery of care and improvement so that voice and community are intrinsic to everyday work.

The following description is adapted from the S&R website [32]:

The core of the S&R approach is a digital platform called LENS™ (*Learning and ENgagement System*), an interactive electronic replacement of the white board where staff gather daily to define issues, develop plans, receive updates, celebrate achievements, and recognize contributions. It enables physical and virtual rounds, huddles, and improvement work so that leaders and managers can effectively communicate and visibly "close the loop" on ideas and concerns shared by frontline teams. This enables real-time coordination and improvement as well as alignment and coordination within a unit and collaboration across multiple teams. Frontline teams have "voice, visibility, and ownership" in shaping their unit's culture and performance.

A key element is SCORE, a system that obtains survey data and provides analysis to support LENS. It builds on and expands the earlier surveys of patients and providers developed by Sexton, AHRQ, and others but differs by being correlated with outcomes based on data from over 700 organizations. SCORE includes questions on culture, engagement, burnout, resilience, patient experience, physician satisfaction, and Magnet. It maps to AHRQ/SOPS, SAQ, and other surveys, thus enabling use of previous data to benchmark and show

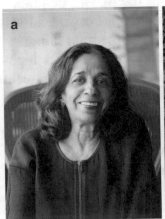 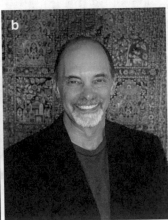 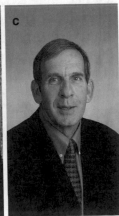

(a) Uma Kotagal, (b) Allan Frankel, and (c) Mike Leonard.

improvement. Data are presented graphically and automated to show unit results and trends across the organization.

S&R team of experts provides guidance for becoming a high-reliability organization. The goal is to generate organizational capacity and a sustainable architecture for excellence by empowering leaders, managers, and teams to clearly understand what they must measure and improve across their transformation journey. The S&R approach holds great promise. It seeks to change the culture by changing behavior at all levels. To the extent that includes engaging top management and the boards in the transformation, the changes should be sustained.

As of this writing, 12 systems of care, representing dozens of hospitals and hundreds of care units, are working with S&R to create safe and cost-effective health care. Time will tell if they succeed.

Making It Happen

What will it take to get hospitals and health-care systems nationwide to implement the VMMC, CCHMC, or S&R models to make the transformations needed to change their cultures? As the experiences of VMMC and CCHMC show, the CEO must have the vision and skills to make it happen and the passion and commitment to carry through. The Board must share that commitment and provide the resources and the backup when the going gets tough.

Perhaps exposure to advanced thinking about leadership, quality, and patient safety, such as by the initiative of the ACHE, combined with increasing evidence of success by peer health-care organizations, will motivate more leaders of organizations to "do the right thing."

But the motives of others engaged in reform may be less high-minded. For a decade or so, CEOs have been bombarded by a stream of articles in the Harvard Business Review and elsewhere about the power of Reliability Science to improve efficiency, including occasional examples in health care. They are beginning to realize that managing the complexity of care demands standardization and simplification of services and that these changes require employee engagement.

So, to be financially sound and deliver safe care, they have joined the trend to embrace reliability science and Lean. The "in" thing is to become an HRO. Many major health-care organizations now have a process engineering office and black belt leaders. The employee focus has advanced from satisfaction to engagement, resilience, and wellness. Resistance to change has lessened as the fraction of younger physicians has increased and the values of autonomy and hierarchy are being replaced by cooperation, teamwork, and respect.

This is an encouraging trend, but there is a dark side. The major trend is directed at the bottom line: consolidation. In our profit-oriented fee-for-service health-care system, market share is everything. Across the country, the big guys are swallowing up the little guys. Some are long-standing, national in scope, and huge, such as HCA (186 hospitals), Ascension Health (151), and Trinity Health (104), and span large geographic areas. Others, such as MGH Brigham (14) in Boston and Northwell (23) in Long Island, are expanding regional monopolies. Others are doing the same thing.

The primary objective of consolidation is financial success. National systems implement standardized practices to increase profits by improving efficiency and reducing costs. Regional monopolies also seek to eliminate competition in order to guarantee market share and raise prices.

In fairness, it is important to note that some large consolidated systems have been leaders in quality improvement and safety. In the current milieu, they can be an effective way to spread systems changes such as Lean and worker engagement. We have the "Ascension Way," the "Trinity Way," etc. that, when well directed, can result in significant changes.

Nonetheless, in most systems, the CFO keeps management focused on the bottom line. The demand for productivity and profits competes with quality and safety, and usually wins, as evidenced by the high burnout rates among physicians and nurses in many of these hospitals. Safety is not the primary goal.

A Role for Government?

So the big question is what will it take to get all hospital CEOs and Boards motivated to make the culture change we need to make care safe and efficient? To make patient safety "job one"? There is no clear answer, but several possibilities come to mind.

One would be federal oversight. Congress could create an FAA equivalent for health care, a Federal Patient Safety Agency, FPSA, to set standards and monitor and enforce compliance. In addition to setting standards for physician competence as described in Chap. 20, the Agency would develop standards for all aspects of health-care delivery in collaboration with representatives from hospitals and health-care systems, the Joint Commission, professional societies, and experts in quality and safety. As noted earlier, participation by stakeholders in developing standards ensures relevance and buy-in with a higher likelihood of compliance.

Specifically for safety, the Agency would set standards for practice, including training in quality and safety, data collection, working conditions, coordination of care, transparency, and reporting. It would require reporting of all serious reportable events. Failure to report would have consequences, such as prohibiting reimbursement of a hospital for any charges for an admission with a SRE. Repeat offenders could be fined and face loss of accreditation.

Given the current political climate, indeed, the climate of the past several decades, it seems highly unlikely there would be Congressional support for significantly increased regulation. A lesser measure, such as requiring *enterprise liability* in which the health-care organization is held accountable for a patient injury rather than the physician, might be possible and would be useful, but also seems unlikely.

Can nongovernmental oversight, such as by the Joint Commission, provide sufficient pressure to motivate health-care organizations to change their cultures? Perhaps. Over the past few years, the Joint Commission has steadily increased requirements for accreditation to promote quality and safety, including implementation of safe practices, reporting of SRE, adherence to core measures of quality, ensuring physician competence, patient engagement, and assessment of patient experience. (See Chap. 12.) Joint Commission Patient Safety Goals have been internalized by many hospitals. These measures have had an impact on the cultures.

However, the ability of the Joint Commission to expand its requirements is limited by its vulnerability to competition. CMS also accepts accreditation of hospitals by other organizations to receive the essential "deemed status" that enables them to receive payments from Medicare and Medicaid. Because these alternative programs are less demanding, they are an attractive "way out" if TJC gets too tough. This could, of course, be turned around if CMS gave the Commission sole accrediting authority, subject to CMS oversight.

A "Burning Platform"?

Some believe that health-care organizations will not change in the absence of an existential threat, a "burning platform." That our dysfunctional system has to get worse before it can get better. To really be threatening, that threat has to be financial.

Many, your author included, believe that the fundamental cause of the dysfunction of the American health-care system is the way hospitals and doctors are paid. The USA is the only advanced economy that runs health care as a business. That business is based on the fee-for-service (FFS) system for paying for health care. The primary goal of any business is to make a profit. In a fee-for-service system, the more services hospitals or doctors provide, the better they do.

The ramifications and nuances of this system are far too complex to be dealt with here, but the implications are clear: in a FFS payment system, the need to focus on productivity and profit is a major deterrent to hospitals making quality of care and patient safety their core mission. Changing to a risk-adjusted capitated system, such as an accountable care organization, with oversight to ensure that standards of appropriateness, quality, and safety are met, would give new meaning to the "bottom line." By itself, changing the payment system would not change the culture, but it would remove the major barrier and provide the right incentives.

Will the COVID-19 pandemic be the "burning platform" that forces change? Under its stress, our health-care system collapsed. Increasing demand for highly expensive COVID care, coupled with a decline in demand for routine services, led to crippling financial losses that have driven substantial numbers of hospitals and office practices into bankruptcy, especially rural and safety net hospitals. In our FFS business model, when markets collapse, so do providers [33].

The pandemic also significantly undermined the system of funding of health care for patients. Millions lost their employment-based health insurance when they lost their jobs [33]. Government subsidies were insufficient to make up for these losses.

As of this writing, it is impossible to know how things will turn out. However, the crisis has increased the national will for universal coverage and for insurance that is not work-related. A substantial majority of Americans now embrace the concept that health care should be a right. All of the approaches to achieve that goal require significant long-term federal outlays, as well as a huge infusion of funds short-term to prevent further collapse of the system.

Will this unprecedented requirement to fund coverage also lead to the recognition of the need to redesign the health-care system to eliminate unnecessary, harmful, and wasteful care? To design a system to meet patient needs, not to make money? Will it be what it takes to move Congress to change the financing of health care from fee-for-service to capitation, from for-profit care to patient-centered accountable care? Will this be what it takes to make patient safety a reality? If so, our suffering will not have been in vain.

References

1. Dixon-Woods M, Bosk CL, Aveling EL, et al. Explaining Michigan: developing an ex post theory of a quality improvement program. Milbank Q. 2011;89:167–205.
2. Leape LL. Error in medicine. JAMA. 1994;272:1851–7.
3. Kohn KT, Corrigan JM, Donaldson MS, editors. To err is human: building a safer health system. Washington: National Academy Press; 1999.
4. Schein EH. Organizational culture and leadership. 4th ed. San Francisco: Jossey-Bass; 2010.
5. Edwards JRD, Davey J, Armstrong K. Returning to the roots of culture: a review and re-conceptualisation of safety culture. Saf Sci. 2013;55:70–80.
6. Glendon AI, Stanton NA. Perspectives on safety culture. Saf Sci. 2000;34:193–214.
7. Vincent C. Patient safety. 2nd ed. Chichester: BMJ Books; 2010.
8. Reason JT. Managing the risks of organizational accidents. Aldershot, Hants; Brookfield: Ashgate; 1997.
9. Frankel A, Haraden C, Federico F, Lenoci-Edwards J. A framework for safe, reliable and effective care. White Paper: Institute for Healthcare Improvement; 2017.
10. Marx D. Patient safety and the "just culture": a primer for health care executives. New York. 17 Apr 2001.

11. Singer S, Lin S, Falwell A, Gaba D, Baker L. Relationship of safety climate and safety performance in hospitals. Health Serv Res. 2009;44:399–421.
12. Roberts KH. New challenges to organizational research: high reliability organizations. Ind Crisis Q. 1989;3:111–25.
13. Weick KE, Sutcliffe KM, Obstfeld D. Organizing for high reliability. Res Organ Behav. 1999;21:81–123.
14. Chassin MR, Loeb JM. The ongoing quality improvement journey: next stop, high reliability. Health Aff. 2011;30:559–68.
15. Roberts K, Stout S, Halpern J. Decision dynamics in two high reliability military organizations. Man Sci. 1994;40:614–24.
16. Institute of Medicine (US) Committee on Quality of Health Care in America. Crossing the quality chasm: a new health system for the 21st century. Washington: National Academies Press; 2001.
17. Top U.S. "Non-profit" hospitals & CEOs are racking up huge profits. 26 June 2019. Accessed October 3, 2020, at https://www.forbes.com/sites/ada-mandrzejewski/2019/06/26/top-u-s-non-profit-hospitals-ceos-are-racking-up-huge-profits/#33444d019dfb.
18. Leape LL, Berwick DM. Five years after "to err is human", what have we learned? JAMA. 2005;293:2384–90.
19. Singer SJ, Falwell A, Gaba DM, et al. Identifying organizational cultures that promote patient safety. Health Care Manag Rev. 2009;34:300–11.
20. Vincent C, Amalberti R. Safer healthcare: strategies for the real world. Cham: Springer; 2016.
21. Shanafelt TD, Schein E, Minor LB, Trockel M, Schein P, Kirch D. Healing the professional culture of medicine. Mayo Clin Proc. 2019;94:1556–66.
22. Edmondson AC. Psychological safety, trust, and learning in organizations: a group-level Lens. In: Kramer R, Cook K, editors. Trust and distrust in organizations: dilemmas and approaches. New York: Russell Sage Foundation; 2004. p. 239–72.
23. American College of Healthcare Executives and IHI/NPSF Lucian Leape Institute. Leading a culture of safety: a blueprint for success. Boston: American College of Healthcare Executives and Institute for Healthcare Improvement; 2017.
24. Ohno T, Bodek N. Toyota production system: beyond large-scale production. 1st ed. Portland: CRC Press; 1988.
25. Rizzardo D, Brooks R. Understanding Lean Manufacturing: Maryland Technology Enterprise Institute; 2003.
26. Womack JP, Jones DT. Lean thinking. 2nd ed. New York: Simon & Schuster, Inc.; 2003.
27. Kenney C. Transforming health care: Virginia Mason Medical Center's pursuit of the perfect patient experience. Boca Raton: CRC Press; 2011.
28. Kenney C. A leadership journey in health care: Virginia Mason's story. London: CRC Press; 2015.

29. Plsek PE. Accelerating health care transformation with lean and innovation: the Virginia Mason experience. Boca Raton: CRC Press; 2014.
30. Gabow PA, Mehler PS. A broad and structured approach to improving patient safety and quality: lessons from Denver Health. Health Aff. 2011;30:612–8.
31. Gabow PA, Goodman PL. The lean prescription: powerful medicine for our ailing healthcare system. Boca Raton: Productivity Press; 2015.
32. Safe & Reliable Healthcare. Accessed 3 Oct 2020, at https://safeandreliablecare.com/.
33. Blumenthal D, Fowler EJ, Abrams M, Collins SR. Covid-19 — implications for the health care system. N Engl J Med. 2020;383:1483–8.

Correction to: Everyone Counts: Building a Culture of Respect

Correction to: Chapter 21 in: L. L. Leape, *Making Healthcare Safe*, https://doi.org/10.1007/978-3-030-71123-8_21

A scientific error had been introduced in Chapter 21, page 365.

"The two papers came out in the **Annals of Internal Medicine** in July 2012 and were well received. The earliest most obvious impact in our hospitals was that several tightened up their procedures and fired some of their most outrageous offenders, physicians whom colleagues had complained about for years" has been corrected to

"The two papers came out in the **Academic Medicine** in July 2012 and were well received. The earliest most obvious impact in our hospitals was that several tightened up their procedures and fired some of their most outrageous offenders, physicians whom colleagues had complained about for years."

The updated version of the chapter can be found at https://doi.org/10.1007/978-3-030-71123-8_21

© The Author(s) 2021
L. L. Leape, *Making Healthcare Safe*,
https://doi.org/10.1007/978-3-030-71123-8_24

Index

© The Author(s) 2021
L. L. Leape, *Making Healthcare Safe*,
https://doi.org/10.1007/978-3-030-71123-8

Printed in the United States
by Baker & Taylor Publisher Services